Pharmacotherapy of Child and Adolescent Psychiatric Disorders

Pharmacotherapy of Child and Adolescent Psychiatric Disorders

EDITED BY

David R. Rosenberg MD

Miriam L. Hamburger Endowed Chair of Child Psychiatry and Professor & Chief of Child
Psychiatry and Psychology at Wayne State University and the Children's Hospital of Michigan,
Detroit, MI, USA

Samuel Gershon MD

Emeritus Professor of Psychiatry, University of Pittsburgh, PA, USA

THIRD EDITION

FOREWORD BY NEAL RYAN MD

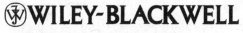

WILEY-BLACKWELL

A John Wiley & Sons, Ltd., Publication

Library of Congress Cataloging-in-Publication Data

Pharmacotherapy of child and adolescent psychiatric disorders / [edited by] David Rosenberg and Samuel Gershon. – 3rd ed.
    p. ; cm.
  Includes bibliographical references and index.
  ISBN 978-0-470-97376-9 (cloth)
  I. Rosenberg, David R. II. Gershon, Samuel.
  [DNLM: 1. Psychotropic Drugs–therapeutic use. 2. Adolescent. 3. Child. 4. Mental Disorders–drug therapy. 5. Psychotropic
Drugs–pharmacology. QV 77.2]
  LC classification not assigned
  618.92′8918–dc23
                                                                                                2011029295

A catalogue record for this book is available from the British Library.

This book is published in the following electronic formats: ePDF 9781119958321; Wiley Online Library 9781119958338; ePub 9781119961000; Mobi 9781119961017

Set in 9.5/13pt Meridien by Aptara Inc., New Delhi, India

First Impression 2012

To J, Isa, the Henster and Foo—the reasons I smile inside and out.

David R. Rosenberg

Contents

List of Contributors

David A. Axelson MD
University of Pittsburgh School of Medicine
Western Psychiatric Institute and Clinic
University of Pittsburgh Medical Center
3811 O'Hara St
Pittsburgh, PA 15213
USA

Boris Birmaher MD
University of Pittsburgh School of Medicine
Western Psychiatric Institute and Clinic
University of Pittsburgh Medical Center
Bellefield Towers, Room 605
100 North Bellefield Avenue
Pittsburgh, PA 15213
USA

Heidi R. Bruty MD
Department of Psychiatry
University of Texas Southwestern
Medical Center
5323 Harry Hines Blvd.
Dallas, TX 75390-8589
USA

Barbara J. Coffey MD, MS
New York University Langone School of
Medicine and Nathan Kline Institute for
Psychiatric Research
NYU Child Study Center
577 First Avenue
New York, NY 10016
USA

Paul Croarkin DO
Department of Psychiatry
University of Texas Southwestern
Medical Center
5323 Harry Hines Blvd.
Dallas, TX 75390-8589
USA

C. Lindsay DeVane PharmD
Department of Psychiatry and Behavioral
Sciences
Medical University of South Carolina
173 Ashley Avenue
Children's Research Institute, Room 405B
Charleston, SC 29425
USA

David J. Edwards PharmD
School of Pharmacy
University of Waterloo
200 University Avenue West
Waterloo
Ontario
Canada N2L 3G1

Graham J. Emslie MD
Department of Psychiatry
University of Texas Southwestern Medical
Center
5323 Harry Hines Blvd.
Dallas, TX 75390-8589
USA

Robert L. Findling MD
Department of Psychiatry
Case Western Reserve University
10524 Euclid Avenue, Suite 1155A
Cleveland, OH 44106
USA

Anna M. Georgiopoulos MD
Department of Child and Adolescent
Psychiatry
Massachusetts General Hospital
Yawkey 6900
55 Fruit Street
Boston, MA 02114
USA

Samuel Gershon MD
University of Pittsburgh
Clinical Research Building
1120 N.W. 14th Street
Suite 1464
Miami, FL 33136
USA

Kareem D. Ghalib MD
Department of Psychiatry
Columbia University/New York State
Psychiatric Institute
1051 Riverside Drive, Unit 74
New York, NY 10032
USA

Charlotte M. Heleniak BA
Department of Psychiatry
Columbia University/New York State
Psychiatric Institute
1051 Riverside Drive, Unit 74
New York, NY 10032
USA

John L. Hertzer MD
Department of Psychiatry
Case Western Reserve University
10524 Euclid Avenue, Suite 1155A
Cleveland, OH 44106
USA

Aron Janssen MD
NYU/Bellevue Department of Child and
Adolescent Psychiatry
577 1st Avenue
New York, NY 10016
USA

Gagan Joshi MD
Department of Child and Adolescent
Psychiatry
Massachusetts General Hospital
Yawkey 6900
55 Fruit Street
Boston, MA 02114
USA

Tejal Kaur MD
Department of Psychiatry
Columbia University/New York State
Psychiatric Institute
1051 Riverside Drive, Unit 74
New York, NY 10032
USA

Joan Luby MD
Washington University School of Medicine
Department of Psychiatry, Child Division
Early Emotional Development Program
Campus Box 8134
660 S Euclid
St. Louis, MO 63110
USA

Tushita Mayanil MD
Pediatric Brain Research and Intervention
Center
University of Illinois at Chicago
1747 West Roosevelt Street
Chicago, IL 60607
USA

**Christopher-Paul Milne DVM,
MPH, JD**
Center for the Study of Drug Development
Department of Public Health and Community
Medicine
Tufts University School of Medicine
75 Kneeland Street
Boston, MA 02111
USA

Mani Pavuluri MD, PhD
University of Illinois at Chicago
1747 West Roosevelt Street
Chicago, IL 60607
USA

Steven R. Pliszka MD
Division of Child and Adolescent Psychiatry
Department of Psychiatry
The University of Texas Health Center at
San Antonio
7703 Floyd Curl Drive MC 7792
San Antonio, TX 78229-3900
USA

David R. Rosenberg MD
Department of Child Psychiatry and
Psychology
Wayne State University and the Children's
Hospital of Michigan
4201 Street Antoine Boulevard
Detroit, MI 48201
USA

Brieana M. Rowles MA
Department of Psychiatry
Case Western Reserve University
10524 Euclid Avenue, Suite 1155A
Cleveland, OH 44106
USA

Moira A. Rynn MD
Department of Psychiatry
Columbia University/New York State
Psychiatric Institute
1051 Riverside Drive, Unit 74
New York, NY 10032
USA

Daniel J. Safer MD
Departments of Psychiatry and Pediatrics
Johns Hopkins University School of Medicine
6 Hadley Square North
Baltimore, MD 21218
USA

Dara Sakolsky MD, PhD
University of Pittsburgh School of Medicine
Western Psychiatric Institute and Clinic
University of Pittsburgh Medical Center
Bellefield Towers, Room 515
100 North Bellefield Avenue
Pittsburgh, PA 15213
USA

Lawrence David Scahill MSN, PhD
Yale Child Study Center
230 S. Frontage Rd
New Haven, CT 06520
USA

Richard I. Shader MD
The Center for the Study of Drug
Development
Tufts University School of Medicine,
Suite 1100
75 Kneeland Street
Boston, MA 02111
USA

Jess Shatkin MD
New York University School of Medicine
577 First Avenue
New York, NY 10016
USA

Garrett M. Sparks MD
Western Psychiatric Institute and Clinic
University of Pittsburgh Medical Center
3811 O'Hara St
Pittsburgh, PA 15213
USA

Mini Tandon DO
Washington University School of Medicine
Department of Psychiatry, Child Division
Early Emotional Development Program
Campus Box 8134
660 S Euclid
St. Louis, MO 63110
USA

Julie Magno Zito PhD
Department of Pharmaceutical Health
Services Research and Department of
Psychiatry
School of Pharmacy and School of Medicine
University of Maryland, Baltimore
Baltimore, MD 21201
USA

Amanda L. Zwilling BA
Tics and Tourette's Clinical and Research
Program
New York University Langone School of
Medicine
NYU Child Study Center
577 First Avenue
New York, NY 10016
USA

Foreword

It has been a decade since the publication of *Pharmacotherapy for Child and Adolescent Psychiatric Disorders*, Second Edition, by David Rosenberg, Pablo Davanzo and Samuel Gershon. New research over this decade has significantly changed the pharmacological and psychotherapeutic approaches to our most significant child psychiatric disorders. This new edition, therefore, has much that is new and important in our day-to-day clinical work.

Advanced psychopharmacology in children and adolescents is hampered by the paucity of studies and the relatively limited information that each separate study provides. Studies are expensive, research is difficult, and children are more complex to study than adults. Therefore, most but not all studies in youth address acute treatment in children with little comorbidity. Even in the most straightforward studies, we do not have the very large sample sizes that would give us narrow confidence intervals and the ability to ask meaningful questions about which subpopulations do best with which treatments. We also have little data on the comparative efficacy of treatments, even as first-line treatment of the acute disorder.

The questions that are more vexing and a larger part of our practice are, however, questions about how to treat refractory disorders, how to treat recurrent disorders, how to manage chronic medication use over years, and the risks of potential rare but serious side-effects. Studying these questions with adequate sample sizes is much harder and much more expensive. Guided by a few groundbreaking studies attempting to answer this sort of question in youth over the past decade, we will, nevertheless, frequently be forced to extrapolate from acute studies and from studies in adults. Not perfect but, like in most of medicine, we choose between Scylla and Charybdis. Most of us choose to extrapolate rather than nihilistically refusing to offer potential treatment to the difficult comorbid refractory youth that make up the majority of patients who come to us.

There has been remarkable progress in our field over the past decade. Few areas have been as fertile and active as the study of bipolar disorder in youth. We now have well-specified studies examining where the boundaries of this condition lie, testing the acute efficacy of a number of treatments particularly atypical antipsychotics, and comparing efficacy between different treatments. Research with antipsychotics in adults is causing the field to question whether today's atypical antipsychotics are indeed superior to first-generation compounds. We are starting to see psychotherapy studies in youths with bipolar disorder.

The past decade has brought us two large studies examining the combination of psychotherapy and pharmacotherapy in adolescent unipolar depression, a study of the treatment of adolescent unipolar depression, and a study of the treatment of adolescent depression refractory to initial SSRI treatment. We have also seen much more discussion of how to interpret studies with small effect sizes, questions about what the high acute placebo effect seen in unipolar depression throughout the lifespan means for our treatment strategies, and much thought given to the publication bias against negative studies and the (past) unavailability of data from negative studies on correctly understanding the aggregate meaning of studies. In addition, challenging questions have been raised about a potential increase in suicide with SSRIs and with other psychopharmacologic agents in youth.

Attention-deficit hyperactivity disorder has been a rich area of study over the decade. While stimulants are remarkably effective, other recent therapies including new long-acting stimulant preparations, atomoxetine, clonidine, and guanfacine, all have a role to play. Here, as in other areas of psychopharmacology, safety monitoring during treatment has received considerable attention.

This book examines in depth critical overarching questions for the field, including the pharmacoepidemiology of psychotropic use in youth, the use of medications for off-label indications, the role of advertising in consumer demand and medication use, and the question of possible use of medication treatment in prevention of disorders before first onset of the full syndromic picture.

Perhaps in another decade, Professor Rosenberg and colleagues will be able to tell us about new pharmacological treatments brought forth from bench-to-bedside translational research and about how genotyping or imaging approaches will truly let us tailor treatments to the individual. Until then, I expect this book will provide us with information critical to the care of youth with serious psychiatric disorders.

Neal Ryan MD
Joaquim Puig-Antich Professor of Psychiatry
University of Pittsburgh

CHAPTER 1
Historical Perspectives on Child and Adolescent Psychopharmacology

Samuel Gershon
University of Pittsburgh, Pittsburgh, USA

The psychiatric treatment of children with drugs was essentially taboo until the 1990s, possibly due to the still major influence of psychodynamic views. This attitude presented a double-sided problem: there was a disinclination to administer pharmacotherapy to children who needed it and would benefit from it and, equally concerning, there was a vocal movement for mass treatment, underscoring a profound cultural shift. The media reported this widely, for example, in the article "Paxil, Prozac, Ritalin—are these drugs safe for kids???" [1]. It was thus commonplace to read that parents and schools were just searching for a quick fix for behaviors that fell outside the "norm." Ritalin had been available since 1954, and so perhaps the acceptance of psychopharmacology as an intervention sped the clock on the acceptability of pharmacological agents to deal with behaviors outside the new cultural norms. These treatment options claimed to offer the possibility for any child who fell outside these behavioral "norms" to be "improved." Thus, a market force developed that underpins the efforts of pharmaceutical companies to develop their products. Although controversial, these concepts have expanded recently to suggest that early diagnosis of psychiatric disorders such as schizophrenia and bipolar disorder may warrant the initiation of pharmacotherapy at the earliest manifestation of "prodromata" of these conditions.

Stimulants may well have been the first entrants into child pharmacotherapy. Amphetamine was resynthesized in the US in the 1920s and had been employed as a respiratory stimulant for narcolepsy and as an appetite suppressant. By 1937 it was shown to be an effective treatment for hyperactivity in children by Charles Bradley [2]. Later others also reported on the efficacy of Ritalin in children with hyperactive states. Its

---

Pharmacotherapy of Child and Adolescent Psychiatric Disorders, Third Edition.
Edited by David R. Rosenberg and Samuel Gershon.
© 2012 John Wiley & Sons, Ltd. Published 2012 by John Wiley & Sons, Ltd.

effectiveness led to the acceptance of the concept of minimal brain dysfunction, which in 1980 in DSMIII was categorized as attention-deficit hyperactivity disorder (ADHD).

Psychopharmacological treatments have been introduced in large part as the result of serendipitous events. The earliest agents included lithium, chlorpromazine, and imipramine. They gradually developed a role in the treatment of adult patients and then were tried in pediatric patients by deduction of the possible similarity of these behaviors to those established in adults. There are many assumptions in this last step to the treatment of children. For example, imipramine and related compounds were indeed quite effective for major depressive disorder in adults. However, their translation to children implied an essential assumption that the depression seen in children was analogous to that seen in adults, and that the underlying substrate would respond similarly. Whatever the assumptions, the outcome belied these assumptions, as the careful studies of Ryan et al. [3] clearly demonstrated. Here we had a cautionary tale and we have not fully explained this outcome and the assumptions inherent therein. Thus we must move cautiously before we presume such simple projections from adults to children.

Then there developed a period of major enthusiasm for two new classes of psychotropic agents: the selective serotonin reuptake inhibitors (SSRIs) and the atypical second-generation antipsychotics (SGAs). As before, their usage was explored initially in adults with the SSRIs becoming widely employed for depressive disorders and pretty much completely displacing the tricyclics. Both classes of drugs were then extensively prescribed for children and adolescents. Following the FDA's warnings, with black-box and bold-print cautions, there has been a significant reduction in their prescriptions. Associated with this is the hotly debated issue of suicidality associated with these antidepressants.

Some of the SGAs have also caused serious concern because of the increased risk of metabolic syndrome with significant weight gain and the concurrence of type-II diabetes. These adverse effects produce a very special risk in developing children. These few instances provide adequate warning about a transfer of psychopharmacological drug prescribing from adults to children. There is now clearly the need, which has been recognized, for the careful clinical evaluation of new agents for specific indications in children.

The prevention and treatment of emotional and behavioral problems affects about one in five children and is the major mental health problem in the United States. Most major mental health problems begin during adolescence. Therefore, this is the critical period for their identification, prevention and often their treatment. Suicide among the young has become an increasing concern over the past several decades. It is important

to consider, within this context, the high rate of suicide in the young in-
ductees in the armed forces. Another aspect of this issue has come up over
the past 10 years and that has been the possible effects of administering
antidepressant drugs to children and adolescents and the concerns that
were raised about possible increase in suicidal outcomes. All these questions have increased the importance of the optimal methods of treatment
of depression in these populations.

This third edition of pharmacotherapy for child and adolescent disorders
is being published 10 years after the first edition. Although the field has
advanced considerably, the fact that we are dealing with a still-developing
nervous system presents both special options and serious cautions. The
use of psychotropic agents in adults has become well established since the
1960s and the picture of their clinical indications and side effect profile
has become much clearer. These issues are still not so well defined in children, as their diagnostic entities are still being delineated and thus specific
therapies are also under debate. The social and cultural background for
the acceptance of psychotropic interventions has altered over the years.
Initially, they were considered inappropriate, dangerous and treatments
of last resort for children. Society has changed its attitude dramatically
and now there is a serious concern of overmedication of children. Thus,
although the field has progressed significantly, the appropriate administration of psychoactive medications to children requires training, skill and
ongoing interaction with the patient and family throughout the course
of treatment.

This is especially the case as many more drugs have been introduced
and their indications and profile of actions are still in progress. The basic
research studies on their mode and site of action will continue to provide
the field with knowledge, which will help considerably in their more targeted usage. The question of early usage of therapeutic interventions in
some of these conditions has been raised, offering the possibility of preventive value. This early and possibly long-term usage raises new and
important questions in regard to short- and long-term possible adverse
effects on developing systems.

Early intervention for all medical or psychiatric disorders is essentially
always considered beneficial. However, with psychiatric disorders in children, especially in the younger age groups, the prospective identification
of prodromata has been and still is problematic. Various investigators have
presented studies on this problem, such as the proposal of "ultra high
risk" (UHR) criteria [4]. One still unresolved problem is the potential effects of the various psychotropic drugs on the developing nervous system
and other organ systems, especially if administered long term, as is often necessary in a number of disorders. Adverse neurocognitive effects
of psychotropic medications have been reported [5, 6]. For example,

GABAergic agonists have been demonstrated to interfere with both mood and memory, as well as attention and psychomotor speed.

Thus, there is a debate about early psychopharmacologic intervention in children. Specifically, it concerns the issue of whether the impact and consequences of lack of treatment outweigh the potential for prematurely labeling children with emotional disturbances. In this population of children and adolescents, early clinical features can also be difficult to distinguish from benign conditions and normal experience. These concerns cannot easily or speedily be resolved. The question of the diagnosis of these psychiatric disorders is still being evaluated for DSM V. Good data on the long-term use of psychotropic agents both on body organs and the central nervous system are still incomplete in young developing systems. Therefore, we believe we can only raise a cautionary note and await further data on both aspects of this question. Hopefully we will have a resolution by the time we come to the fourth edition of this volume.

All of these activities in the field have contributed to the creation of this third edition. It is hoped that this volume will serve as a valuable guide to the treatment of patients 18 years of age and under with psychiatric disorders. This volume is presented as a practical guide to the clinical psychiatrist. The book also provides valuable material for other health care professionals in the management of children and adolescents with psychiatric conditions. The material presented here is in a format readily available for psychologists, social workers, therapists, nursing staff and students, as well as medical students, pediatricians and family practitioners. We felt that a brief historical review of the background of the development of psychopharmacological interventions in children could provide a frame of reference for the developments and practices in the field today. It should also provide a perspective that the field is and should be changing. We have delineated what is known currently on the basis of a critical review of controlled trials available. We have also attempted to integrate the basic neuroscience available to help guide clinical decision making.

References

1 Kalb C: Drugged-out toddlers. A new study documents an alarming increase in behavior altering medication for preschoolers. *Newsweek* 2000; **135**: 53.
2 Bradley C: The behavior of children receiving benzedrine. *Am J Psychiatry* 1937; **94**: 577–585.
3 Ryan N, Puig-Antich J, Ambrosini P et al.: The clinical picture of major depression in children and adolescents. *Arch Gen Psychiatry* 1987; **44**: 854–61.
4 Yung AR, Phillips LJ, Yuen HP et al.: Risk factors for psychosis in an ultra high risk group. Psychopathology and Clinical Features. *Schiz. Res* 2004; **67**: 131–42.

5 Henin A, Mick E, Biederman J, Fried R et al.: Is psychopharmacological treatment associated with neuropsychological deficits in bipolar youth? *J Clin Psychiatry* 2009; **70:** 1178–85.
6 Donaldson S, Goldstein LH, Landau S et al.: The Maudsley Bipolar Disorder Project: the effect of medication, family history, and duration of illness on IQ and memory in bipolar I disorder. *J Clin Psychiatry* 2003; **64:** 86–93.

CHAPTER 2

Pharmacoepidemiology of Psychotropic Medications in Youth

Daniel J. Safer[1] & Julie Magno Zito[2]
[1] Johns Hopkins University School of Medicine, Baltimore, USA
[2] University of Maryland, Baltimore, USA

Introduction

Pharmacoepidemiology

A major function of pharmacoepidemiology is to analyze large computerized datasets in order to reveal patterns of medication treatment in community populations. Such analyses are commonly used to estimate prevalence, persistence of use, correlates, and trends in treatment. These measures of utilization are developed from various sources including: (1) Medicaid reimbursement claims [1–3] and state children's health insurance program (s-CHIP) claims from higher income public insurance enrollees [4]; (2) Health Maintenance Organization (HMO) records [5–7]; (3) commercial insurance data from multiple data files [8] and from pharmacy benefit managers (PBMs) [9, 10]; (4) national population surveys of office visits, such as National Ambulatory Medical Care Surveys (NAMCS) [11, 12] and population surveys of patient-reported service use, such as Medical Expenditure Panel Surveys (MEPS) [13]; (5) school and community surveys [14, 15]; (6) state controlled substance data bases [16]; (7) federal production quota data on controlled substances [17]; (8) prescription sales data [18]; and (9) population-based cohort studies to assess treatment outcomes [19, 20]. Finally, data on the unintended effects of medications can be analyzed from the FDA Adverse Drug Event (ADE) Reporting System (AERS), which consists of voluntary reports of ADEs from physicians, manufacturers and the community [21]. Collectively, these sources produce a mosaic of U.S. patterns of psychotropic use and treatment-emergent adverse events which may differ across region,

Pharmacotherapy of Child and Adolescent Psychiatric Disorders, Third Edition.
Edited by David R. Rosenberg and Samuel Gershon.
© 2012 John Wiley & Sons, Ltd. Published 2012 by John Wiley & Sons, Ltd.

socioeconomic class, and other broad dimensions of population health that are not reflected in clinical trial populations or in case series reports.

Strengths of pharmacoepidemiology

Community datasets include all eligible, enrolled or surveyed individuals, not only those who seek treatment. Thus, total enrollees are all those surveyed from the denominator, which is the foundation for the prevalence of use in a population-based estimate. Demographic information, outpatient services, and other relevant variables are commonly linked to the medication dataset. The linkage permits stratification on numerous correlates including race and ethnicity (from Medicaid and federal surveys only), age group, gender, region of residence, Medicaid eligibility category, private insurance, and the presence of psychiatric or chronic comorbidities. Various outcomes beyond summary prevalence measures are being used—for example, measuring concomitant between- and within-drug class treatment. (more than one psychotropic class or drug entity simultaneously), assessing drug-related laboratory monitoring data, and measuring persistence (days) of treatment.

New methods used in pharmacoepidemiology

In the last decade, new methods have been applied to drug data alone and linked to other health services. First, in contrast to prevalent user methods, new user methods measure newly initiated drug therapy [22,23] and this approach has been increasingly used to more precisely assess the temporal effect of regulatory changes, for example boxed warnings on antidepressant labels [23]. Second, multivariate data analyses can correct for extrinsic influences on practice patterns and establish odds ratios (measuring the probability of use relative to a reference group). Third, the persistence of drug treatment is a measure of duration of use from large datasets as a surrogate for medication adherence.

Focus of this update

This chapter will focus on: (1) psychotropic medication trends in relation to psychiatric diagnosis; (2) frequently or increasingly used classes, for example, stimulants, antidepressants and antipsychotics; (3) the use of several classes concurrently (concomitant treatment); (4) the preschool age group; and (5) international differences in prevalence of medication use.

Prevalence and trends for medications prescribed for ADHD

From parent reports in the National Health Interview Survey conducted by the Center for Disease Control (CDC) in 2003 and 2007, the prevalence of medication treatment for youth aged 4–17 who had been diagnosed with ADHD was 4.3% in 2003 [24] and 4.8% in 2007 [25]. In the 2003 survey, 56.3% of youth who had been diagnosed with ADHD were being treated with medication for that disorder [24]. In the 2007 survey, 66.3% of youth currently diagnosed with ADHD were being medicated for that disorder [25]. These data indicate that an additional estimated 285,000 youth in the United States were being treated with medication for ADHD in 2007 compared with 2003.

In recent prevalence studies, the annual U.S. rates of medication treatment for ADHD are as follows: (1) stimulants—atomoxetine: 4.6% in Florida Medicaid youth aged 0–19 in 2003–4 [2]; 4.4% in commercially insured youth aged 0–19 years in 2005 [26]; (2) stimulants: 3.7% in Vermont Medicaid for youth aged 0–18 in 2007 [27].

The prevalence of medication treatment of ADHD in U.S. youth since the 1990s has expanded according to published claims data [2, 7, 28] as well as in a MEPS study [29]. However, the latter report indicated that the use of stimulant medications for youth had reached a plateau in the period from 1997–2002 [29], a widely quoted finding that is not consistent with increased use from other data sources. In a mid-Atlantic U.S. state, Medicaid data revealed that the prevalence for stimulants in youth less than 20 years old was 3.8% in 1996 [1] and 6.6% in 2000 [4]. In an HMO population in California, Habel et al. [7] reported that stimulant use rose slightly in youth aged 2–18 years from 1.86% in 1996 to 1.93% in 2000. In Vermont Medicaid, the stimulant prevalence for youth less than 19 years grew 9% from 3.3% in 1997 to 3.6% in 2007 [27]. Whereas the rate of increase in stimulant treatment for youth with ADHD has indeed slowed in recent years, the overall prevalence of pediatric medications for ADHD continues to climb [25].

By examining stratified prevalence rates, demographic and clinical differences can be shown. For example, stimulant prevalence has been lowest in western U.S. states and highest in southern U.S. states [9, 13]. It is *higher* in: White youth (compared to African American and Hispanic youth) [1, 13]; youth who receive special education services [15]; foster children and disabled youth who qualify for supplemental security income payments (SSI); youth aged 10–14 years [1, 4]; Medicaid-insured compared to privately insured youth [30, 31] and in higher income families [9, 32, 33]. The gender ratio (M:F) has narrowed steadily over the past few decades. For example, in the Vermont Medicaid study of youth less than 19 years, the M:F ratio for stimulant treatment was 3.3:1 in 1997 but it dropped to 2.4:1 in 2007 [27].

In the last 15 years, the use of medication treatments for ADHD (which include stimulants and atomoxetine) has grown in certain subpopulations. These include older teenagers, [25] African-American youths [2, 13, 25]

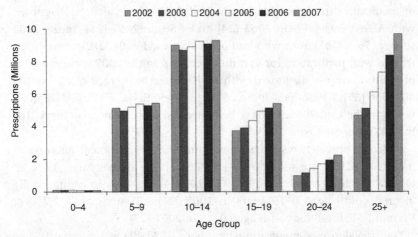

Figure 2.1 Amphetamine and methylphenidate stimulant medications: projected number of total prescriptions dispensed by U.S. retail pharmacies, 2002–7.
Source: SDI, Vector One® National (VONA), extracted January 2008.

and youth with public health insurance [13]. Although it is outside the scope of a chapter focused on treatment of youth, it is of note that that the increase in medication treatment for ADHD by adults in the last decade has been profound. It appears that as much as 40% of these medications are now prescribed for adults [26,34,35]. This trend is evident in the figure representing U.S. age-grouped rates of prescriptions for stimulant medications between 2002 and 2007 [35] (see Figure 2.1).

In 2009, stimulant treatment (methylphenidate and amphetamine salts) comprised approximately 85%–90% of medications prescribed specifically for the treatment of ADHD [36]. Whereas methylphenidate was the primary stimulant prescribed until 2000, its market share has since proportionally decreased, now being split with amphetamine salts [37]. By 2005, over 40% of stimulants were amphetamines [26,34,36]. Also since 2002, the use of long-acting forms of stimulant medication has become dominant over immediate release forms [26,36–38].

The major specialty of the prescribers of stimulants is pediatrics [6,7,39,40]. Since the 1990s, nurse practitioners have been prescribing an increasing proportion of the total ADHD drugs prescribed [15].

The persistence of use of medications over time for ADHD varies a great deal from study to study and according to the study population. Most U.S. studies show that the average persistence is well under one year [2,26,41]. In the Marcus et al. [42] study, the median persistence of stimulant treatment by California Medicaid-insured youth was 90 days. Habel et al. [7] found a similar level of stimulant persistence in a California HMO population. Persistence is often intermittent, but at least 20% of those who initiate stimulant medication in childhood remain on these medications well into adolescence [2, 43].

Several studies used cohort designs to longitudinally track the regional experience of youth from a large systematically assessed youth population. For example, Barbaresi et al. [44] followed a birth cohort over 14 years and found that 87% of those with a well defined ADHD diagnosis had been dispensed medication (primarily stimulants) for that disorder. This study of an upper middle-class, largely white, stable population in Rochester, Minnesota, has limited generalizability, although the investigation including the assessment and measures of outcomes has been pioneering. Stimulant use persisted in these Rochester youth for a median duration of 33.8 months [19]. By contrast, Zima et al. [20] followed 530 youth aged 5–11 years old in a Medicaid managed care longitudinal cohort in Los Angeles County for two years (2004–6) and found that stimulant refill persistence for youth with ADHD was only 40% over a six-month period.

Nonstimulant medications for ADHD

Atomoxetine use for ADHD grew following its approval for the treatment of ADHD in 2002. However, use of this noradrenergic reuptake inhibitor has since leveled off and this drug in 2009 comprised approximately 10% of the medication treatments indicated for ADHD [26, 36]. In one study, atomoxetine was primarily coprescribed (61%) with stimulants [45]. Recently, two long-acting alpha-agonist preparations have been approved for the treatment of ADHD: guanfacine extended release and clonidine extended release. These drug entities will be discussed in the alpha-agonist section.

Antidepressant medication

Prevalence

From 1987 through 2003, antidepressant treatment prevalence for youth rose steadily in Medicaid, commercially-insured, and in HMO populations [1, 5, 10, 27, 46]. For example, in a national commercially insured population, the prevalence of antidepressants in youth aged 18 years and younger rose from 1.6% in 1998 to 2.4% in 2002 [10]. In a HMO population in California, the prevalence of antidepressants in youth aged 5–17 rose from 1.0% in 1994 to 2.1% in 2003 [5]. In a mid-Atlantic Medicaid population of youth aged 2–19 years, the prevalence of antidepressant treatment increased from 1.9% in 1994 to 3.6% in 2000 [4, 47]. In a national survey (MEPS) of the parents of children less than 19 years old, the prevalence of antidepressant treatment rose from 1.3% in 1997 to 1.8% in 2002 [48].

In March 2004, the FDA issued an advisory—followed by a boxed warning for antidepressant product labeling in October 2004—to express concern and then to warn prescribers and the public about the increased risk for suicidal ideation or suicidal behavior in youth who take antide- pressant medication [49]. After the 2004 publicity, which followed the FDA decision, the rate of prescriptions for antidepressants dropped for youth in most analyses. In the Vermont Medicaid dataset covering youth less than 19 years old, antidepressant dispensing dropped from an an- nual prevalence of 5.2% in 2002 to 4.0% in 2007 [27]. Other analyses also revealed this decline [23, 50]. The FDA warning led to a particularly prominent decline in the prescription prevalence of paroxetine [18, 51]. In a commercially insured population, there was a slight increase in youth of dispensed fluoxetine, which was the only antidepressant approved at that time for the treatment of depression in youth [52]. When separated by diagnostic subgroup, there was no change in antidepressant use pre- to post-FDA warning for commercially insured youth with a diagnosis of major depressive disorder [23]. The finding suggests that the drop in use occurred for indications that had less well established evidence of benefits.

In the 1990s, the prevalence of antidepressant medication for Medicaid- insured youth was at least as high for youth 10–14 years of age as for youth aged 15–17 years [1, 53]. Also at that time, boys aged 10–14 years were prescribed antidepressants at a higher prevalence than girls that age in a MEPS parent-reported survey [13] as well as for Medicaid-insured youth [1, 27]. However, in commercially-insured youth, antidepressant use *overall* was more prevalent in girls than boys [10], as was also the case in HMOs [1, 5]. Since the late 1990s, in commercially insured and in federal survey studies, teenage girls have been the dominant users of antidepres- sants [10, 54].

Antidepressant treatment prevalence has consistently been higher for White as compared to African-American and Hispanic youth [1, 13, 48]. Medicaid-insured youth have had a higher prevalence of use of these med- ications than HMO and commercially-insured youth [12, 13, 47]. Youth in higher income families have had a greater prevalence of antidepressant use [48, 54].

Antidepressant subclasses and off-label use

Selective serotonin reuptake inhibitors (SSRIs) became the predominantly prescribed antidepressant subclass for youth from the mid-1990s [5, 48]. Beginning at that time, the use of tricyclic antidepressants (TCAs) went into a precipitous decline [5, 46]. Antidepressant prescriptions for youth have been written primarily by nonpsychiatrists. In 2003, 44% of the prescribers of antidepressant medications for youth were psychiatrists [50]. During the period from 1998–2005, 29% of the youth prescribed antidepressants in a national claims, employer-based healthcare database were treated by psychiatrists [55]. Much of the antidepressant medication prescribed is for off-label use, particularly for behavior disorders [47, 52]. In cases where it is prescribed for depression in youth, the most common diagnosis associated with antidepressant use is depressive disorder, NOS, not major depressive disorder [56]. The persistence of antidepressant medication treatment in Medicaid and HMO-insured youth has been reported to average 3 to 4 months [5, 53].

Antipsychotic medication

The annual prevalence of antipsychotic medication dispensed for youth has risen dramatically since the 1980s. In a national survey of parents, the prevalence of antipsychotic medication prescribed for youth less than 20 years old was 0.2% in 1987 [13]. In a mid-Atlantic state, the annual prevalence for Medicaid-insured youth aged less than 20 years old was 0.15% in 1987 and 0.8% in 1996 [1]. In physician visit data from NAMCS, youth aged less than 21 years had an annual antipsychotic medication visit rate of 0.33% in 1993, but of 1.44% in 2002 [12]. In Vermont, the annual prevalence of antipsychotic medication for Medicaid-insured youth less than 20 years old rose from 0.3% in 1997 to 2.0% in 2007 [27]. For youth aged 6–17 years in a Medicaid 7-state dataset, antipsychotic medication prevalence rose from 2.7% in 2001 to 4.2% in 2004 [57].

As is true for antidepressants and stimulants, the prevalence of antipsychotic medication is highest for Medicaid youth and far lower for the HMO- and commercially insured. During the years 1987 through 1996, the annual HMO antipsychotic prevalence in the Kaiser Permanente northwest region among youth aged <20 years averaged one-third of that of the annual prevalence of Medicaid-insured youth in a mid-Atlantic U.S. state [1]. In 2001, youth enrolled in a southern commercially insured managed care organization had an antipsychotic medication prevalence one-fourth that of Medicaid-insured youth [58]. In a 2004 comparison of antipsychotic medication prevalence for youth, Crystal et al. [57] reported that those covered by Medicaid insurance (in seven U.S. states) were more than four times more likely to be prescribed antipsychotic drugs than youth covered by private insurance.

Antipsychotic medications are more likely to be prescribed to older ($\geq$10 years) and to White youth [1, 12, 59]. The male:female ratio of use has ranged from 1.6:1 to 2.3:1 [57, 58, 60]. The proportion of users of antipsychotic medications less than 10 years of age was 23% for Medicaid-insured [58], 24% for a commercially insured population [61], and 29% for those in a managed care organization in 2001 [58]. The proportion of youth aged 10–14 dispensed antipsychotic medication has been similar to that for youth aged 15–19 years [58, 61, 62].

The great majority of physician diagnoses made in conjunction with antipsychotic medication treatment have been ADHD and conduct disorders [11, 12, 39, 60, 62]. In recent years, the prescribing of antipsychotic medication to outpatient youth has increasingly been associated with the diagnosis of bipolar disorder. For example, in Texas Medicaid-insured youth less than 20 years old, the prevalence of this diagnosis in relation to antipsychotic treatment rose from 9.5% in 1998 to 14.5% in 2001 [63]. Antipsychotic medication linked to a diagnosis of psychosis was reported in less than 10% of youth during physician office visits in 2000–2 [12], for only 7% of privately-insured Missouri youth treated between 2002–5 with antipsychotics [64], and in 6% of youth visits with prescribed antipsychotics from 1996–2007 [60]. Antipsychotic use in Medicaid-insured youth is strikingly higher (over tenfold) for those in foster care and those who qualify for Supplemental Security Income (SSI) compared to those who qualify because of low family income [4]. Similarly, antipsychotic medication prevalence is much higher for those diagnosed with autism spectrum disorder [65, 66]. In a national registry study of youth with autism spectrum disorder aged less than 19 years, 67% who were simultaneously diagnosed with bipolar disorder were reported by their parents to be taking an antipsychotic medication in 2007–8 [67].

By the year 2001, over 90% of antipsychotic medications in the United States were of the atypical subclass [68]. The rank order of atypical antipsychotic medication use among Florida Medicaid-insured youth in 2002–5 was as follows: risperidone, quetiapine, olanzapine, aripiprazole, and ziprasidone [69]. This rank order was similar to that reported by Curtis et al. [61]. By 2005–9, aripiprazole sales and usage among Medicaid-insured youth had moved up to second or third place [36, 62]. Since 2002, olanzapine treatment for Medicaid-enrolled youth has also prominently decreased [62, 69].

A majority of complex psychotropic regimens for youth that include antipsychotic medication are prescribed by psychiatrists [11, 60, 70]. The average persistence of antipsychotic medication treatment in a Medicaid-insured population of youth is slightly less than three months [71]. In a study of Medicaid-insured youth with a diagnosis of bipolar disorder, only 23% remained on antipsychotic medication at the six-month assessment [72].

Alpha-agonists

Alpha-agonist medications such as clonidine and guanfacine were rarely prescribed for psychiatric use in school-aged, Medicaid-insured youth in the 1980s and 1990s (0.004% in 1987 and 0.66% in 1996) in a mid-Atlantic state [1]. The prevalence of use of these drugs is likely to expand more since long-acting formulations of these drugs were recently approved by the FDA for the treatment of ADHD, namely, guanfacine in 2009 and clonidine in 2010.

Anticonvulsant "mood stabilizers"

The annual prevalence of anticonvulsant "mood stabilizers" in youth in an HMO doubled from 0.34% in 1994 to 0.69% in 2003 [5]. In a mid-Atlantic U.S. state, the anticonvulsant "mood stabilizer" prevalence in Medicaid - insured youth aged <20 rose from 0.02% in 1987 to 1.28% in 1996 [1]. These drugs are more likely to be used in males, White youth, youth in foster care, and youth who qualified for SSI [73]. It is of note that anticonvulsant drugs were primarily used for seizure disorders in youth in the early 1990s [74] but by the year 2000, only 19% of prescribed anticonvulsants in the Medicaid analysis of one U.S. state were associated with a seizure diagnosis [73]. In 2000, 12.1% of these drugs in a Medicaid dataset were prescribed for bipolar disorder [73]. In 2003, 31% of anticonvulsant "mood stabilizers" in an HMO population of youth aged 5–17 years of age were prescribed for bipolar disorder [5]. There is recent evidence from physician office visit data that the prevalence of anticonvulsant mood stabilizers for youth has significantly declined since 2004 [60]. This may be partly because published trial findings on the efficacy of anticonvulsant mood stabilizers for pediatric bipolar disorder have been discouraging [75].

Concomitant psychotropic medication

A review of concomitant medication treatment for youth written in 2001 primarily reported data from case series studies because these were the primary data available [76]. Since then, a good deal more data has become available. Comer et al. [60] using physician-visit reports found that, among those with a current mental health diagnosis, the percentage of visits with two or more concomitant psychotropic class use increased from 22% in 1996–9 to 32% in 2004–7. Also from physician visit data, Bhatara et al. [77] compared the prevalence of concomitant psychotropic medication including stimulant treatment for children with ADHD from 1993 to 1998, and reported a fivefold concomitant medication increase over that time period. McIntyre and Jerrell [3] assessed Medicaid claims data from one U.S. state and linked it with outpatient diagnoses from physician visits and found a sixfold increase from 1996 to 2005 in the use of 2 or more concomitant psychotropic medications for the treatment of youth with major depressive disorder.

Comer et al. [60] reported that psychotropic medication class combinations increasingly used for youth between 1997 and 2006 were antidepressants with antipsychotics, and stimulants with antipsychotics. McIntyre and Jerrell [3] found that drug combinations for youth commonly included stimulants with antidepressants during the 1996–2001 period, whereas drug combinations predominantly included antipsychotics during the 2002–5 period.

In physician-visit data, Comer et al. [60] found that psychiatrists were the prescribers in 70% of two or more drug-class concomitant psychotropic visits, but in only 28% of single-class psychotropic visits. Comer et al. [60] also reported that youth given comorbid diagnoses were most likely to receive concomitant psychotropic medications; that mood disorder was diagnosed in only 16% of single class psychotropic visits but was diagnosed in 45% of two or more class psychotropic visits, and that antipsychotics had the greatest increase from 1996 to 2007 in multiclass psychotropic visits (odds ratio = 4.4. CI = 2.50–7.65).

In a survey of U.S. psychiatrists treating 392 youth in routine psychiatric practice during the period from 1997–9, Duffy et al. [78] reported that 52% of children treated by psychiatrists received concomitant psychotropic medication. In an outpatient report on the psychotropic medication treatment of youth diagnosed with autism spectrum disorder, Gerhard et al. [65] reported that 42% of the physician outpatient visits in 2001–5 involved two or more concomitant psychotropic medication classes. In an analysis of outpatient treatment for Texas foster care youth in 2004, Zito et al. [79] reported that 72% of these youth were prescribed two or more classes of psychotropic medications concomitantly during physician outpatient visits. In a community survey of parents of children diagnosed with bipolar disorder, Bhangoo et al. [80] reported that the average number of psychotropic medications prescribed to these children (aged 6–17) at the time of contact was 3.4 medications. In autism spectrum disorder registry data, 51% of parents of youth with comorbid bipolar disorder reported that their child was receiving three or more psychotropic medications concurrently [67].

Duffy et al. [78] found that youth receiving concomitant psychotropic medication prescribed by psychiatrists were more often characterized by the following: a diagnosis of bipolar disorder, prior inpatient status, having a comorbid psychiatric disorder, and having co-existing medical impairments. Similarly, Comer et al. [60] reported that youth prescribed two or more concomitant psychotropic medications during physician office visits were more commonly characterized by the following: teen age status; being recipients of public as opposed to private insurance; having psychiatrist prescribers; having two or more psychiatric diagnoses; and being diagnosed with mood, anxiety and adjustment disorders.

Multiple class studies

Several studies have reported on youth who received—during a given year—multiple classes of psychotropic medication, which were not necessarily prescribed at the same time. Generally, the investigators of these studies reported the same variables that were more characteristic of those who received concomitant medication. The investigators include: (1) Martin et al. [81], using a 1999 Connecticut Medicaid managed care dataset, who found multiples more likely in White youth, males, youth in state custody and older youth; (2) dosReis et al. [82] using data from two Medicaid states on youth less than 20 years old who found multiples more likely in males, youth aged 10–14, those on SSI, and those in foster care, and (3) McIntyre and Jerrell [3] using Medicaid data from a southern state covering the period 1996–2005 who identified polypharmacy to be more likely in males, non-African-American youth, those diagnosed with ADHD, bipolar disorder, or psychosis, and those with co-morbid psychiatric diagnoses.

Preschool psychotropic medication use

Two U.S. studies focused on psychotropic medication prevalence trends in preschool youth [8, 83]. Zito et al. [83] found that stimulant dispensing in Medicaid-enrolled youth aged two to four years in a mid-Atlantic and a mid-Western state rose threefold and 1.8-fold, respectively, from 1991 to 1995. Olfson et al. [8] reported that antipsychotic medication use in privately insured children aged two to five years doubled between 1999–2001 and 2007. A follow-up study by Zito et al. [84], which covered the same aged youth in the mid-Atlantic state Medicaid population found that by 2001, the annual prevalence of receiving any psychotropic medication doubled (from 1995), reaching an annual rate of 2.3%.

As in studies with other age groups, the psychotropic medication prevalence of the commercially and HMO-insured preschoolers was lower than that of Medicaid-insured preschoolers [6] and behavior problems were the primary symptoms that led to preschool youths being placed on psychotropic medication [6, 8]. In an editorial on the Olfson et al. [8] paper, Egger [85] expressed major concerns about the minimal level of evidence supporting the use of antipsychotic medication to treat preschoolers.

International patterns of psychotropic medication for youth

Compared to Western Europe, youth in the United States have a far higher prevalence of all the major classes of psychotropic medication except hypnotics and anxiolytics [86,87]. Prevalence of use in the United States is particularly prominent for stimulants and antidepressants, and somewhat less so for antipsychotics. Unlike in the United States, it is not a common practice in Western Europe to use anticonvulsants as "mood stabilizers" or to use alpha-agonists for psychiatric indications. Lithium was infrequently used for youth in the United States, but almost never prescribed for youth in Western Europe. Preschoolers in the U.S. are dispensed stimulants at a rate far exceeding that in other country, but antipsychotic medications are more likely to be prescribed to preschoolers in Germany and the Netherlands than in the United States. The prevalence of concomitant psychotropic medication practice is two to three times higher in the United States than in Western Europe [87].

Cross-national psychotropic medication prevalence differences for youth are influenced by numerous cultural, state regulatory, marketing, insurance, and price restriction factors [86]. Diagnostic differences also influence cross-national prescribing patterns. For example, pediatric bipolar disorder is diagnosed far more frequently in the United States where the diagnosis is highly associated with the frequent prescription of atypical antipsychotic medications [63,88].

Conclusion

From the early 1990s, pharmacoepidemiologic research on child and adolescent medication patterns became popular methods to assess both medical [89] and behavioral/emotional drug therapies from community-based populations. Such data carry several important limitations (for example, concerning the reliability of diagnoses, and unknown patient consumption) but when interpreted appropriately they produce a valuable public health perspective on the role of medication in the pediatric population. In addition, these data can generate hypotheses for further studies to assess the effectiveness and safety of psychotropic medication.

References

1 Zito JM, Safer DJ, dosReis S et al.: Psychotropic practice patterns for youth. *Arch Pediatr Adolesc Med* 2003; **157**: 17–25.
2 Winterstein AG, Gerhard T, Shuster J et al.: Utilization of pharmacologic treatment in youths with attention deficit/hyperactivity disorder in Medicaid database. *Ann Pharmacotherap* 2008; **42**: 24–31.
3 McIntyre RS, Jerrell JM: Polypharmacy in children and adolescents treated for major depressive disorder: a claims database study. *J Clin Psychiatry* 2009; **70**: 240–6.

4 Zito JM, Safer DJ, Zuckerman JH et al.: Effect of Medicaid eligibility category on racial disparities in the use of psycotropic medicatons among youths. *Psychiat Serv* 2005; **56**: 157–63.

5 Hunkeler E, Firemen B, Lee J et al.: Trends in use of antidepressants, lithium, and anticonvulsants in Kaiser Permanente-insured youths, 1994–2003. *J Child Adolesc Psychophamacol* 2005; **15**: 26–39.

6 DeBar LL, Lynch F, Powell J et al.: Use of psychotropic agents in preschool children. *Arch Pediatr Adolesc Med* 2003; **157**: 150–7.

7 Habel LA, Schaefer CA, Levine P et al.: Treatment with stimulants among youths in a large California health plan. *J Child Adolesc Psychopharmacol* 2005; **15**: 62–7.

8 Olfson M, Crystal S, Huong C, Gerhard T: Trends in antipsychotic drug use by very young, privately insured children. *J Am Acad Child Adolesc Psychiatry* 2010; **49**: 13–23.

9 Cox ER, Motheral BR, Henderson RR et al.: Geographic variation in the prevalence of stimulant medication use among children 5–14 years old: results from a commercially insured US sample. *Pediatrics* 2003; **111**: 237–43.

10 Delate T, Gelenberg AJ, Simmons VA et al.: Trends in the use of antidepressants in a national sample of commercially insured pediatric patients, 1998–2002. *Psychiat Serv* 2004; **55**: 387–91.

11 Cooper WO, Arbogast PG, Ding H et al.: Trends in prescribing of antipsychotic medications for U.S. children. *Ambul Pediatr* 2006; **6**: 79–83.

12 Olfson M, Blanco C, Liu L et al.: National trends in the outpatient treatment of children and adolescents with antipsychotic drugs. *Arch Gen Psychiatry* 2006; **63**: 679–85.

13 Olfson M, Marcus SC, Weissman MM, Jensen PS: National trends in the use of psychotropic medications by children. *J Am Acad Child Adolesc Psychiatry* 2002; **41**: 514–21.

14 Rowland AS, Skipper B, Rabiner DL: The shifting subtypes of ADHD: classification depends on how symptom reports are combined. *J Abnorm Child Psychol* 2008; **36**: 731–43.

15 Safer DJ, Malever M.: Stimulant treatment in Maryland public schools. *Pediatrics* 2000; **106**: 533–9.

16 Rappley MD, Gardiner JC, Jetton JR et al. The use of methylphenidate in Michigan. *Arch Pediatr Adolesc Med* 1995; **149**: 675–9.

17 Safer DJ, Krager JM: Effect of a media blitz and a threatened lawsuit on stimulant treatment. *JAMA* 1992; **268**: 1004–7.

18 Pamer CA, Hammad TA, Wu Y et al.: Changes in US antidepressant and antipsychotic prescription patterns during the period of FDA actions. *Pharmcoepidemiol Drug Safety* 2010; **19**: 158–74.

19 Barbaresi WJ, Katusic SK, Colligan RC et al.: Long-term stimulant medication treatment of attention-deficit/hyperactivity disorder: results from a population-based study. *J Dev Behav Pediatr* 2006; **27**: 1–10.

20 Zima BT, Bussing R, Tang L et al.: Quality of care for childhood attention-deficit/hyperactivity disorder in a managed care Medicaid program. *J Am Acad Child Adolesc Psychiatry* 2010; **49**: 1225–37.

21 Woods SW, Martin A, Spector SG, McGlashan TH: Effects of development on olanzapine-associated adverse events. *J Am Acad Child Adolesc Psychiatry* 2002; **41**: 1439–46.

22 Cooper WO, Hickson GB, Fuchs C et al.: New users of antipsychotic medications among children enrolled in TennCare. *Arch Pediatr Adolesc Med* 2004; **158**: 753–9.

23 Valluri S, Zito JM, Safer DJ et al.: Impact of the 2004 Food and Drug Administration pediatric suicidality warning on antidepressant and psychotherapy treatment for new-onset depression. *Medical Care* 2010; **48**: 947–54.

24 Visser SN, Lesesne CA, Perou R. National estimates and factors associated with medication treatment for childhood attention-deficit/hyperactivity disorder. *Pediatrics* 2007; **119** (Suppl 1): s99–s106.

25 Visser SN, Bitsko RH, Danielson ML et al.: Increasing prevalence of parent-reported attention-deficit/hyperactivity disorder among children—United States, 2003 and 2007. *MMWR* 2010; **59**: 1439–43.

26 Castle L, Aubert RE, Verbrugge RR et al. Trends in medication treatment for ADHD. *J Atten Disord* 2007; **10**: 335–42.

27 Pandiani J, Carroll B. Psychotropic medications received by Medicaid enrolled youth 1997–2007. Unpublished report, 2008. Available at http://psychrights.org/states/Vermont/KidDrugging/08-02-29VtKidDruggingReport.pdf, accessed July 27, 2011.

28 Pastor P, Reuben CA: Diagnosed attention deficit hyperactivity disorder and learning disability: United States, 2004–2006. National Center for Health Statistics, *Vital Health Stat* 2008; **10** (237): 1–14. Available at www.cdc.gov/nchs/data/series/sr_10/Sr10_237.pdf, accessed July 27, 2011.

29 Zuvekas SH, Vitiello B, Norquist GS. Recent trends in stimulant treatment use among U.S. children. *Am J Psychiatry* 2006; **163**: 579–85.

30 Martin A, Sherwin T, Stubbe D et al.: Use of multiple psychotropic drugs by Medicaid-insured and privately insured children. *Psychiat Serv* 2002; **53**: 1508.

31 Safer DJ, Zito JM, Gardner JF: Comparative prevalence of psychotropic medications among youths enrolled in the SCHIP and privately insured youths. *Psychiat Serv* 2004; **55**: 1049–51.

32 Froelich TE, Lanphear BP, Epstein JN et al. Prevalence, recognition, and treatment of attention-deficit/hyperactivity disorder in a national sample of US children. *Arch Pediatr Adolesc Med* 2007; **161**: 857–64.

33 Fulton BD, Scheffler RM, Hinshaw SP et al. National variation of ADHD diagnostic prevalence and medication use: health care providers and education policies. *Psychiat Serv* 2009; **60**: 1075–83.

34 Brinker A, Mosholder A, Schech SD et al. Indication and use of drug products used to treat attention-deficit/hyperactivity disorder: a cross-sectional study with inference on the likelihood of treatment in adulthood. *J Child Adolesc Psychopharmacol* 2007; **17**: 328–33.

35 Swanson JM, Volkow ND: Psychopharmacology: concepts and opinions about the use of stimulant medications. *J Child Psychol Psychiat* 2009; **50**: 180–93.

36 Grohol JM: Top 25 psychiatric prescriptions for 2009. http://psychcentral.com/lib/2010/top-25-psychiatric-prescriptions-for-2009, accessed 27 July, 2011.

37 Olfson M, Marcus SC, Wan G. Stimulant dosing for children with ADHD: a medical claims analysis. *J Am Acad Child Adolesc Psychiatry* 2009; **48**: 51–9.

38 Scheffler RM, Hinshaw SP, Modrek S, Levine P: The global market for ADHD medications. *Health Affairs* 2007; **26**: 450–7.

39 Chen C, Gerhard T, Winterstein AG: Determinants of initial pharmacological treatment for youths with attention-deficit/hyperactivity disorder. *J Child Adolesc Psychopharmacol* 2009; **19**: 187–95.

40 Zarin D, Tanielian TL, Suarez AP et al.: Treatment of attention-deficit hyperactivity disorder by different physician specialties. *Psychiat Serv* 1998; **49**: 171.

41 Perwien AR, Hall J, Swensen A et al.: Stimulant treatment patterns and compliance in children and adults with newly treated attention-deficit/hyperactivity disorder. *J Managed Care Pharm* 2004; **10**: 122–9.

42 Marcus SC, Wan GJ, Kemner JE et al. Continuity of methylphenidate treatment for attention-deficit/hyperactivity disorder. *Arch Pediatr Adolesc Med* 2005; **159**: 572–8.

43 Safer DJ, Zito JM, Fine EM. Increased methylphenidate usage for attention deficit disorder in the 1990s. *Pediatrics* 1996; **98**: 1084–8.

44 Barbaresi WJ, Katusic SK, Colligan RC et al.: How common is attention-deficit/hyperactivity disorder? *Arch Pediatr Adolesc Med* 2002; **156**: 217–24.

45 Bhatara VS, Aparasu RR. Pharmacotherapy with atomoxetine for US children and adolescents. *Ann Clin Psychiatry* 2007; **19**: 175–80.

46 Ma J, Lee KV, Stafford RS. Depression treatment during outpatient visits by U.S. children and adolescents. *J Adolesc Health* 2005; **37**: 434–42.

47 Zito JM, Safer DJ, dosReis S et al. Rising prevalence of antidepressants among U.S. youths. *Pediatrics* 2002; **109**: 721–9.

48 Vitiello B, Zuvekas SH, Norquist GS. National estimates of antidepressant medication use among U.S. children, 1997–2002. *J Am Acad Child Adolesc Psychiatry* 2006; **45**: 271–9.

49 Hammad TA, Laughren T, Racoosin J. Suicidality in pediatric patients treated with antidepressant drugs. *Arch Gen Psychiatry* 2006; **63**: 332–9.

50 Nemeroff CB, Kalali A, Keller MB et al. Impact of publicity concerning pediatric suicidality data on physician practice patterns in the United States. *Arch Gen Psychiatry* 2007; **64**: 466–72.

51 Olfson M, Marcus SC, Druss BG: Effects of Food and Drug Administration warnings on antidepressant use in a national sample. *Arch Gen Psychiatry* 2008; **65**: 95–101.

52 Thomason C, Riordan H, Schaeffer J et al.: Antidepressant prescribing practices prior to and after black-box warnings. Poster presented at the annual meeting of the Am Acad Child Adolesc Psychiatry. San Diego, CA, October 2006.

53 Richardson LP, DiGiuseppe D, Christakis DA et al.: Quality of care for Medicaid-covered youth treated with antidepressant therapy. *Arch Gen Psychiatry* 2004; **61**: 475–80.

54 Olfson M, Gameroff M, Marcus SC et al. Outpatient treatment of child and adolescent depression in the United States. *Arch Gen Psychiatry* 2003; **60**: 1236–42.

55 Morrato EH, Libby AM, Orton HD et al. Frequency of provider contact after FDA advisory on risk of pediatric suicidality with SSRIs. *Am J Psychiatry* 2008; **165**: 42–50.

56 DeBar LL, Clarke GN, O'Connor E, Nichols GA. Treated prevalence, incidence, and pharmacotherapy of child and adolescent mood disorders in an HMO. *Mental Health Services Research* 2001; **3**: 73–83.

57 Crystal S, Olfson M, Huang C et al.: Broadened use of atypical antipsychotics: safety, effectiveness, and policy challenges. *Health Affairs* 2009; **28**: w770–w781.

58 Patel NC, Crismon ML, Hoagwood K et al. Trends in the use of typical and atypical antipsychotics in children and adolescents. *J Am Acad Child Adolesc Psychiatry* 2005; **44**: 548–56.

59 Townsend L, Gerhard T, Huang C et al.: Psychotropic prescription rates and psychiatric diagnoses among publicly insured foster youth in 45 states. Poster presented at the annual mtg. of the Am Acad Child Adolesc Psychiat, NYC, October 2010.

60 Comer JS. Olfson M, Mojtabai R. National trends in child and adolescent psychotropic polypharmacy in office-based practice,1996–2007. *J Am Acad Child Adolesc Psychiatry* 2010; **49**: 1001–10.

61 Curtis LH, Masselink LE, Ostbye T et al.: Prevalence of atypical antipsychotic drug use among commercially insured youths in the United States. *Arch Pediatr Adolesc Med* 2003; **159**: 362–6.

62 Pathak P, West D, Martin BC et al.: Evidence-based use of second-generation antipsychotics in a state Medicaid pediatric population, 2001–2005. *Psychiat Serv* 2010; **61**: 123–9.

63 Patel NC, Crismon ML, Shafer A. Diagnoses and antipsychotic treatment among youths in a public mental health system. *Ann Pharmacother* 2006; **40**: 205–11.

64 Halloran DR, Swindle J, Takemoto SK: Use of atypical antipsychotics in privately-insured Missouri youth: 45. *Pediatr Res* 2006; **60**: 498.

65 Gerhard T, Chavez B, Olfson M et al.: National patterns of the outpatient pharmacological management of children and adolescents with autism spectrum disorder. *J Clin Psychopharmacol* 2009; **29**: 307–10.

66 Witwer A, Lecavalier L: Treatment incidence and patterns in children and adolescents with autism spectrum disorders. *J Child Adolesc Psychopharmacol* 2009; **15**: 671–81.

67 Rosenberg RE, Mandell DS, Farmer JE et al. Psychotropic medication use among children with autism spectrum disorders enrolled in a national registry, 2007–2008. *J Autism Dev Disord* 2010; **40**: 342–51.

68 Aparasu RR, Bhatara V: Antipsychotic prescribing trends among youths, 1997–2002. *Psychiat Serv* 2005; **56**: 904.

69 Constantine R, Tandon R. Changing trends in pediatric antipsychotic use in Florida's Medicaid program. *Psychiat Serv* 2008; **59**: 1162–8.

70 Patel NC, Crismon ML, Hoagwood K et al.: Physician specialty associated with antipsychotic prescribing for youths in the Texas Medicaid program. *Medical Care* 2006; **44**: 87–90.

71 Sleath B, Domino ME, Wiley-Exley E et al. Antidepressant and antipsychotic use and adherence among Medicaid youths: differences by race. *Community Ment Health J* 2010; **46**: 265–72.

72 Case BG, Marcus SC, Olfson M, Siegel CE: Patterns of first medication treatment for publicly insured youth diagnosed with bipolar disorder. Poster presented at the annual meeting of the American Academy of Child and Adolescent Psychiatry, New York, October 2010.

73 Zito JM, Safer DJ, Gardner JF et al. Anticonvulsant treatment for psychiatric and seizure indications among youths. *Psychiat Serv* 2006; **57**: 681–5.

74 Cooper WO, Federspiel CF, Griffin MR et al. New use of anticonvulsant medications among children enrolled in the Tennessee Medicaid program. *Arch Pediat Adolesc Med* 1997; **151**: 1242–6.

75 Correll CU, Sheridan EM, DelBello MP: Antipsychotic and mood stabilizer efficacy and tolerability in pediatric and adult patients with bipolar mania: comparative analysis of acute, randomized, placebo-controlled trials. *Bipolar Disord* 2010; **12**: 116–41.

76 Safer DJ, Zito JM, dosReis S: Concomitant psychotropic medication for youths. *Am J Psychiatry* 2003; **160**: 438–49.

77 Bhatara VS, Feil M, Hoagwood K et al.: Trends in combined pharmacotherapy with stimulants for children. *Psychiat Serv* 2002; **53**: 244.

78 Duffy FF, Narrow WE, Rae DS et al.: Concomitant pharmacotherapy among youths treated in routine psychiatric practice. *J Child Adolesc Psychopharmacol* 2005; **15**: 12–25.

79 Zito JM, Safer DJ, Sai D et al.: Psychotropic medication patterns among youth in foster care. *Pediatrics* 2008; **121**: e157–e163.

80 Bhangoo RK, Lowe CH, Myers FS et al. Medication use in children and adolescents treated in the community for bipolar disorder. *J Child Adolesc Psychopharmacol* 2003; **13**: 515–22.

81 Martin A, Van Hoof T, Stubbe D et al. Multiple psychotropic pharmacotherapy among child and adolescent enrollees in Connecticut Medicaid managed care. *Psychiat Serv* 2003; **54**: 72–7.

82 dosReis S, Zito JM, Safer DJ et al.: Multiple psychotropic medication use for youths: a two-state comparison. *J Child Adolesc Psychopharmacol* 2005; **15**: 68–77.

83 Zito JM, Safer DJ, dosReis S et al. Trends in the prescribing of psychotropic medications to preschoolers. *JAMA* 2000; **283**: 1025–30.

84 Zito JM, Safer DJ, Valluri S et al.: Psychotherapeutic medication prevalence in Medicaid-insured preschoolers. *J Child Adolesc Psychopharmacol* 2007; **17**: 195–203.

85 Egger H: A perilous disconnect: antipsychotic drug use in very young children. *J Am Acad Child Psychiatry* 2010; **49**: 3–6.

86 Safer DJ, Zito JM: International patterns of pediatric medication for emotional and behavioral disorders. In: Martin A, Scahill L, Kratochvill CJ (eds): *Pediatric Psychopharmacology* 2nd edn. New York, NY: Oxford University Press, 2011, pp. 763–74.

87 Zito JM, Safer DJ, van den Berg LT et al.: A three-country comparison of psychotropic medication prevalence in youth. *Child Adolesc Psychiat Ment Health* 2008; **2**: 26.

88 Moreno C, Laje G, Blanco C et al. National trends in the outpatient diagnosis and treatment of bipolar disorder in youth. *Arch Gen Psychiatry* 2007; **64**: 1032–9.

89 Korelitz JJ, Zito JM, Mattison D, Gavin N: Frequency of medication use in the pediatric population: NICHD contract no. GS-23F-8144H. Task Order No. HHSN275200403388C, 2005–9. Available through the NICHD.NIH web site at http://bpca.nichd.nih.gov/resources/reviews/index.cfm, accessed July 27, 2011.

CHAPTER 3

Off-Label Prescribing of Drugs in Child and Adolescent Psychiatry

C. Lindsay DeVane
Medical University of South Carolina, Charleston, USA

Introduction

The approval of drugs for marketing in the United States, and the accompanying label describing their approved uses, are regulated by the Food and Drug Administration (FDA). The FDA is one of eleven divisions of the Cabinet-level Department of Health and Human Services, which is the federal government's principal agency for protecting the health of Americans. As implied by its title, the FDA has broad regulatory responsibilities over a variety of consumer products. These include cosmetic additives, dietary supplements, packaged foods, pet foods, vaccines, blood components, medical devices, and other products. Over-the-counter (OTC) and prescription drugs, including generic drugs, are regulated by the FDA's Center for Drug Evaluation and Research (CDER). The role of CDER is to assure that all OTC and prescription drugs are safe and effective. This is primarily accomplished by the regulation of drug marketing. The FDA does not regulate prescribing or medical practice. Applications for FDA approval to sell drugs in the United States must provide sufficient data to support claims of efficacy and safety. Thus, the availability of a drug by prescription implies that its labeling and advertisement have undergone an FDA evaluation for accuracy of all claims. An important concept discussed in this chapter is that the use of drugs inconsistent with the approved labeling should be practiced with recognition that FDA scrutiny for efficacy and safety has not been exercised to the same degree compared to the review performed in the process of approving drug indications.

The term "drug label" refers to the prescribing information that accompanies all drugs available by prescription in the United States. "Off-label" prescribing is commonly thought of as the use of an approved drug for an

---

Pharmacotherapy of Child and Adolescent Psychiatric Disorders, Third Edition.
Edited by David R. Rosenberg and Samuel Gershon.
© 2012 John Wiley & Sons, Ltd. Published 2012 by John Wiley & Sons, Ltd.

unapproved use [1]. Off-label prescribing is a much broader concept and occurs in multiple ways. Examples are provided in Table 3.1. Some forms of off-label prescribing, such as splitting tablets to ease administration or lower costs, may usually be regarded as minor deviations compared to prescribing a drug for an unstudied use. However, breaking apart some dosage forms may alter their subsequent drug absorption characteristics or provide an incorrect dose, and only infrequently results in cost-savings [2]. Either deviation can represent an off-label practice. Thus, off-label prescribing carries certain potential benefits as well as risks. Substantial evidence of efficacy may exist for an indication that is not discussed in the drug labeling. For example, evidence for efficacy of fluvoxamine in the treatment of major depression is unequivocal, but fluvoxamine is not approved by the FDA as a treatment for depression. Another example of off-label prescribing is employing a more rapid upward titration of drug dosage than recommended in the labeled information; however, certain situations may benefit from such a practice. For seriously ill patients, rapid dose increases for some drugs may attain a therapeutic benefit sooner than would be expected by following the recommended titration schedule. Hospitalization may be avoided, or minimized, and convenient scheduling of patient visits for evaluation may represent other potential benefits from individualized titration. A legitimate concern for off-label prescribing is for the occurrence of a serious adverse event that could prompt an accusation of inappropriate prescribing. If this situation occurs, previous positive patient experiences associated with off-label prescribing may be regarded as non-blinded and

Table 3.1 Forms and examples of "off-label" prescribing of drugs

Form	Example
Prescribing for an indication not approved in the labeling	Antipsychotic prescribing for borderline personality disorder
A prescribed dosage outside of the approved range or outside the range recommended by weight	Prescribing fluvoxamine for adolescent OCD in a dose of 350 mg/day
Dosage titration faster than recommended in the labeling	Increasing the initial aripiprazole dose in autistic disorder in less than four days
A different dosage form	Breaking apart enteric-coated tablets to incorporate into apple sauce or orange juice for children
Prescribing a different route of administration	Using ophthalmic drops for optic administration; or using an intramuscular formulation by the intravenous route
Use in an age range below the approved range	Use of aripiprazole in a 3 year old with autism
Use in an age range above the approved range	Use of risperidone in a 30-year-old adult patient with autism

uncontrolled anecdotal reports that provide minimal scientific evidence of efficacy and safety.

The outcome of drug treatment can never be completely assured. Whether on-label or off label, pharmacotherapy may be beneficial, inconsequential, and sometimes harmful. Prescribing clozapine for some adults with schizophrenia can provide dramatic improvement in recalcitrant psychoses but carries a risk of agranulocytosis for all patients. Prescribing clozapine for an adult with bipolar disorder would be outside of the approved labeling of clozapine's indications. Prescribing clozapine for an adolescent with PTSD would be outside the approved label for both indications and age. However, neither of these two applications would be outside of legal medical practice. Supportive data describe the successful use of clozapine in children [3,4]. When pharmacotherapy is used to treat mental illness, an improvement in symptoms is usually satisfactory evidence to both prescriber and patient that drug treatment was required for a beneficial response. The issue of off-label prescribing is often an unimportant concern unless a serious adverse reaction occurs.

A view emerges from the literature pertaining to off-label prescribing that it is a necessary aspect of practicing child and adolescent psychiatry. The American Medical Association, other professional groups, as well as the FDA, have all endorsed the practice of off-label prescribing in certain circumstances [5]. The following position of the FDA is taken from its regulatory guidance related to "off-label" uses of drugs: "If physicians use a product for an indication not in the approved labeling, they have the responsibility to be well informed about the product, to base its use on firm scientific rationale and on sound medical evidence, and to maintain records of the product's use and effects" [6]. This chapter will review evidence for the extent of off-label prescribing, discuss issues that lead to this practice, and note recent regulations that encourage drug development for children and adolescents. Finally, guidelines are suggested for decision making when confronted with situations where prescribing within approved labeling appears inadequate for the treatment needs of children and adolescents with mental disorders.

Extent of off-label prescribing

Drug prescribing for children and adolescents can be considered in the larger context of drug and chemical exposure as a life-long experience. It usually begins *in utero* with the placental passage of drugs taken by the mother before birth, from chemicals present in her food, or contaminants in the environment. Undoubtedly, most people die with drug residues in their body. This phenomenon of drug exposure across the lifespan has increased in prevalence as drug development for treatment of human disease is increasingly directed toward prevention of susceptible illness. For example, supportive evidence exists for the reduction in all-cause mortality by the statin class of anti-hyperlipidemics when taken by people without established cardiovascular disease but who have cardiovascular risk factors [7]. Low-doses of aspirin are taken by millions of people around the world for a beneficial anti-platelet effect. The trend toward prophylactic pharmacotherapy is likely to accelerate with further identification of genetic biomarkers for predisposition to disease. Adding recreational drug use in the form of caffeine and alcohol further contributes to lifetime drug exposure. In general, most of the lifespan exposure to legal drugs is socially acceptable as a societal norm. One area that has generated substantial concern for the potential of unknown harm is the use of psychoactive drugs in children and adolescents [8–10]. Table 3.2 lists psychoactive drugs by their earliest approved use for a psychiatric indication.

Data of qualitative and quantitative psychoactive drug exposure of children presents a view that pediatric drug consumption is increasing [11]. In 1998, Greenhill [12] found less than a dozen controlled efficacy studies of psychoactive drugs in children in the preschool age-group. The only area in which a substantial number of controlled studies supported efficacy and safety for school-age children was the use of psychostimulants for ADHD [13]. However, the extensive use of psychostimulants has alarmed some authors. By the mid-1990s, epidemiological data indicated 2.8% of U.S. children aged 5 to 18 were receiving methylphenidate [14].

Our review in 1996 of the published use of selective serotonin reuptake inhibitors (SSRI) in children found only three controlled clinical trials [15]. These trials reported drug experience in a total of 65 patients. Eighteen additional open-label trials included 322 patients and 23 case reports were available documenting use in a variety of unapproved indications. The bulk of this literature would not constitute strong evidence for efficacy and safety in 1996. At this same time, the evidence base was increasing for the efficacy of SSRIs in the treatment of adult anxiety disorders. The better tolerability and safety in overdose compared to the tricyclic class of antidepressants made the off-label use of SSRI in children an attractive treatment option [16]. Earlier controlled trials of tricyclics in children had not provided substantial evidence for their efficacy in childhood depression [17]. As would be subsequently learned through controlled clinical trials of SSRI in adolescents [18] these drugs created a liability of suicidal thinking and behavior in adolescents [19]. This effect is currently noted in the SSRI labeling with a black-box warning, the FDA's strongest indication of a potential adverse event.

Off-label prescribing for children with developmental disabilities has a substantial documentation [20–23]. Off-label use in preschool children

Table 3.2 Psychoactive drugs approved by the FDA according to earliest age of labeled use and indication

Minimal age in years according to label	Drug	Approved indications	Comments
No defined minimum age	Carbamazepine	Anticonvulsant	This drug has no approved psychiatric indication in children; treatment of seizures is indicated in children; bipolar I is an adult indication for carbamazepine
2	Thioridazine	Various behavioral symptoms	Thioridazine sold as Mellaril was discontinued worldwide in 2005 by its manufacturer Novartis
	Divalproex sodium, oxcarbazepine	Anticonvulsant	
3	Haloperidol; amphetamine; dextroamphetamine	Schizophrenia; control of Tourette's syndrome ADHD	Haloperidol injectable forms are not approved for children or for Tourette's syndrome for any age
5	Risperidone	Irritability associated with autistic disorder	Efficacy and safety was demonstrated in autistic disorder and not in autistic spectrum disorders (Asperger's or ASD-NOS); approved age range is 5 to 17
6	Aripiprazole Imipramine sertraline Amphetamine (as Dextrostat), Amphetamine (extended release as Adderal XR) Methylphenidate (long acting as Concerta), Methylphenidate patch, Dexmethylphenidate (Focalin or Focalin XR), Methamphetamine, Atomoxetine Lisdexamfetamine, Guanfacine,	Irritability associated with autistic disorder Enuresis Obsessive compulsive disorder Attention-deficit hyperactivity disorder*	Approved age range is 6 to 17

(continued)

Table 3.2 (*Continued*)

Minimal age in years according to label	Drug	Approved indications	Comments
8	Fluvoxamine Fluoxetine	Obsessive compulsive disorder Depression	
10	Aripiprazole, Risperidone; Quetiapine, clomipramine (før OCD only)	Bipolar mania and mixed episodes Obsessive compulsive disorder	
12	Pimozide Escitalopram Doxepin; Lithium	Tourette's disorder Major depressive disorder Depression Manic episodes of bipolar disorder	
13	Risperidone, quetiapine, aripiprazole Olanzapine	Schizophrenia Second line treatment for manic or mixed episodes of bipolar disorder; schizophrenia	
18	All other psychoactive drugs, including benzodiazepines used as anti-anxiety agents, monoamine-oxidase inhibitors, remaining antidepressants, traditional and atypical antipsychotic drugs, clozapine, gabapentin, topiramate, lamotrigine	Various adult indications; "adult" not always defined in labeling but presumed to be 18 and older Labeling may also exclude elderly	Does not include injectable benzodiazepines (midazolam) used as an anesthetic or diazepam as an anticonvulsant

*Approval of ADHD products and some generic drugs may differ across branded products according to age.

with an Axis I disorder has been estimated as high as 12% [21]. The practice of prescribing psychoactive drugs to children off-label is international in scope. In Australia, a survey of 187 child and adolescent psychiatrists indicated that over 40% had prescribed off-label and 10% had prescribed a combination of psychoactive drugs for children less than three years old [24]. Prescription data documented a doubling of SSRI use over a four-year period in Germany with the highest use in adolescent girls age 15–19 [25]. In summary, the literature supports an impression that child and adolescent psychiatrists engage extensively in off-label prescribing, but also suggests this activity constitutes a necessary element of contemporary practice.

Need for psychoactive drug treatments for children and adolescents

There is an unequivocal need for continued research to define effective treatments of mental disorders in children and adolescents. Many chapters in this volume provide this documentation. The presence of mental illness is often apparent in the first two decades of life and many psychiatric disorders can be reliably diagnosed in children. Epidemiological studies support continuity between child and adult psychopathology. In a study extending over 14 years, Hofstra et al. [26] found an approximate two- to sixfold increased risk for adult DSM-IV diagnoses from a sample of 1578 Dutch children and adolescents. In a sample of 86 children characterized with a DSM-IV manic episode, the average age was 10.8 ± 2.7 years [27]. When re-examined every six months for four years, those subjects diagnosed with prepubertal and early adolescent bipolar disorder were characterized with long-episode durations having a time to recovery of 60.2 weeks.

Given the chronic clinical course of major mental disorders in adults, there is a valid need for studies to determine the efficacy of treating mental illness in children and adolescents. A major issue is to determine whether early intervention with pharmacotherapy produces benefits in adults by altering the course of illness in childhood. A lack of evidenced-based data to address some of these issues leaves the child/adolescent psychiatrist at a disadvantage in employing pharmacotherapy. Off-label prescribing is a logical treatment alternative especially when evidence exists for efficacy and safety. When drugs are first available for prescribing, they are often labeled for only a single FDA-approved use although an abundance of supportive data may exist for other indications. As noted above, this situation does not preclude legally prescribing for off-label uses.

Economic considerations contribute to drug development for a single indication. For a drug with a modest market potential of approximately half-a-billion dollars a year, a delay in FDA approval represents a potential revenue loss of greater than $1 million per day. Few companies can postpone seeking FDA approval for an initial use to await additional data to support other indications. The incentive exists to submit for FDA approval as soon as sufficient data supports a single use. Economic incentives also support filing an application for approval of an already accepted indication rather than for a novel use. Unfortunately for pediatric psychopharmacology, this situation has historically created further disincentive to collect data from children and adolescents out of concern that the appearance of new adverse events may influence approval for adult use. An influential example is provided by the development of bupropion as an antidepressant. The FDA originally approved the drug for depression in 1985 but marketing was delayed following the report of seizures in four of 55 bulimic, nondepressed, patients [28]. The seizure rate was eventually shown not to exceed that of other antidepressants when the daily dose was kept below 450 mg. However, the issue of seizures delayed marketing until 1989. This experience promoted a concern that research into secondary indications may pose an unnecessary risk during drug development while simultaneously seeking FDA approval for a primary indication.

All of the SSRIs originally approved for depression were eventually shown to be useful for obsessive-compulsive disorder. Thus, it may have been logical to assume at some point, when one or two SSRIs were approved for OCD, that the remaining SSRIs would have similar efficacy for this indication. While this specific assumption has been proven true, to assume that all members of a class of drugs possess an interchangeable pharmacology is risky. The SSRIs have shown differences in adverse events across individual drugs in adults for common events [29] and for producing a discontinuation syndrome [30]. A similar situation applies to the atypical antipsychotics as they do not all share an equal risk of producing weight gain or metabolic syndrome.

Both aripiprazole and risperidone are FDA approved in the treatment of patients with autism for control of behavioral irritability. Both of these drugs may increase metabolic effects and precipitate undesirable increases in body weight that make them intolerable for some patients. Assuming that ziprasidone, another member of the class of atypical antipsychotics, has similar efficacy, but lower liability for weight gain, has some basis for support from adult data [31]. However, other pharmacological differences, such as cardiac conduction effects, cannot be assumed to be the same in children and adults and requires specific investigation in younger populations. Pimizide and haloperidol are used to treat tics associated with Tourette's disorder but both carry a risk of seizures and production of tardive dyskinesia. The experience in adults with risperidone and aripiprazole suggests that both of these drugs should be safer than the older alternatives in Tourette's disorder [32] but neither has FDA approval for this use. Unfortunately, when a patent for exclusive marketing is about to expire, an economic incentive for pediatric drug development also disappears.

If drug development in adults could adequately inform how to use psychoactive drugs in children, there would be no need for clinical trials in children and adolescents. However, there are multiple reasons why adult results do not always translate to children and adolescents. An abundance of data exists that documents physiological differences between children and adults that impacts drug disposition and effects justifying separate drug development programs according to age [33]. Merely extrapolating an adult dose to a child on the basis of lower weight may result in either inadequate exposure or overexposure based on adult dosage recommendations. Most dosage regimens for adults have been developed in a fairly narrow range of body weights, often assuming an average weight of 170 lb. When the same mg dose is converted into mg/kg and applied to children, they may receive less than an adequate dose. Children generally have a greater ratio of liver weight to total body mass than adults and may require doses higher than an adult when normalized to body weight to be effective as hepatic drug clearance can exceed adult values. This is more likely to apply to drugs that are highly metabolized than those with a substantial renal excretion. Unfortunately, these considerations do not appear to be equally applicable to all drugs and must be individually tested. In addition, the young patient may have different receptor sensitivities from an adult. For example, plasticity in dopamine neurotransmission has been shown to occur well into adolescence [34]. Just as some elderly patients become more sensitive to drug effects for this reason, it is reasonable to expect such differences also exist in children and adolescents.

Legislation supporting pediatric drug development

The pharmaceutical industry has incentives to generate reliable, objective evidence concerning new uses of approved drugs. They can expand the market for a product by conducting supplementary research necessary to seek the FDA's approval for an off-label use. This reduces product liability risks by obtaining FDA approval for revised labeling to include new indications. Overall, they can respond to a marketplace where healthcare professionals and institutions, managed care organizations, and insurers utilize objective evidence of a product's benefits as a basis for making treatment and reimbursement decisions.

Despite incentives, development of drug treatments for children and adolescents with mental disorders has been a relatively neglected priority of the pharmaceutical industry. Rarely have psychoactive drug development programs been initiated with the expressed goal of achieving initial FDA approval to treat a mental disorder of children. Some notable exceptions include the psychostimulants for ADHD and the current development of various drugs for fragile X syndrome. Consequently, the use of the majority of drugs in child and adolescent psychiatry has evolved from prior developments in adults and off-label uses in children and adolescents. The FDA Modernization Act in 1997 authorized a pediatric exclusivity process to encourage the study of drugs in pediatrics. Pediatric studies conducted by the industry and specifically designated by the FDA can be rewarded by a 6 month exclusivity extension in patent rights. Between 1998 and 2004, this provision in the law resulted in 253 studies submitted to the FDA [35]. Further legislation has encouraged drug development for children and adolescents. On September 27, 2007, President George W. Bush signed into law H.R. 3580, the Food and Drug Administration Amendments Act of 2007, which significantly enhanced the authority of the FDA and provided additional resources needed to conduct the comprehensive reviews necessary to evaluate new drugs and devices. The Best Pharmaceuticals for Children Act (BPCA) and the Pediatric Research Equity Act (PREA) were both designed to encourage more research into, and more development of, treatments for children.

One provision of the 1997 FDA Modernization Act regulated advertising of unapproved uses of drugs. The FDA does not prohibit a drug manufacturer from providing information about off-label use when this information is requested by the prescriber. What is prohibited is allowing a manufacturer to freely distribute unsolicited information about off-label uses of approved products that significantly focuses on that manufacturer's product. In reality, this is a difficult policy to maintain. In 2007, for example, the FDA received for review greater than 70 000 pieces of promotional material [36]. Given the volume of work, periods of months may elapse in the review process before the FDA determines that promotional materials, advertising campaigns, direct-to-consumer advertising, or other promotions may be in violation. It then has the authority to issue warning letters to cease specific practices, or to confiscate mislabeled products. Ultimately, through the Department of Justice, civil penalties may be levied in egregious cases. A recent example occurred in May 2004 when Pfizer, Inc. agreed to a settlement of $430 million for the alleged off-label promotion of Neurontin (lamotrigine) for various uses including bipolar disorder, various pain disorders and attention-deficit disorder. In September 2007, Bristol-Myers Squibb agreed to a settlement of $515 million for alleged off-label promotion of Abilify (aripiprazole) for dementia with psychoses and for pediatric use for which it was not labeled at the time.

In contrast to the extreme examples of alleged off-label promotion above, the FDA encourages the industry to submit scientific evidence about new uses by allowing supplemental applications with the aim of revising the product labeling. Neurontin (lamotrigine) has been subsequently labeled for use as maintenance therapy in adults with bipolar I disorder and Abilify (aripiprazole) is approved for manic and mixed episodes in bipolar I disorder in adolescents aged 10 to 17 and for children aged 6 to 17 for irritability associated with autistic disorder. The amount of data required by the FDA for supplemental approval varies according to specific circumstances.

Recommendations to follow when considering off-label prescribing

When the current drug therapy management of a behavioral problem within labeling guidelines (dose, length of dosing) is inadequate or problematic in some way, off-label prescribing may be an option. The following guidelines should be considered when confronted with this situation.

1 Ensure that current management is inadequate or problematic.
2 Identify potential "off-label" treatments.
3 Understand a theoretical basis for benefit.
4 Evaluate the strength of the existing evidence: theoretical < in vitro or animal studies < uncontrolled case reports < case series < non-blinded clinical trials < randomized controlled trials.
5 Identify target symptoms or behaviors to indicate benefit.
6 Develop a plan for management of adverse events and drug discontinuation if necessary.
7 Discuss alternatives with family, caregivers, and patients.
8 Seek and document informed consent.
9 Identify any mitigating circumstances influencing drug disposition or pharmacodynamics.
10 Design a dosage regimen to achieve a therapeutic benefit if one exists.

The particular patient situation could take a number of different forms, including drug-drug interactions interfering with other necessary therapeutic regimens, the lack of dosage forms that the child can take, or the appearance of unacceptable adverse events in the face of a continued need for treatment. Specifically identified circumstances should exist that lead to a decision for off-label prescribing. When off-label treatments are considered, several choices may be available. An alternative with substantial evidence for efficacy and safety should be preferred. Whatever choice is made, the prescriber should have a basis for off-label use. This could consist of a pharmacological argument that a drug will produce a certain action on neuronal circuits or receptors thought to be involved with the pathophysiology of the disorder. Most often evidence for efficacy and safety in adults will exist although substantial documentation of similar benefits in children may be lacking. When multiple choices are available, an evaluation of the existing evidence should be considered. If double-blind controlled studies are available, this situation often presents a sound basis for a decision. The use of any pharmacotherapy should be accompanied by identification of target symptoms or desirable outcomes before the initiation of treatment. Even though parents and physicians often use global assessments in determining whether drug therapy was beneficial or not, the extent to which specific behaviors to monitor can be identified will aid in the subsequent assessment of the success or failure of an off-label treatment. In addition, potential adverse events, based on known pharmacology, identified at the same time as target symptoms for benefit, will simplify subsequent decisions related to changes in dosing or discontinuation decisions. Ideally, some pre-thought should be given to contingency planning for adverse events and or drug discontinuation.

One concern of clinicians when prescribing off label is whether untoward events could lead to patient harm. Patients, parents, and relatives all assume that prescribed treatments follow from evidence of efficacy and safety evaluated by a competent clinician. When off-label use of drugs in children and adolescents is being considered, a transparent discussion of the need is recommended. Recognizing the inadequacy of a current treatment, setting out the available evidence for trying alternatives, and planning for contingencies, all constitute components of good medical practice. In this regard, seeking informed consent, and assent from the child or adolescent when desirable, is recommended documentation. Lastly, follow-up documentation of the results of off-label prescribing is also recommended as a part of clinical practice and has a potential benefit for supporting similar prescribing in subsequent patient encounters.

References

1 Stafford RS: Regulating off-label drug use-rethinking the role of the FDA. *New EnglMed* 2008; **358**: 1427–9.
2 Bachynsky J, Wiens C, Meinychuk K: The practice of splitting tablets: cost and therapeutic aspects. *Pharmacoeconomics* 2002; **20**: 339–46.
3 Gogtay N, Rapoport J.: Clozapine use in children and adolescents. *Expert Opinion on Pharmacotherapy* 2008; **9**: 459–65.
4 US Food and Drug Administration: "Off-label" and investigational use of marketed drugs, biologics, and medical devices—information sheet. Available at http://www.fda.gov/RegulatoryInformation/Guidances/ucm126486.htm, accessed July 27, 2011.
5 Kant R, Chalansani R, Chengappa KNR et al.: The off-label use of clozapine in adolescents with bipolar disorder, intermittent explosive disorder, or posttraumatic stress disorder. *J Child AdolescPsychopharmacol* 2004; **14**: 57–63.
6 Dresser R, Frader J: Off-label prescribing: a call for heightened professional and government oversight. *J Law Medicine, and Ethics* 2009; **37**: 476–85. http://www.fda.gov/RegulatoryInformation/Guidances/ucm126486.htm, accessed March 23, 2011.
7 Brugts JJ, Yetgin T, Hoeks SE et al.: The benefits of statins in people without established cardiovascular disease but with cardiovascular risk factors: meta-analysis of randomized controlled trials. *Brit Med J* 2009; **338**: 2376.
8 Zito JM, Safer DJ, DosReis S et al.: Psychotropic practice patterns for youth: a 10-year perspective. *Arch Pediatr Adolesc Med* 2003; **157**: 17–25.
9 Conrad P: Prescribing more psychotropic medications for children, What does the increase mean? *Arch PediatrAdolesc Med* 2004; **158**: 829–30.

10 Thomas CP, Conrad P, Casler R et al. Trends in the use of psychotropicmedications among adolescents, 1994–2001. *Psych Serv* 2006; **57**: 63–9.

11 Editorial: Increased medication use in attention-deficit hyperactivity disorder: regressive or appropriate? *JAMA* 1988; **260**: 2270–2.

12 Greenhill LL: The use of psychotropic medication in preschoolers: indications, safety and efficacy. *Can J Psychiatry* 1988; **43**: 576–81.

13 Spencer T, Biederman J, Wilens T et al.: Pharmacotherapy of attention-deficit hyperactivity disorder across the life cycle. *J Am Acad Child Adolesc Psychiatry* 1996; **35**: 409–32.

14 Safer DJ, Zito JM, Fine EM: Increased methylphenidate usage for attention deficit disorder in the 1990s. *Pediatrics* 1996; **98**: 1084–8.

15 DeVane CL, Sallee FR: Serotonin selective reuptake inhibitors in child and adolescent psychopharmacology: a review of published experience. *J Clin Psychiatry* 1996; **57**: 55–66.

16 Daly JM, Wilens T: The use of tricyclic antidepressants in children. *Pediatr Clin NA* 1998; **45**: 1123–35.

17 Kye CH, Waterman GS, Ryan ND: A randomized controlled clinical trial of amitryptyline in the acute treatment of adolescent major depression. *J Am Acad Child Adolesc Psychiatry* 1996; **35**: 1139–44.

18 Keller MB, Ryan ND, Strober M et al.: Efficacy of paroxetine in the treatment of adolescent major depression: a randomized, controlled trial. *J Am Acad Child Adolesc Psychiatry* 2001; **40**: 762–72.

19 Gibbons RD, Brown CH, Hur K et al.: Early evidence on the effects of regulators suicidality warnings on SSRI prescriptions and suicide in children and adolescents. *Am J Psychiatry* 2007; **164**: 1356–63.

20 Aman MG, Lam KSL, Van Bourgondien ME: Medication patterns in patients with autism: temporal, regional, and demographic influences. *J Child Adolesc Psychopharmacol* 2005; **15**: 116–26.

21 Luby JL, Stalets MM, Belden A: Psychotropic prescriptions in a sample including both healthy and mood disruptive disordered preschoolers: relationships to diagnosis, impairment, preschooler type and assessment methods. *J Child Adolesc Psychopharmacol* 2007; **17**: 205–12.

22 Bildt A, Mulden EJ, Sheens T et al.: Pervasive developmental disorder, behavioral problems, and psychiatric drug use in children and adolescents with mental retardation. *Pediatrics* 2006; **118**: 1860–6.

23 Hanft A, Hendren RL: Pharmacotherapy of children and adolescents with pervasive developmental disorders. *Essential Psychopharmaacol* 2004; **6**: 12–23.

24 Efron D, Hiscock H, Sewell JR et al.: Prescribing of psychotropic medications for children by Australian pediatricians and child psychiatrists. *Pediatrics* 2003; **111**: 372–5.

25 Fegert JM, Kolch M, Zito JM et al.: Antidepressant use in children and adolescents in Germany. *J Child Adolescent Psychopharmacol* 2006; **16**: 197–206.

26 Hofstra MB, van der Ende J, Verhulst FC: Child and adolescent problems predict DSM-IV disorders in adulthood: a 14 year follow-up of a Dutch epidemiological sample. *J Am Acad Child Adolesc Psych* 2002; **41**: 182–9.

27 Geller B, Tillman R, Craney JL et al.: Four-year prospective outcome and natural history of mania in children with a prepubertal and early adolescent bipolar disorder phenotype. *Arch Gen Psych* 2004; **61**: 459–67.

28 Horne RL, Ferguson JM, Pope HG: Treatment of bulimia with bupropion: a multi center controlled trial. *J Clin Psychiatry* 1988; **49**: 262–6.

29 DeVane CL: Comparative safety and tolerability of selective serotonin reuptake inhibitors. *Hum Psychopharmacol* 1995; **10:** 185–93.

30 Rosenbaum J, Fava M, Hoog SL: Selective serotonin reuptake inhibitor discontinuation syndrome: a randomized trial. *Bio Psychiatry* 1998; **44:** 77–87.

31 Allison DB, Mentore JL, Moonseong H. Antipsychotic induced weight gain: a comprehensive research synthesis. *Am J Psychiatry* 1999; **156:** 686–96.

32 Bruggeman R, Van der Linden C, Buitelaar JK: Risperidone versus pimozide in Tourette's Disorder: a comparative double-blind parallel group study. *J Clin Psychiatry* 2001: **62:** 50–6.

33 Abdel-Rahman SM, Reed MD, Wells TG et al.: Considerations in the rational design and conduct of Phase I'II pediatric clinical trials: avoiding the problems and pitfalls. *Clin Pharm Ther* 2007; **81:** 483–94.

34 Anderson SL, Teicher MH: Sex differences in dopamine receptors and the relevance to ADHD. *Neurosci and Neurobehav Rev* 2000; **24:** 137–41.

35 Benjamin DK, Smith PB, Murphy MD et al.: Peer-reviewed publication of clinical trials completed for pediatric exclusivity. *JAMA* 2006; **296:** 1266–73.

36 GAO-08-835. Prescription Drugs, DA's Oversight of the Promotion of Drugs for Off-Label Uses. Report to the Ranking Member, Committee on Finance, U.S. Senate, United States Government Accountability Office, 2008. Available at: http://www.gao.gov/new.items/d08835.pdf, accessed July 27, 2011.

CHAPTER 4

The Use of Generic Drugs in Pediatric Psychopharmacology

Richard I. Shader & Christopher-Paul Milne

Center for the Study of Drug Development, Tufts University School of Medicine, Boston, USA

What is a generic drug?

A generic drug is a copy of an original, brand-named, or innovative drug that has lost its patent protection. It has the same active ingredient(s) as the original drug, but it differs in its inactive constituents. Current patent laws allow for patent protection for a new formulation, exclusive of its active moiety.

Why are we discussing generic drugs?

First, we believe that the use of generic drugs will increase rapidly in the coming years because of expanding healthcare coverage for children and increasing pressures to contain and restrain healthcare expenditures. We recently noted that approximately 77% of all psychotropic drugs prescribed in the United States are generic [1]. Unfortunately, we were unable to determine whether there was any difference in this proportion for children as compared to adults. Because generic manufacturers do not bear the burden of drug development and can piggyback on the advertising and name recognition of the brand-named agent, the costs of generics can be substantially lower than those of the original product. Consumers and third-party payers benefit from competition when more than one generic version of a product is available. Not surprisingly, dispensing pharmacies prefer generic drugs because their mark-up (profit margin) can be higher because their base cost is lower than that of innovator products.

Another reason for explicating this topic is that many prescribing clinicians confuse relative differences in pharmacokinetics and pharmacodynamics in adults and children with differences in generic versus

Pharmacotherapy of Child and Adolescent Psychiatric Disorders, Third Edition.
Edited by David R. Rosenberg and Samuel Gershon.
© 2012 John Wiley & Sons, Ltd. Published 2012 by John Wiley & Sons, Ltd.

innovator drugs. It is clear that children differ from adults on many parameters and that these parameters change as children develop and mature. Examples include: amount and type of plasma binding proteins, fat and body water proportions, glomerular filtration rate, membrane permeability, as well as transporter proteins in the gut wall (for example, p-glycoprotein) and hepatic metabolizing enzymes such as CYP 3A4 versus 3A7 and some conjugating enzymes such as glucuronosyltransferases [2]. Although no published studies could be found that compare drug absorption in children versus adults, a recent study by the Food and Drug Administration (FDA) examined 2070 unpublished reports from their files conducted in adults over a 12-year period comparing the rate and extent of absorption of innovator drugs versus their generic equivalents. As the difference between them was approximately 3.5%, the findings supported the claim of similarity between these formulations on absorption parameters [3]. Another review of nine types of cardiovascular agents from 38 randomized controlled trials found clinical equivalence in all but three of the studies [4]. The authors of that report concluded that there was no evidence for the superiority of innovator drugs over their generic equivalents. However, they did note an unfavorable or skeptical view of generics in over half of 43 editorials accompanying these trials.

On the other hand, the FDA recently passed the bioequivalence data rule (see Final Rule, "Requirements for Submission of Bioequivalence Data," Federal Register, 16 January, 2009), which requires sponsors submitting an abbreviated new drug application (ANDA) to include all bioequivalence studies the applicant has conducted on the drug product formulation under review. The FDA noted that in the past ANDA applicants typically failed to submit studies, including ones that did not show their product meeting bioequivalence criteria [5].

Basic requirements for generic drugs

In order to gain approval from the FDA for marketing, a generic drug must meet the following criteria: contain the same active ingredient; be identical in strength, dosage form, and route of administration; have the same use indications; be bioequivalent (same amount of active ingredient delivered to site of action at same rate within certain parameters); meet the same batch requirements for identity, strength, purity and quality; and, be manufactured under the strict standards of the good manufacturing regulations. In other words, bioequivalence means that the generic product has comparable pharmacokinetic and pharmacodynamic properties to the original product. In practical terms, the area under the concentration versus time curve (AUC), the peak concentration (C_{MAX}), the time to peak concentration (T_{MAX}), and the absorption lag time (t_{LAG}) of the generic copy must be within 80% to 125% of the original product taken in the fasting state [6].

However, the FDA does accept some chemical differences in the active ingredient. For example, there may be different salts or esters. We recently expressed concern about a hydrobromide generic equivalent of an antidepressant and antismoking aid, bupropion hydrochloride [7]. Due to the potential for bromide salts to cause central nervous system (CNS) toxicity and the particular vulnerability of children to CNS toxicity, this is one of the rare instances in which generic substitution could potentially cause clinically meaningful problems in children.

Inactive ingredients may be different—inactive ingredients are called excipients. They are considered to be pharmacologically inactive ingredients that serve a variety of purposes. Excipients include, but are not limited to: stabilizers, coatings, binders, sweeteners and other flavorings, fillers, moisture-proofing sorbents, preservatives, and lubricants.

Although most prescribing clinicians never think about excipients, they are the major ingredients that distinguish generic from innovator drugs. The size, color, shape, or sweetness of a pill can make it more appealing or palatable to children, a consideration that may be less relevant for adults.

Excipients may also have an impact on shelf life. For example, a generic version of lorazepam deteriorated to a powdery clump within six months while still in its original plastic container. That version is no longer marketed.

Two excipients are worthy of particular mention for children. One is lactose, because of the prevalence of lactose intolerance in children. Lactose intolerance begins to appear at around age six even though the lactase enzyme typically begins to decline after age two [8]. Another is the possibility of allergic responses to dyes used as colorants. Fortunately, a major producer of rashes, tartrazine (yellow dye # 5) is no longer used in prescription medicines (although it may still be present in some over-the-counter products).

The status of regulations regarding generic drugs and children

There has been significant evolution of the requirement that drug and biological product developers conduct assessments of their products for pediatric use, even when the adult population is the main market target. That mandate originated from recognition over time that a significant amount of the therapy administered to children consisted of "off-label" use of adult products, which entailed a host of problems such as suboptimal utilization of adult drugs for children, adverse safety events in children from poor dosing adjustment, as well as safety, efficacy, and compliance problems resulting from the lack of child-friendly formulations. Those circumstances have been redressed to some extent over the last decade or so, beginning with the inception of the Pediatric Studies Initiative in the late 1990s in the US, followed soon after by a similar program in Europe, and gradually spreading in some way, shape, or form to other major regulatory bodies throughout the world. In the United States, the essential components were called the "carrot and the stick" because of the combination of a mandatory and voluntary program, initially designed to address distinct aspects of the problem that are now more complementary. Nonetheless, gaps remain. One of these gaps is how to provide incentives for the performance of pediatric assessments for off-patent drugs and for studies leading to pediatric labeling for generic drugs.

Abbreviated new drug application (ANDA) requirements

In 1984, the Drug Price Competition and Patent Term Restoration Act, informally known as the "Hatch-Waxman Act," was passed, which authorized the submission of an abbreviated new drug application (ANDA) for generic drugs.

There are three types of submissions for generic drugs:
- A full NDA, s. 505(b)(1) of FDCA—applies when the sponsor of the innovator or pioneer drug, also called the reference listed drug (RLD), has generated all the preclinical and clinical study data (almost by definition not the path to approval typically taken by the generic applicant except in the case of certain so-called "branded generics" when the FDA approves a salt or ester of an already-approved drug or versions of the same off-patent original drug with the identical active ingredient and they are given brand names by their manufacturers);
- 505 (b)(2) NDAs are granted under the following situations: (i) applicant is unable to submit an ANDA because the modified drug differs in some substantial way from the innovative drug, and, (ii) the pharmacology and toxicology data, for example, are derived from the literature, but the clinical studies are performed by the sponsor; or (iii) to support a new indication, for example, when the sponsor relies on the findings of the FDA on safety and effectiveness for the drug from a prior approval, but may submit other data (this type of NDA is considered a cross between a generic and innovator drug approval because it may not require review of data other than BA or BE studies or data from limited confirmatory testing, and may be used even if the product is eligible for an ANDA);

- ANDAs under s. 505 (j) of FDCA are granted in the following situations: (i) when the generic drug version is the same as the innovative version in all material respects based on CMC and bioequivalence data, or (ii) the generic version is different from the pioneer drug in any significant respect, but the generic applicant has submitted a "suitability petition" to the FDA. An ANDA suitability petition is a petition (request) to the FDA to permit the filing of an ANDA for a drug that differs from the innovator [9].

Pediatric assessments of adult drugs (history up to current status)

How did we get to where we are today? Seminal events in the regulation of pediatric drugs start with the 1902 Biologics Control Act, which was passed after a diphtheria antitoxin was contaminated with tetanus spores, killing 13 children, and with the Pure Food and Drug Act, which followed in 1906. The latter prohibited the manufacture, sale, or transport of adulterated or misbranded drugs and was proposed in response to deaths among patients due to medications containing dangerous substances. Examples include Mrs. Winslow's Soothing Syrup (used for teething), which contained high amounts of alcohol and morphine, leading to coma, addiction, and death among infants.

The next landmark in regulatory scrutiny of drugs was reached in 1938 with the passage of the Food, Drug, and Cosmetic Act that gave the FDA authority to oversee the safety of food, drugs, and cosmetics. Its introduction was influenced by 107 deaths, many among children, reported to be caused by the ingestion of Elixir Sulfanilamide. The elixir contained diethylene glycol, a solvent in antifreeze that causes renal toxicity. The act required drug firms to prove to the FDA that any new drug was safe before it could be marketed. The 1962 Kefauver–Harris Amendment was a response to the number of severe birth defects caused by the sleeping aid thalidomide. Before the passage of this amendment, a sponsor's New Drug Application had only to demonstrate that their drug was safe. Under this amendment, a New Drug Application was required to demonstrate that the drug was effective as well as safe [10].

Many of the incidents prompting the above legislation involved children, but the resulting laws mostly benefited adults. In 1979 the FDA issued a requirement that labels note specifically whether safety and efficacy had been established in pediatric populations. The 1994 Pediatric Labeling Rule, another FDA regulation, requested that the pharmaceutical industry submit literature and other data providing additional information on the use of drugs in pediatric patients. The 1998 pediatric rule (Federal

Register 2 December 1998) required manufacturers to assess the safety and effectiveness of new drugs and biological products in pediatric patients. The FDA extended this requirement to marketed drugs and biological products whenever they are used in a substantial number of pediatric patients for their labeled indications or when they would provide a meaningful therapeutic benefit over existing treatments for pediatric patients or when the absence of adequate labeling could pose significant risks to pediatric patients. Because regulatory approaches had met with limited success over the years, in 1997 Congress preemptively passed the pediatric studies provision as part of the Food and Drug Administration Modernization Act (FDAMA), offering incentives for sponsors to test drugs in pediatric populations voluntarily: six months of additional marketing exclusivity and patent protection when studies are performed in children as requested by the FDA [10].

Best Pharmaceuticals for Children Act

The patent exclusivity of FDAMA was extended through 2007 with the Best Pharmaceuticals for Children Act (BPCA), passed in 2002. As a complement to the incentives offered by BPCA, the Pediatric Research Equity Act (PREA), passed in 2003, imposed a requirement that pharmaceutical companies test a new drug likely to be used in children [10].

The Best Pharmaceuticals for Children Act, signed into law January 2002, established a process for the study of on-patent and off-patent drugs for use in pediatric populations. It addressed collaboration on scientific investigation, clinical study design, weight of evidence, and ethical and labeling issues. As noted above, BPCA also renewed FDAMA's six months of marketing and patent protection for drugs whose sponsors perform the studies and produce the reports requested by the act. This six-month extension was offered not only for a drug that was studied in pediatric populations but also for any of the sponsor's formulations, dosage forms, and indications that contain the same active part, or moiety, of a molecule and have existing marketing exclusivity or patent life. For example, if a company markets an oral formulation and a topical cream containing the same moiety but submits a pediatric study for only one of the formulations, the six months of marketing exclusivity is added to patent protection for both products.

For the study of a drug that is still on patent, a company will typically submit a Proposed Pediatric Study Request to the FDA. The FDA will determine whether there is a public health benefit to support pediatric studies. BPCA also allows the FDA to initiate a study through a Written Request. If the FDA issues such a request, the drug's sponsor has 180 days to respond.

If the sponsor decides to conduct the study, results are submitted to the FDA. If the sponsor does not conduct the requested study, a process is in place by which the FDA can refer on-patent products to the Foundation for the National Institutes of Health (FNIH), which works to advance research by linking private-sector donors and partners to National Institutes of Health (NIH) programs. The FNIH will either fund the study or, if it lacks sufficient funding, refer the drug to NIH. If funding is available, NIH will issue a Request for Proposals (RFPs) from third parties to conduct the needed studies.

Incentives under BPCA do not apply to biologic, generic, or off-patent drugs, or to other drugs that lack marketing exclusivity or patent protection. For those products, BPCA provides a contract mechanism through which NIH can fund pediatric studies (again contingent on available funding). The NIH publishes in the *Federal Register* a list of drugs for which additional pediatric studies are needed. The list is compiled by a consensus group of representatives from the National Institute of Child Health and Human Development, the FDA, and others. The FDA issues a Written Request for the needed studies, and a product's sponsor has 30 days to respond. If the sponsor agrees to conduct the study, its results are submitted to the FDA. If not, the FDA refers the Written Request to NIH. As described above for on-patent drugs, NIH issues a Request for Contracts (RFCs) and awards a contract on a competitive basis to a third-party investigator [10]. Since BPCA went into effect, the FDA has issued about 20 RFCs and Requests for Proposals (RFPs) for studies of off-patent drugs with an equal number pending. No further action was to be taken until 2009, when the NIH announced that studies of drugs in 34 conditions or therapeutic areas were in the works [11, 12].

Pediatric Research Equity Act

The Pediatric Research Equity Act amends the federal Food, Drug, and Cosmetic Act to authorize the FDA to require pediatric studies of drugs or biologics when other approaches are insufficient to ensure that the products are safe and effective for use in children. Under PREA, the FDA can require pediatric studies of a product for which a New Drug Application is submitted if the agency determines the product is likely to be used in a substantial number of pediatric patients, or if it would provide meaningful benefits for children over existing treatments.

The PREA restores some important aspects of the 1998 Pediatric Rule, which was enjoined in 2002. Unlike BPCA, under which the FDA can issue a Written Request for any indication, PREA restricts the FDA to the specific indication contained in the submission to the agency. However,

PREA applies to any application for a new ingredient, new indication, new dosage form, new dosage regimen, or new route of administration. In addition, while the results of BPCA-initiated studies are disseminated publicly through the FDA's web site, PREA information is not routinely released to the public.

Under the PREA, a pediatric assessment is required for new applications, except when waived or deferred, and is designed to provide data needed to evaluate the safety and efficacy of a drug or biologic and to support dosing and administration for each pediatric subpopulation for which the product has been found safe and effective. A waiver to the requirement for a pediatric assessment is granted when the necessary studies are impossible or highly impractical, when there is strong evidence suggesting the product would be ineffective or unsafe, or when the product does not represent a meaningful therapeutic benefit over existing therapies and is unlikely to be used in a substantial number of pediatric patients. Partial waivers may also be granted for a specific pediatric subpopulation (for example, adolescents or neonates). A partial waiver may be granted as well if a product's specific formulation cannot be effectively altered. For example, if the chemical properties of a medication prevent its production as a liquid, it may be waived from study in newborns or children under five years of age, who would require a liquid formulation [10].

In the 1998 Pediatric Rule, pediatric study requirements were not imposed on ANDAs for exact generic copies of approved drugs. In 2003, when the Pediatric Rule was essentially resurrected as the PREA, it stayed true to the 1998 Pediatric Rule in providing that ANDAs would not have to include a pediatric assessment unless triggered by the Suitability Petition process. However, in a "Catch-22" not atypical in government regulatory schemes, an ANDA Suitability Petition (to make a change to active ingredient, dosage form, or route of administration) would trigger the necessity of a pediatric assessment. Yet, such a pediatric assessment cannot be performed because PREA dictates that the Suitability Petition must be denied, since by definition ANDAs do not contain clinical investigations (see basic requirements for ANDAs). Therefore, under the PREA, generic drug manufacturers are faced with Hobson's choice; make changes to the innovator label or conduct costly and time-consuming pediatric clinical investigations [13].

Intersection of requirements for generics and pediatric assessment

At a recent meeting of the American Academy of Pediatrics, Dr. Diane Murphy, Director of the Office of Pediatric Therapeutics, outlined the basic issues from the FDA's perspective. If the innovator product (the original or reference labeled drug—RLD) does not have a pediatric indication, neither will the generic. If the reference innovator has a pediatric indication, then the generic product will have the same indication and the same information on pediatrics. However, a generic product may not be developed for all the dosing forms that the innovator developed [14].

The FDA's major operational premise is that the innovator is already known to be safe and effective and the generic is the same drug in a similar formulation. Thus, safety and effectiveness do not need to be demonstrated again. The focus for generic approval is on trials showing bioequivalence and pharmaceutical equivalence. Little transparency exists for the who, what and where of these trials, however, clinical trials for bioequivalence in generic drug applications were not intended by the authors of the FDAAA to be listed in ClinicalTrials.gov under the provision that excluded phase 1 studies from mandatory listing. Furthermore, the IND regulations 21 CFR 312.2(b)(1) (i) exempt most bioequivalence studies from IND requirements because it would disclose their development plans to competitors and discourage generic drug entry [15].

Among the basic regulatory requirements for an ANDA is that the generic must have the "same" label as the innovator. However, generics may delete portions of labeling protected by patents or exclusivity. As already noted, generics may differ in excipients and to a limited degree in PK data. There may also be differences in the How Supplied information. Section 11 of the BPCA of 2002 amended the FDA Act to add a new provision, which was reauthorized in the 2007 FDAAA. The new provision provided that an ANDA submitted in the wake of relabeling an innovator after addition of labeling information resulting from studies performed for pediatric exclusivity may omit a pediatric indication or other aspect of labeling. The generic must, however, include a statement that because of marketing exclusivity the drug is not labeled for pediatric use, and enumerate any appropriate pediatric contraindications, warnings, or precautions that the Secretary considers necessary. The FDA subsequently spelled out in amendments to the prescription drug labeling regulations under 21 CFR s. 201.56(d) (5) that this means risk information contained in the Contraindications, Warnings and Precautions, or Use in Special Populations sections of the label must be included [16]. Together with the presence of the same amount of active ingredient acting in a bioequivalent manner, another requirement for ANDA approval is that the generic product should contain acceptable inactive ingredients. Or, if they are not the same as the innovator, information must be provided that the inactive ingredients used will not change the safety and/or efficacy of the product. It is usually found acceptable if the ingredient has previously been used in another drug product for the same route of administration and in the same or higher daily amount [14].

Future directions

The situation is somewhat conflicted in the US and perhaps it would be simpler to do as they do in Europe, where generics are excluded from the Pediatric Regulation, and therefore no Pediatric Investigation Plan is needed [17]. Nonetheless, back in the US, under the BPCA, as renewed in 2007, generic drug manufacturers typically would have little incentive to provide pediatric data, although the FDA is still trying to work through the NIH program to secure data. However, generics could pursue a Suitability Petition for generic drugs known to be used in children, and then under the PREA trigger they would have to perform a pediatric assessment. But in so doing, they would potentially qualify for three years of exclusivity under Hatch–Waxman, and, if they also "volunteer" to answer a Written Request issued under the BPCA, they could get an additional six months of exclusivity [13]. How often this is likely to happen is uncertain, but failing this route, there is little incentive, mandatory or voluntary, for clinical assessment of off-patent pediatric drugs.

As Dr. Murphy noted, we are still waiting for the first pediatric label from the NIH program to study off-patent products or products for which industry has declined the Written Request from the FDA. However, she maintains that it is not fair to deny approval of a generic because the reference innovator has less than optimal safety or efficacy. We cannot hold generics to a higher standard than the reference innovator, and, since safety and effectiveness have already been shown for the innovator, the generic only has to meet bioequivalence criteria.

Nonetheless, as noted by Dr. Wayne Snodgrass, Chairman of the Committee on Drugs for the American Academy of Pediatrics, this leaves patients and practitioners in the lurch. For off-patent or older agents, NIH lacks sufficient resources to conduct the needed pediatric studies. He cited morphine as an example. Information is lacking on the optimal use of morphine, or even on the drug's basic kinetics, in various age groups and with different disease processes [10]. In fact, morphine was listed as on-patent in the latest NIH priority drug listing, but it had to be referred to the Foundation for NIH to address the Written Request, which is under way for neonates. This is evidence of the critical need to resolve this gap in the system for off-patent, generic, or on-patent but unsponsored drugs. Morphine is a very effective, but also potentially dangerous, weapon in the practitioner's armamentarium, yet it can only be wielded clumsily despite years of clinical use due to the continuing lack of resources and willpower.

Concluding thoughts

At the present time, we have (except for rare exceptions such as different salts or other esters) few, if any, significant findings that suggest that children of an age that is appropriate for the use of psychotropic drugs would handle a generic drug differently from the way they would handle an innovator drug. It is interesting that such a concern should arise given that use of generic drugs is commonplace among prescribing clinicians who treat children. Does anyone think twice about prescribing generic diphenhydramine or erythromycin? The authors welcome any examples from our readers that would alter this conclusion.

References

1 Greenblatt DJ, Harmatz JS, Shader, RI: Psychotropic drug prescribing in the United States. *J Clin Psychopharmacol* 2011; **31:** 1–3.
2 Oesterheld J, Shader RI, Martin A: *Clinical and Developmental Aspects of Pharmacokinetics and Drug Interactions.* In: Martin A, Volkmar FR: *Lewis's Child and Adolescent Psychiatry,* 4th edn. Philadelphia, PA: Walters Kluwer/Lippincott Williams & Wilkins, 1997, pp. 742–53.
3 Davit BM, Nwakama PE, Buehler GJ et al. Comparing generic and innovator drugs: a review of 12 years of bioequivalence data from the United States Food and Drug Administration. *Ann Pharmacother* 2009; **43:** 1583–97.
4 Kesselheim AS, Misono AS, Lee JL et al.: Clinical equivalence of generic and brand-name drugs used in cardiovascular disease *JAMA* 2008; **300:** 2514–26.
5 USDHHS, FDA, CDER, Office of Generic Drugs, *Guidance for Industry: Submissions of Summary Bioequivalence Data for ANDAs,* April 2009. Available at http://www.fda.gov/downloads/Drugs/GuidanceComplianceRegulatoryInformation/Guidances/UCM134846.pdf, accessed July 27, 2011.
6 Center for Drug Evaluation and Research. Guidance for Industry: Bioavailability and Bioequivalence Studies for Orally Administered Drug Products—General Considerations. United States Food and Drug Administration, 2003. http://www.fda.gov/downloads/Drugs/GuidanceComplianceRegulatoryInformation/Guidances/ucm070124.pdf. Accessed January 2, 2011.
7 Shader, RI: Antidepressants as hydrobromide salts: are they a cause for concern? *J Clin Psychopharmacol* 2009; **29:** 317–18.
8 Guandalini S, Frye RE, Rivera DM et al. Lactose intolerance. http://emedicine.medscape.com/article/930971-overview. Accessed January 4, 2011.
9 Milne C-P and Cairns C: Generic drug regulation in the US under the Hatch–Waxman Act. *Pharmaceutical Development and Regulation* 2003; **1**(1): 11–27.
10 *Addressing the Barriers to Pediatric Drug Development: Workshop Summary.* Institute of Medicine (US) Forum on Drug Discovery, Development, and Translation. Washington (DC): National Academies Press (US), 2008.
11 Current Status of Drugs that have been Listed by NIH (NICHD) for BPCA as of March 28, 2007. http://bpca.nichd.nih.gov/about/process/status.cfm. Accessed January 4, 2011.

12 Priority List of Pediatric Therapeutic Needs as of September 1, 2009. http://
bpca.nichd.nih.gov/about/process/status.cfm. Accessed January 4, 2010.

13 Cotrell S, Goldstein B. Regulatory considerations for study of generic drugs under
Best Pharmaceuticals for Children Act: NICHD and FDA collaboration. In: Mulberg,
A, Silber, S, van den Anker, J: *Pediatric Drug Development: Concepts and Applications*.
Wiley-Blackwell: Hoboken, NJ, 2009, pp. 165–71.

14 Murphy D. Director, Office of Pediatric Therapeutics, Office of the Commissioner,
FDA, American Academy of Pediatrics Meeting: Section on Clinical Pharmacology
and Therapeutics Program, October 19, 2009. http://www.fda.gov/ScienceResearch/
SpecialTopics/PediatricTherapeuticsResearch/ucm189451.htm. Accessed January 4,
2011.

15 Kishore, R, Tabor, E. Overview of the FDA Amendments Act of 2007: its effect on
the drug development landscape. *Drug Information Journal* 2010; **44:** 469–75.

16 Karst KR. BPCA Section 11 and Pediatric Labeling; revised Labeling Carve-Out
Citizen Petition Scorecard, June 22, 2009, FDA Law Blog of Hyman, Phelps, and
McNamara, P.C. Available at http://www.fdalawblog.net/fda_law_blog_hyman_phelp
s/2009/06/bpca-section-11-and-pediatric-labeling-revised-labeling-carveout-citizen-
petition-scorecard.html, accessed July 27, 2011.

17 European Medicines Agency, 5 October 2010, *Report—Workshop on Paediatric Formulations for Assessors in National Regulatory Agencies*. Available at http://www.ema.euro
pa.eu/docs/en_GB/document_library/Minutes/2010/10/WC500097497.pdf, accessed
July 27, 2011.

CHAPTER 5

Psychoactive Drug Use in Children: Basic Concepts in Clinical Pharmacology

David J. Edwards

School of Pharmacy, University of Waterloo, Waterloo, Ontario, Canada

Introduction

It has been said that children are not miniature adults when it comes to the pharmacotherapy of disease. Differences in body size and maturation between children and adults make it challenging to determine the optimal dosing regimen of many drugs [1–4]. A lack of research on the disposition and effects of drugs in the pediatric population compounds this problem. In response to disasters, such as grey baby syndrome, associated with chloramphenicol use [5], infants and children were excluded from most clinical trials of new medications for many years even when it was likely that the drug could be used to treat pediatric conditions. Pediatricians have been forced to prescribe drugs tested exclusively on adults with little or no labeling information to guide the selection of dose in children. Fortunately, recent changes in attitudes and regulations have promoted an increase in the volume of research related to the clinical pharmacology of drugs in the pediatric population.

Up to 10% of children have conditions such as attention-deficit hyperactivity disorder (ADHD), depression or anxiety that are potentially responsive to pharmacotherapy [6]. The effectiveness of drug therapy depends on the selection of the correct therapeutic agent as well as the choice of an appropriate dosing regimen. This chapter will review the pharmacokinetic parameters that are used to characterize drug disposition and discuss the influence of ontogeny, pharmacogenomics, drug interactions, and body size in designing optimal dosing regimens of drugs in children.

Pharmacotherapy of Child and Adolescent Psychiatric Disorders, Third Edition.
Edited by David R. Rosenberg and Samuel Gershon.
© 2012 John Wiley & Sons, Ltd. Published 2012 by John Wiley & Sons, Ltd.

Basic concepts in pharmacokinetics

The science of pharmacokinetics is concerned with the rates of absorption, distribution, metabolism and elimination (ADME) of drugs in the body. This information is essential in selecting an appropriate dose and dosing interval for a patient. The primary pharmacokinetic parameters that characterize the disposition of drugs are bioavailability, clearance, volume of distribution and half-life. These parameters control the degree of exposure that a patient will have to a specific dose and allow for characterization of the relationship between dose and plasma concentration.

Absorption and bioavailability

Medications are most commonly taken by mouth in both children and adults. In order to exert an effect, orally administered psychoactive agents must pass from the gastrointestinal tract through the liver and into the systemic circulation for delivery to the central nervous system. Bioavailability (F) represents the fraction of the administered dose reaching the systemic circulation relative to an intravenous dose. Drugs that are acid-labile may degrade in the acidic environment of the stomach. Dissolution of the drug molecule in fluids of the gastrointestinal tract is also a requirement for absorption and may be influenced by gastric pH or administration with meals. Food may enhance dissolution through the presence of lipid in the meal or by delaying gastric emptying [7]. The oral bioavailability of ziprasidone is increased about twofold when given with food accompanied by significantly less variability compared with the fasting state [8]. Buspirone also shows a doubling in bioavailability when administered with food [9].

Most psychoactive drugs are highly lipophilic, which slows dissolution but promotes movement across biological membranes such as the intestinal wall. However, even if a drug possesses the requisite physical and chemical characteristics for absorption, there is no guarantee of systemic bioavailability. Cytochrome P450 enzymes, particularly CYP3A4, can extract a substantial fraction of the dose on first-pass through the intestinal wall and liver [10, 11]. In addition, P-glycoprotein, the product of the MDR1 gene, is expressed in high concentration in the enterocyte and transports substrates back into the intestinal lumen contributing to poor bioavailability [10–12]. Chlorpromazine, thioridazine, fluphenazine, haloperidol, moclobemide, protriptyline, imipramine, nefazodone, fluvoxamine, buspirone, paroxetine, fluoxetine and sertraline are examples of drugs used in the treatment of psychiatric conditions that are subject to extensive first-pass extraction [9, 13–16].

Distribution

The distribution of a drug in the body is influenced by its chemical characteristics as well as binding to plasma proteins. The volume of distribution (V) is the pharmacokinetic parameter used to measure drug distribution. It is defined as the ratio of the amount of drug in the body to the concentration in the blood. V can be infinitely large and does not correlate with a real physiological space. As an example, the selective serotonin reuptake inhibitor (SSRI) fluoxetine has a volume of distribution of 1500–2000 l in children [17]. Many drugs are highly bound to plasma proteins with albumin being the most important binding protein due to its high concentration (4–5 g/100 ml) as well as affinity for binding both acidic and basic drugs. Alpha-1-acid glycoprotein also contributes to the binding of many basic drugs. Despite a high degree of plasma protein binding, many antipsychotic and antidepressant drugs have a large volume of distribution due to their lipophilicity and affinity for tissue binding sites.

Distribution into the central nervous system is a prerequisite in order for psychoactive drugs to exert a pharmacologic effect. This requires penetration of the drug through the blood-brain barrier. Transporters such as P-glycoprotein serve a protective function in limiting the entry of potentially toxic compounds into the brain. A number of drugs used in psychopharmacology are P-glycoprotein substrates including chlorpromazine, fluphenazine, fluvoxamine, haloperidol, imipramine, paroxetine, sertraline and quetiapine [18]. Cerebral concentrations of risperidone are tenfold higher in knockout mice that lack functional P-glycoprotein in the blood-brain barrier [19]. Inhibitors of P-glycoprotein may increase penetration of drug into the brain while inducers (such as St. John's wort) would be expected to have the opposite effect.

Clearance

Clearance (Cl) is the volume of plasma from which a drug is irreversibly removed per unit time and represents the efficiency of removal of drug from the blood. Renal clearance is the net effect of filtration at the glomerulus plus active tubular secretion minus reabsorption of the drug. Factors such as the lipophilicity of the drug molecule, degree of plasma protein binding, molecular size and urinary pH can influence renal elimination of drug. Most psychoactive drugs are lipophilic and highly bound to plasma proteins resulting in limited glomerular filtration and efficient reabsorption. As a result, renal clearance tends to be minimal.

Hepatic clearance is primarily mediated through Phase I and Phase II metabolism. Phase I reactions involve the formation of a more polar metabolite that may be eliminated renally or further metabolized via conjugation with endogenous substrates such as sulfate, acetate and glucuronic acid (Phase II). Phase I metabolism is usually mediated by one or more of the cytochrome P450 enzymes. The cytochrome P450 system consists of a number of families and subfamilies of enzymes that differ in terms of substrate specificity, polymorphic expression in the population and susceptibility to inhibition and induction [20–24]. The most important with respect to drug metabolism are CYP1A2, CYP2C8/9/10, CYP2C19, CYP2D6 and CYP3A4. Although present in a number of tissues throughout the body, expression is greatest in the liver. CYP3A4 is responsible for the metabolism of 40-50% of all drugs and represents about 40% and 80% of the total cytochrome P450 content of the liver and intestine respectively [20, 24, 25]. Metabolism does not always result in a less active species. Many psychotherapeutic agents have active metabolites including fluoxetine (norfluoxetine), imipramine (desipramine), amitriptyline (nortriptyline), thioridazine (mesoridazine) and risperidone (hydroxyrisperidone).

Half-life

The elimination half-life of a drug is the time required for plasma concentrations to decline by 50% and reflects the persistence of drug in the plasma. It is dependent on clearance and volume of distribution. A low value for clearance or a large volume of distribution will result in a long half-life. It should be noted that the half-life of most drugs tends to be shorter in children compared with adults [26]. In 20 children between two and six years of age, buspirone half-life averaged 1.6 hours [27] compared with typical values of 2–3 hours in adults [9].

Since half-life reflects the persistence of the drug in the body, it is not surprising that it is a primary determinant of the duration of effect. This may account for the observation by Smith [28] that the risk of suicidal ideation or behavior is highest for antidepressants with a short half-life and lowest for drugs like fluoxetine whose half-life may exceed 100 hours. As a general principle, drugs that have a longer half-life will have a longer duration of action and can be dosed less frequently. Longer dosing intervals are preferred in order to enhance patient convenience and adherence to the medication regimen. The short half-life of drugs such as methylphenidate used in the treatment of ADHD is problematic because multiple daily doses are required and symptom coverage can be uneven as drug concentrations rise and fall over the dosing interval [29]. This problem has been addressed by new modified-release formulations of methylphenidate and amphetamine salts that release the drug over an extended period of time [29].

Dosing considerations for psychoactive drugs in children

Dosing strategies with chronic administration of drugs are based on achieving and maintaining plasma concentrations within a range known to be associated with beneficial therapeutic effects and minimal toxicity. This information comes almost entirely from studies conducted in adults. Stephenson [30] has suggested that the response of children to medications in most diseases should be similar to adults since the basic physiologic and cellular processes that influence drug effect are similar irrespective of age. The impression that children are more sensitive to the effect of drugs may be more related to pharmacokinetic differences that result in more exposure to some medications.

The area under the plasma concentration-time curve (AUC) under steady-state conditions is the most appropriate measure of the degree of exposure of a patient to a dosing regimen. Alternatively, exposure can be estimated from the average drug concentration under steady state conditions:

$$C_{ss,av} = \frac{F \times Dose}{Cl \times \tau} \tag{5.1}$$

where τ is the dosing interval. Since bioavailability (F) in children is generally comparable to that in adults, the primary challenge is accounting for the difference in clearance between children and adults. Clearance is influenced by a number of factors, some of which are unique to pediatric patients (development, body size) while others (drug interactions, genetic effects) are common to dosing patients of any age.

Effect of development on drug disposition in children

The development of the processes affecting drug disposition in newborns, infants and children have been extensively reviewed [1–4, 31]. At birth, gastric pH is elevated, gastric emptying is slow and peristalsis is irregular. However, the processes governing both passive absorption and active transport of drugs tend to mature by four months of age resulting in slower but otherwise comparable absorption between children and adults [1–4]. Oral bioavailability of drugs that are subject to a high degree of first-pass metabolism may be increased in newborns due to immaturity of drug metabolizing enzymes. Topical administration of drugs to infants can result in substantially increased plasma concentrations due to a thinner stratum corneum, greater hydration of the epidermis and a much higher ratio of surface area to body mass [1].

Infants have a higher proportion of total body water than adults (75% versus 55%) and extracellular fluid (40% versus 20%). They also have less fat, less muscle and lower (20%) concentrations of albumin [1–4]. The volume of distribution of hydrophilic compounds such as gentamicin is higher in infants compared with adults as a result of these differences. However, there appear to be few clinically significant differences in volume of distribution between older children and adults. The glomerular filtration rate also increases rapidly in the first month of post-natal life and reaches adult values (when normalized for body surface area) by the age of one.

The ontogeny of drug metabolism is of interest because most psychoactive drugs are eliminated by this mechanism. CYP3A7 is the predominant P450 enzyme at birth but declines quickly thereafter and is undetectable in most adults. Other important P450 enzymes including CYP3A4, CYP2D6 and CYP2C enzymes are present at low concentrations in newborns but surge within the first week reaching 20–30% of adult values within the first month of post-natal life. CYP1A2 is the last important drug-metabolizing enzyme to develop. Adult values for cytochrome P450 activity appear to be achieved within the first year of life. The glucuronidation of many substrates is impaired at birth. Jaundice in newborns due to reduced glucuronidation of bilirubin by UGT1A1 is common, and grey baby syndrome has been attributed to an inability to efficiently glucuronidate chloramphenicol [5, 31]. The presence of numerous isoforms of uridine glucuronosyltransferase (UGT), the enzyme responsible for glucuronidation, with overlapping substrate specificity makes it difficult to draw general conclusions concerning the development of glucuronidation. However, it appears safe to assume that full maturity of these enzymes is reached by four years of age [2].

Immaturity in the development of renal function and drug metabolism in newborns and infants coupled with wide variability in maturity between patients of similar postnatal age makes it difficult to design appropriate dosing regimens in this population. However, psychoactive medications are rarely used in patients under the age of five. By this age, it can be assumed that the basic physiologic processes that govern drug disposition are reasonably mature and the primary challenge in drug dosing is accounting for the difference in body size between children and adults.

Pharmacogenetics of drug metabolism

Genetic differences between patients can influence both the pharmacokinetics and the response of a patient [32]. A number of studies have examined the genetic variability in ADHD drug targets such as the dopamine transporter, dopamine receptor, and norepinephrine transporter [32–34]. At present, it is not possible accurately to predict response to medications used in ADHD from the patient's genetic profile but a number of promising associations have been identified.

Much research has been devoted to the pharmacogenetics of the cytochrome P450 enzymes CYP2D6 and CYP2C19 [20, 23]. Both enzymes are involved in the metabolism of many psychoactive drugs with one study reporting that 52% of psychiatric patients were treated with at least one drug metabolized by CYP2D6 [35]. Over 70 different mutated alleles for CYP2D6 have been identified and these occur with varying frequency in different ethnic groups [20, 23, 36–39]. Individuals possessing two copies of the wild type allele will be phenotypic extensive metabolizers (EMs). Nonfunctional or reduced function alleles occur in approximately 25–30% of Caucasians resulting in 5–10% of the population having the poor metabolizer (PM) phenotype. Less than 2% of Asians are phenotypic PMs while the frequency of African American PMs appears to fall somewhere in between. Gene duplication also occurs with three or more copies of the CYP2D6 gene producing an ultrarapid metabolizer (UM) phenotype. Although relatively uncommon in Caucasians of northern European descent, this phenotype has been reported in up to 10% of individuals in the Mediterranean area and 15–25% of Ethiopians [20, 23, 38, 39].

The clinical consequence of the polymorphic expression of enzymes such as CYP2D6 is not always easy to predict. Certainly, higher plasma concentrations are expected in PMs whereas concentrations may be close to undetectable in UMs given standard doses. Up to a tenfold difference between PMs and UMs is possible for drugs such as risperidone, imipramine, desipramine, and nortriptyline [40, 41]. Complicating the assessment of the impact of genotype, however, is the fact that many antidepressants and antipsychotics have active metabolites that make a substantial contribution to the effects of the drug. While PMs have high concentrations of parent compound and little metabolite, UMs and EMs will have low concentrations of the parent and substantial amounts of active metabolites. Risperidone and venlafaxine are drugs where the pharmacologic effects are due to the combined contributions of parent and metabolites.

Several studies have documented differences in clinical outcomes related to the CYP2D6 genotype. Poor metabolizers taking antidepressants metabolized by CYP2D6 had a 4-fold increased risk of toxicity while UM's were five times more likely to be nonresponders [42]. A study involving 360 patients treated with risperidone found that PMs were more than three times as likely to develop an adverse event and six times more likely to discontinue treatment due to an adverse event compared with EMs [43]. Plasma concentrations of atomoxetine, a CYP2D6 substrate used in the treatment of ADHD, may be as much as tenfold higher in PMs. In ten children with adverse events, 80% were found to have at least one nonfunctional allele for CYP2D6 [44]. Genotyping for CYP2D6 could allow pediatricians to individualize the dosage of a number of psychoactive drugs with improved effectiveness and less toxicity. Although this remains primarily a research tool at present, recent advances in technology have substantially lowered the cost of genotyping and a number of companies are now marketing this test for clinical use.

Drug interactions

A survey of office-based psychiatric practices conducted in 2005–6 found that one-third of all office visits resulted in patients receiving three or more prescriptions for psychotropic medication [45]. This represented a twofold increase compared with data collected in 1996–7 and suggests that polypharmacy with antidepressant and antipsychotic drugs is increasing. Whenever patients are taking more than one medication, the possibility of a drug interaction exists. There are many potential mechanisms by which drugs interact, but the most common involves induction or inhibition of cytochrome P450 enzymes. The most well-known inducers of metabolism are the anticonvulsant drugs phenytoin, phenobarbital and carbamazepine along with the antibiotic rifampin. These compounds induce a broad range of P450 enzymes resulting in increased protein concentration that is maximal 1–4 weeks after starting therapy with the inducer. Induction causes an increase in clearance as well as decreased oral bioavailability of drugs subject to first-pass metabolism. This has the potential to render psychotherapeutic agents ineffective when the effect of the drug is primarily due to the parent compound. St. John's wort is a herbal product that is commonly used for self-treatment of mild depression. It is a potent inducer of cytochrome P450 enzymes and P-glycoprotein. Clinically significant reductions in concentrations of cyclosporine, indinavir and the SSRIs paroxetine, sertraline, and venlafaxine have been reported [46]. Clinicians should be aware of the possibility that parents might administer St. John's wort to their children. A study conducted in Ireland found that one in six children had taken an herbal medicine and some had received St. John's wort [47].

Perhaps a more common cause of drug interactions in psychopharmacology is inhibition of metabolism [48]. A large number of psychoactive drugs have been identified as inhibitors of cytochrome P450 enzymes. Inhibition can be clinically evident even after the first dose and is a primary concern when inhibitors are co-administered with drugs having a narrow therapeutic range. Several SSRIs are potent inhibitors of P450 enzymes [49]. Fluvoxamine inhibits CYP1A2 and CYP2C9 while fluoxetine also decreases CYP2C9 activity. Paroxetine and fluoxetine inhibit CYP2D6, as does haloperidol and the MAO-A inhibitor moclobemide. Excessive sedation and extrapyramidal symptoms associated with up to twentyfold increases in plasma concentrations were observed in subjects given perphenazine in combination with paroxetine [50]. The magnitude of drug interaction with CYP2D6 may be influenced by the genotype of the patient. Since PMs do not have a functional form of the enzyme, inhibitors of CYP2D6 have little or no effect in these individuals.

CYP3A4 is responsible for metabolism of the broadest range of drugs. Potent inhibitors include ketoconazole, itraconazole, diltiazem, erythromycin, and clarithromycin. Plasma concentrations of buspirone are increased more than tenfold when co-administered with potent inhibitors such as itraconazole [51]. Nefazodone and fluoxetine also inhibit CYP3A4 and should be administered with caution in children receiving drugs metabolized by this enzyme.

Body size and drug dosing in children

Although the physiologic processes responsible for drug clearance will generally be mature in a school-aged child receiving treatment with psychoactive medication, the absolute value for drug clearance will be smaller due to the difference in size between children and adults. The daily dose requirement in a child relative to a healthy adult can be estimated according to the following formula:

$$Dose_{child} = Dose_{adult} \times \frac{Cl_{child}}{Cl_{adult}} \tag{5.2}$$

A critical question in predicting the dose for a child relates to how differences in clearance between adults and children should be scaled. Reducing drug dosage on the basis of weight is likely to underestimate the required dose. Takahashi et al. [52] reported that the unbound oral clearance of S-warfarin was 18.1 ml/min/kg in prepubertal children compared with 11.6 ml/min/kg in adults. The clearance of paroxetine [53] and many other drugs has been found to be up to twice as high in children compared with adults when adjusted for body weight. An alternative and widely used approach to account for differences in body size between children and adults is to use body surface area. Surface area is a function of both the height and weight of the child and can be calculated using a simplified formula as follows:

$$SA\ (m^2) = \frac{\sqrt{Ht \times Wt}}{60} \tag{5.3}$$

where height is measured in cm and weight in kg. Drug clearance normalized for surface area is relatively similar in children and adults for many drugs [52, 54].

The science of allometrics relates differences in body size to function. It is widely used in cross-species scaling and these principles have been applied to the problem of drug clearance in children [55–57]:

$$Cl_{child} = Cl_{adult} \times \left(\frac{Wt_{child}}{Wt_{adult}} \right)^{\frac{3}{4}} \tag{5.4}$$

This equation is known as the 3/4 power law and appears to accurately predict drug clearance over a wide range of body weight in children. It is not useful in neonates, infants and young children because it cannot account for the rapid and highly variable development of processes governing drug clearance in these populations. During the early years of rapid maturation, physiologically based models for predicting drug clearance may be more useful [58].

Johnson [59] evaluated several approaches for scaling drug doses for children and concluded that no method was ideal. Doses based on body weight tended to underpredict dose requirements but this more conservative estimate may be appropriate in infants and newborns from a safety perspective. Psychoactive medication use occurs predominantly in children who are at least five years of age. In this population of school-aged prepubertal children, differences in dose between allometric scaling and the use of body surface area are likely to be minimal. Most clinicians are likely to be more comfortable with using the latter approach.

Summary

Appropriate dosing of psychoactive drugs requires an understanding of pharmacokinetic parameters such as bioavailability, clearance and half-life. In addition, the influences of development, genetics, drug interactions and body size must be accounted for in arriving at the most appropriate dosing regimen for an individual child. Expanded application of therapeutic drug monitoring and increasing availability of genetic testing is a positive development that should contribute to more appropriate use of drugs in children. Despite an increasing body of literature on drug disposition and effects in children, more research is needed and clinicians need to continue to be vigilant in monitoring the effects of psychoactive medications in children.

References

1 Kearns GL, Abdel-Rahman SM, Alander SW et al.: Developmental pharmacology—drug disposition, action and therapy in infants and children. *N Engl J Med* 2003; **349:** 1157–67.

2 Pichini S, Papaseit E, Joya X et al.: Pharmacokinetics and therapeutic drug monitoring of psychotropic drugs in pediatrics. *Ther Drug Monit* 2009; **31:** 283–318.

3 Bartelink IH, Rademaker CMA, Schobben FAM et al.: Guidelines on paediatric dosing on the basis of developmental physiology and pharmacokinetic considerations. *Clin Pharmacokinet* 2006; **45:** 1077–97.

4   Anderson GD, Lynn AM: Optimizing pediatric dosing: A developmental pharmaco-
    logic approach. *Pharmacotherapy* 2009; **29:** 680–90.
5   Burns LE, Hodgman JE: Fatal circulatory collapse in premature infants receiving
    chloramphenicol. *N Engl J Med* 1959; **261:** 1318.
6   Riddle MA, Labellarte MJ, Walkup JT: Pediatric psychopharmacology: Problems and
    prospects. *J Child Adolesc Psychopharmacol* 1998; **8:** 87–97.
7   Fleisher D, Li C, Zhou Y et al.: Drug, meal and formulation interactions influenc-
    ing drug absorption after oral administration. *Clin Pharmacokinet* 1999; **36:** 233–
    54.
8   Miceli JJ, Glue P, Alderman J et al.: The effect of food on the absorption of oral
    ziprasidone. *Psychopharmacol Bull* 2007; **40:** 58–68.
9   Mahmood I, Sahajwalla C: Clinical pharmacokinetics and pharmacodynamics of bus-
    pirone, an anxiolytic drug. *Clin Pharmacokinet* 1999; **36:** 277–87.
10 Hall SD, Thummel KE, Watkins PB et al.: Molecular and physical mechanisms of
    first-pass extraction. *Drug Metab Dispos* 1999; **27:** 161–6.
11 Johnson TN, Thomson M: Intestinal metabolism and transport of drugs in children:
    the effects of age and disease. *JPGN* 2008; **47:** 3–10.
12 Chinn LW, Kroetz DL: ABCB1 pharmacogenetics: progress, pitfalls, and promise. *Clin
    Pharmacol Ther* 2007; **81:** 265–9.
13 Mayersohn M, Guentert TW: Clinical pharmacokinetics of the monoamine oxidase-A
    inhibitor moclobemide. *Clin Pharmacokinet* 1995; **29:** 292–332.
14 Fang J, Gorrod JW: Metabolism, pharmacogenetics, and metabolic drug-drug inter-
    actions of antipsychotic drugs. *Cell Mol Neurobiol* 1999; **19:** 491–510.
15 Devane CL: Metabolism and pharmacokinetics of selective serotonin reuptake in-
    hibitors. *Cell Mol Neurobiol* 1999; **19:** 443–66.
16 Greene DS, Barbhaiya RH. Clinical pharmacokinetics of nefazodone. *Clin Pharma-
    cokinet* 1997; **33:** 260–75.
17 Wilens TE, Cohen L, Biederman J et al.: Fluoxetine pharmacokinetics in pediatric
    patients. *J Clin Psychopharmacol* 2002; **22:** 568–75.
18 Linnet K, Ejsing TB. A review on the impact of P-glycoprotein on the penetration of
    drugs into the brain. Focus on psychotropic drugs. *Eur Neuropschopharmacol* 2008; **18:**
    157–69.
19 Doran A, Obach RS, Smith BJ et al.: The impact of P-glycoprotein on the disposition
    of drugs targeted for indications of the central nervous system: evaluation using the
    mdr1a/1b knockout mouse model. *Drug Metab Dispos* 2005; **33:** 165–74.
20 Zhou SF, Liu JP, Chowbay B: Polymorphism of human cytochrome P450 enzymes
    and its clinical impact. *Drug Metab Rev* 2009; **41:** 89–295.
21 Zhou SF, Wang B, Yang LP et al.: Structure, function, regulation and polymorphism
    and the clinical significance of human cytochrome P450 1A2. *Drug Metab Rev* 2010;
    42: 268–354.
22 Zhou Sf, Zhou ZW, Yang LP et al.: Substrates, inducers, inhibitors and structure-
    activity relationships of human cytochrome P450 2C9 and implications in drug de-
    velopment. *Curr Med Chem* 2009; **16:** 3480–675.
23 Zhou SF, Liu JP, Lai XS: Substrate specificity, inhibitors and regulation of human
    cytochrome P450 2D6 and implications in drug development. *Curr Med Chem* 2009;
    16: 2661–805.
24 Rendic S, Guengerich FP: Update information on drug metabolism systems—2009,
    part II: summary of information on the effects of diseases and environmental factors
    on human cytochrome P450 (CYP) enzymes and transporters. *Curr Drug Metab* 2010;
    11: 4–84.

25 Thelen K, Dressman JB: Cytochrome P450-mediated metabolism in the human gut wall. *J Pharm Pharmacol* 2009; **61:** 541–48.

26 Ginsberg G, Hattis D, Miller R et al.: Pediatric pharmacokinetic data: implications for environmental risk assessment for children. *Pediatrics* 2004; **113:** 973–83.

27 Edwards DJ, Chugani DC, Chugani HT et al.: Pharmacokinetics of buspirone in autistic children. *J Clin Pharmacol* 2006; **46:** 508–14.

28 Smith EG: Association between antidepressant half-life and the risk of suicidal ideation or behavior among children and adolescents: confirmatory analysis and research implications. *J Affect Disord* 2009; **114:** 143–8.

29 Connor DF, Steingard RJ: New formulations of stimulants for attention-deficit hyperactivity disorder. Therapeutic potential. *CNS Drugs* 2004; **18:** 1011–30.

30 Stephenson T: How children's responses to drugs differ from adults. *Br J Clin Pharmacol* 2005; **59:** 670–73.

31 Benedetti MS, Whomsley R, Canning M: Drug metabolism in the paediatric population and in the elderly. *Drug Discov Today* 2007; **12:** 599–610.

32 Leeder JS: Developmental and pediatric pharmacogenomics. *Pharmacogenomics* 2003; **4:** 331–41.

33 Kieling C, Genro JP, Hutz MH et al.: A current update on ADHD pharmacogenomics. *Pharmacogenomics* 2010; **11:** 407–19.

34 Stein MA, McGough JJ: The pharmacogenomic era: promise for personalizing attention deficit hyperactivity disorder therapy. *Child Adolesc Psychiatric Clin N Am* 2008; **17:** 475–90.

35 Mulder H, Heerdink ER, van Iersel EE et al.: Prevalence of patients using drugs metabolized by cytochrome P450 2D6 in different populations: a cross-sectional study. *Ann Pharmacother* 2007; **41:** 408–13.

36 Weinshilbaum R. Inheritance and drug response. *N Engl J Med* 2003; **348:** 529–37.

37 Shin J, Kayser SR, Langaee TY. Pharmacogenetics: from discovery to patient care. *Am J Health-Syst Pharm* 2009; **66:** 625–37.

38 Eichelbaum M, Ingelman-Sundberg M, Evans WE. Pharmacogenomics and individualized drug therapy. *Annu Rev Med* 2006; **57:** 119–37.

39 Ingelman-Sundberg M. Genetic polymorphisms of cytochrome P450 2D6 (CYP2D6): clinical consequences, evolutionary aspects and functional diversity. *Pharmacogenomics J* 2005; **5:** 6–13.

40 Xiang Q, Zhao X, Zhou Y et al.: Effect of CYP2D6, CYP3A5, and MDR1 genetic polymorphisms on the pharmacokinetics of risperidone and its active moiety. *J Clin Pharmacol* 2010; **50:** 659–66.

41 Kircheiner J, Rodriguez-Antona C: Cytochrome P450 genotyping. Potential role in improving treatment outcomes in psychiatric disorders. *CNS Drugs* 2009; **23:** 181–91.

42 Rau T, Woholeben G, Wuttke H et al.: CYP2D6 genotype: impact on adverse effects and nonresponse during treatment with antidepressants—a pilot study. *Clin Pharmacol Ther* 2004; **75:** 386–93.

43 De Leon J, Susce MT, Pan RM et al.: The CYP2D6 poor metabolizer phenotype may be associated with risperidone adverse drug reactions and discontinuation. *J Clin Psychiatry* 2005; **66:** 15–27.

44 Ter Laak MA, Temmink AH, Koeken A et al.: Recognition of impaired atomoxetine metabolism because of low CYP2D6 activity. *Pediatr Neurol* 2010; **43:** 159–62.

45 Mojtabai R, Olfson M: National trends in psychotropic medication polypharmacy in office-based psychiatry. *Arch Gen Psychiatry* 2010; **67:** 26–36.

46 Borrelli F, Izzo AA: Herb-drug interactions with St Johns's wort (Hypericum perforatum): an update on clinical observations. *AAPS J* 2009; **11:** 710–27.

47 Crowe S, Lyons B: Herbal medicine use by children presenting for ambulatory anesthesia and surgery. *Paediatr Anaesth* 2004; **14:** 916–19.

48 Ten Eick AP, Nakamura H, Reed MD: Drug-drug interactions in pediatric psychopharmacology. *Pediatr Clin North Am* 1998; **45:** 1233–64.

49 Greenblatt DJ, von Moltke LL, Harmatz JS et al.: Drug interactions with newer antidepressants: role of human cytochromes P450. *J Clin Psychiatry* 1998; **59**(suppl 15): 19–27.

50 Ozdemir V, Naranjo CA, Herrmann N et al.: Paroxetine potentiates the central nervous system side effects of perphenazine: contribution of cytochrome P4502D6 inhibition in vivo. *Clin Pharmacol Ther* 1997; **62:** 334–47.

51 Kivisto KT, Lamberg TS, Kantola T et al.: Plasma buspirone concentrations are greatly increased by erythromycin and itraconazole. *Clin Pharmacol Ther* 1997; **62:** 348–54.

52 Takahashi H, Ishikawa S, Nomoto S et al.: Developmental changes in pharmacokinetics and pharmacodynamics of warfarin enantiomers in Japanese children. *Clin Pharmacol Ther* 2000; **68**: 541–55.

53 Findling RL, Reed MD, Myers C et al.: Paroxetine pharmacokinetics in depressed children and adolescents. *J Am Acad Child Adolesc Psychiatry* 1999; **38**: 952–9.

54 Edwards DJ, Stoeckel K: The pharmacokinetics of new oral cephalosporins in children. *Chemotherapy* 1992; **38**(suppl 2): 2–9.

55 Holford NHG: A size standard for pharmacokinetics. *Clin Pharmacokinet* 1996; **30:** 329–32.

56 Knibbe CA, Zuideveld KP, Aarts LP et al.: Allometric relationships between the pharmacokinetics of propofol in rats, children and adults. *Br J Clin Pharmacol* 2005; **59**, 705–11.

57 Anderson BJ, Holford NHG: Mechanistic basis of using body size maturation to predict clearance in humans. *Drug Metab Pharmacokinet* 2009; **24:** 25–36.

58 Alcorn J, McNamara PJ: Using ontogeny information to build predictive models for drug elimination. *Drug Discov Today* 2008; **13:** 507–12.

59 Johnson TN: The problems in scaling adult drug doses to children. *Arch Dis Child* 2008; **93:** 207–11.

CHAPTER 6

Psychostimulants

Steven R. Pliszka
The University of Texas Health Science Center at San Antonio, San Antonio, USA

Introduction

The negative impact of the symptoms of attention-deficit/hyperactivity disorder (ADHD) on many different aspects of patient and family life is well established [1]. Fortunately, stimulants are a critical and highly efficacious part of the treatment regimen for ADHD. Stimulant treatment is one of the most thoroughly researched topics in the mental health arena. The first use of amphetamine (AMP) in children with disruptive behavior disorders was first described seven decades ago. Thus the treatment of ADHD (albeit under many different names of the disorder) predates the use of antibiotics [2]. In his original paper, Bradley [2, p. 578] described the clinical response of children to stimulants in words that remain true to this day:

> Possibly the most striking change in behavior during the week of Benzedrine therapy occurred in the school activities of many of these patients. Fourteen children responded in a spectacular fashion. Different teachers, reporting on these patients, who varied in age and accomplishment, agree that a great increase of interest in school material was noted immediately . . . The improvement was noted in all school subjects. It appeared promptly on the first day Benzedrine was given and disappeared on the first day it was discontinued.

Since Bradley's seminal work, stimulants have become the most widely prescribed psychopharmacological treatment in children, even as the name of the disorder has morphed from "minimal brain dysfunction" to "hyperkinesis" to ADHD. In recent years, animal studies, functional magnetic resonance imaging (fMRI), electroencephalogram (EEG) techniques, event-related potentials (ERP) and radionucleotide imaging have led to greater understanding of the mechanisms of action of stimulants.

Pharmacotherapy of Child and Adolescent Psychiatric Disorders, Third Edition.
Edited by David R. Rosenberg and Samuel Gershon.
© 2012 John Wiley & Sons, Ltd. Published 2012 by John Wiley & Sons, Ltd.

Effective use of stimulants is essential for any clinician who deals with patients suffering from ADHD.

Epidemiology of stimulant use

There has been a dramatic rise in prescriptions of stimulants from 1 million a year in 1990 to 14 million a year in 2002 [3]. This increase is most likely due to greater awareness of the disorder among parents, increasing comfort of physicians with stimulant treatment, and pharmaceutical company marketing efforts that accompanied the introduction of longer acting stimulants [3]. The Center for Disease Control (CDC) [4] performed a nationwide telephone survey in 2003–4, which showed that 14% and 6% of parents of ten-year-old boys and girls, respectively, reported their child had been diagnosed with ADHD. These parents reported that 9% of boys and 4% of girls were treated with stimulants at some point in their lives, though only about half of those diagnosed with ADHD were being treated at the time of the interview.

Structure and biochemical mechanism of action

The molecular structures of methylphenidate (MPH) and amphetamine (AMP) are shown in Figures 6.1 and 6.2. Methylphenidate acts as a reuptake blocker of both dopamine (DA) and norepinephrine (NE); AMP also has these properties but, in addition, it can reverse the action of the NE/DA transporter to induce release even in the absence of an action potential, and inhibit monoamine oxidase [5, 6]. These additional effects are thought to be the reason AMP is more potent than MPH, but once equivalent doses are given, clinical efficacy appears to be similar between the two classes of agents. In their immediate release forms their serum pharmacokinetic half-lives (T $\frac{1}{2}$) are quite different—2.5 hours for MPH and 12 hours for AMP—but their pharmacodynamic half-lives (the point at which the clinical effects are $\frac{1}{2}$ the maximum are more similar—2 hours for MPH and 3–5 hours for AMP [7].

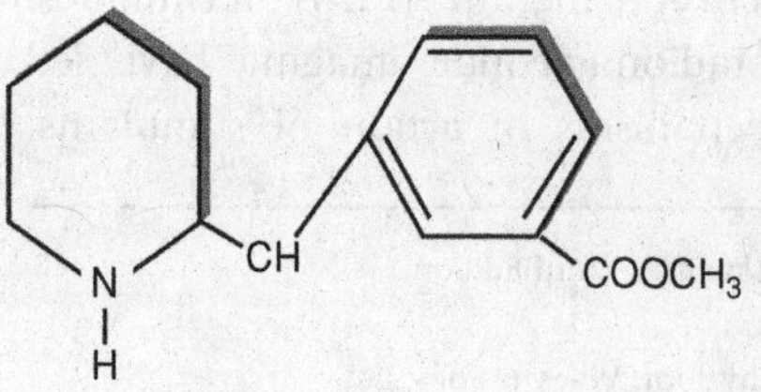

Figure 6.1 Methylphenidate.

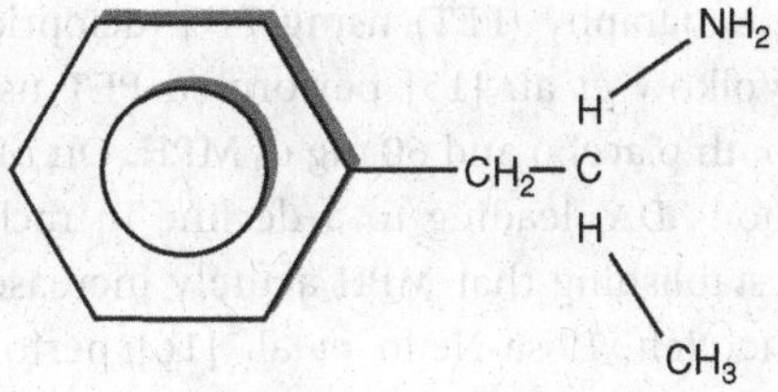

Figure 6.2 Amphetamine.

Basic science studies show that phasic release of catecholamines (dopamine (DA) and norepinephrine (NE)) to relevant stimuli occurs when an animal is alert and interested, while high tonic catecholamine release is associated with feelings of stress and loss of control [8, 9]. The effects of NE and DA on attention and behavior are most likely mediated through interactions with an extensive range of receptors that demonstrate varying affinities for these catecholamines. Dopamine acts at both the D1 (D1- and D5-receptors) and D2 (D2-, D3-, and D4-receptors) families of receptors. Norepinephrine acts chiefly at α_1-, α_2-, and β-receptors; the α_2-receptors are further subdivided as α_{2A}, α_{2B}, and α_{2C}. These subtypes are located presynaptically on noradrenergic neurons, dendrites, or axon terminals, and postsynaptically on neurons receiving noradrenergic input. Although presynaptic receptors are the most recognized, the majority of α_2-receptors in the brain are postsynaptic. NE has the highest affinity for α_2-receptors, with lower affinity for α_1- and β-receptors [10].

In a series of studies with rhesus monkeys, Arnsten and colleagues have attempted to isolate the actions of stimulants on prefrontal cortex (PFC) neurons [9, 11, 12]. Monkeys are trained to do executive function tasks while the activities of PFC neurons are monitored. The $\alpha2$ antagonist yohimbine and the $\alpha1$ agonist phenylephrine abolish the activity of these neurons, while guanfacine enhances their activity, suggesting the NE enhances executive function via stimulation of $\alpha2$ NE receptors. This group has also studied the effects of MPH on DA function. Moderate levels of a D1 agonist improved firing of neurons active during these tasks, while the D1 antagonist SCH23390 abolished the cognitive enhancing effects of MPH. The totality of this work suggests stimulants achieve their therapeutic effects via both dopaminergic and noradrenergic effects.

Neuroimaging studies of stimulant effects

Radio-labeled ligands can be used to study cerebral blood flow, or they can be designed to bind to areas of interest in the brain, particularly the DA transporter [13] or DA receptors [14]. Another approach to examine the effects of MPH in the brain is to image subjects with positron emission tomography (PET) using 11C-raclopride, which binds to DA-2 receptors. Volkow et al. [15] performed PET using this ligand in healthy men on both placebo and 60 mg of MPH. On MPH, subjects released more endogenous DA, leading to a decline in raclopride binding relative to placebo, establishing that MPH acutely increases the amount of DA in the synaptic cleft. Rosa-Neito et al. [16] performed a PET raclopride study with nine adolescents with ADHD; the subjects were scanned both on placebo and again on a therapeutic dose of MPH. The MPH induced a decrease in raclopride binding relative to placebo. The magnitude of the decrease in raclopride binding correlated well with MPH-induced improvements on cognitive testing. Finally, Volkow showed that control subjects had a greater change in raclopride binding (i.e. more release of DA) on MPH than placebo compared to those with ADHD. Interestingly, within the ADHD group, reduced DA release in response to MPH was associated with higher baseline symptoms of ADHD. The study suggested that stimulants enhance DA *in vivo*, but that inherently less DA release is part of the pathophysiology of ADHD.

Another approach that examines stimulant action in the brain is the direct study of the binding of ligands to the DA transporter [13]. Several ligands, including 123I-Altropane, 123I-IPT and 99Tc-TRODAT-1, and 123I-citalopram are available, bind to the DA transporter and give a measure of its binding potential. Typically Single Positron Emission Tomography (SPECT) is used to assess the amount of ligand binding to the receptor, although Altropane can be used with PET [13]. The PET ligand PE2I can also be used to image the DA transporter [17]. In seven studies reviewed by Spencer et al. [13], five showed the DA transporter binding to be increased in subjects with ADHD relative to controls, while two studies showed no difference between the ADHD and control groups. In a more comprehensive study, Volkow et al. [18] used PET to establish that the DA transporter availability is *reduced* in adults with ADHD relative to controls. Despite the inconsistent findings with regard to baseline levels of ADHD, studies can examine the effect of stimulants on DA transporter availability.

Krause et al. [19] obtained SPECT using TRPDAT-1 in a small number of adults with ADHD both at baseline and again after a dose of MPH. They found the DA transporter binding potential to be reduced with treatment, but the SPECT was done 90 minutes after the MPH dose when the medication is expected to be binding to the transporter. Thus it cannot be concluded that MPH down regulated the transporter [13]. Vles et al. [20] also found that DA transporter binding potential was reduced after three months of MPH treatment in six boys with ADHD, but the time of SPECT in relation to the last MPH dose was not reported. When MPH treatment was withdrawn from five children with ADHD, DA transporter binding potential immediately increased to pretreatment values, suggesting that MPH does not induce any long-term down regulation of the transporter [21].

Quantitative EEG (QEEG) and Event Related potential (ERP) measures have also been used to study the response of children with ADHD to medication. In QEEG, EEG activity is examined within specific frequency bands. The complex EEG waveform is decomposed via Fournier analysis into component frequency bands: delta ($<$ 4 Hz), theta (4–7 Hz), alpha (8–12 Hz) and beta ($>$ 13 Hz). The beta band is associated with mental alertness. Most studies have shown that children with ADHD show decreased beta and increased amounts of the other frequencies, particularly in the frontal area [22, 23]. While there is a subgroup of children who show an excess of beta [24], they do not appear to be clinically distinguishable from those with decreased beta. Children with ADHD also show decreased theta/beta and theta/alpha ratios relative to controls; stimulant treatment of ADHD can increase these ratios, "normalizing" the QEEG [25]. Clarke et al. [26] compared 20 children with ADHD who had responded well to MPH to 20 who had responded well to dextroAMP using QEEG power. Theta/beta ratios in the frontal, central, and posterior leads were higher for the MPH responders than the dextroAMP responders, and MPH responders had greater theta/alpha ratios in the frontal leads. Loo et al. [27] found similar results, adding that nonresponders to MPH tended to show decreased beta while on the medication. Increased beta post-treatment also correlated with improvements in ADHD symptoms on parent behavior rating scales. It is important to note, however, that these results represent group averages; at the level of the individual patients, QEEG does not predict stimulant response above the rate predicted by the clinical diagnostic information [23]. Loo et al. [28] compared the MPH response of children with ADHD who were homozygous for the 10-repeat allele of the DA transporter with those who were heterozygous for the 9 repeat allele. The 10-R homozygotes showed increased beta power and increased beta/theta ratios on MPH relative to placebo, while children with ADHD who were 9-repeat allele carriers showed the opposite pattern. In the future, use of QEEG in conjunction with genetic and functional MRI may allow a more comprehensive picture of the neurophysiology of stimulant effects.

With event-related potentials (ERP), the subject performs a repetitive cognitive task and EEG is obtained during each trial. The EEG is then averaged over many trials, canceling out random brain activity and producing a waveform that represents the brain's response to each class of stimuli in the task. In studies of ADHD, oddball auditory ERP tasks and inhibitory tasks, such as the continuous performance test (CPT), have been most utilized [29]. In the auditory oddball task, the subject must detect rare tones among a long string of common tones. Healthy controls produce a larger P300 wave to the oddball tones than to the common tones, but this difference is markedly reduced in children with ADHD [29]. The meaning of this difference in the P300 is debated. The P300, which in these tasks is most prominent over the parietal areas, possibly reflects activity related to evaluation of the stimuli, but may also represent the amount of mental capacity that is invested in the task [30]. In most treatment studies of oddball tasks using ERP, MPH enhances the P300 response to the rare stimuli [31].

Since ADHD (particularly the combined type) has been conceptualized as a disorder of inhibitory control [32], clearer results have emerged from studies using tasks assessing this cognitive domain. When performing the Continuous Performance Test (CPT), the child must respond to target stimuli and avoid responding to other stimuli. In the Go/No Go task, the child responds to a Go stimulus the majority of the time but must refrain from responding when the No Go stimuli are presented. No-Go or stop signals on an inhibitory task are associated with a right lateralized N200, which may signal the triggering of the prefrontal inhibitory processes [33]; this N200 has been shown to be reduced in children with ADHD [34]. When on MPH, the N200 to No Go stimuli of children with ADHD no longer showed any differences from controls [35]. No Go stimuli of inhibitory tasks also elicit a frontocentral P300 (to be distinguished from the parietal P300 discussed above), which is thought to be generated by the anterior cingulate [36]. Seventeen boys with ADHD and controls performed the CPT while ERP was obtained at baseline and then one week later after a 10 mg dose of MPH [37]. P300 to the No Go stimuli was greater than that to the Go stimuli, and the No Go P300 of children with ADHD was significantly increased after treatment with MPH. Twelve children with ADHD performed the Stop Signal Task while ERPs were obtained [38]. Each child completed two testing sessions, once on placebo and again on an individualized dose of MPH, with the order of medication administration counterbalanced. Subjects had to press a button each time a letter appeared on the screen, but withhold their response if the letter "S" appeared after the target stimulus. During successful inhibitions, MPH significantly increased the amplitude of the right frontal N200, while during unsuccessful inhibitions MPH increased the amplitude of the NoGo-P3. Thus, MPH may improve inhibitory control by enhancing brain mechanisms that trigger the inhibitory process and make stopping, a motor act, more probable (reflected by increased N200) and by increasing attentional resources to the task when unsuccessful inhibitions occur (as reflected by increased NoGo-P3).

Functional MRI, which is noninvasive and involves no nuclear radiation, is an expanding research tool. Using primarily measures of inhibitory control, comparisons of ADHD children to controls during fMRI have shown differences in fronto-striatal activity, particularly in the right prefrontal cortex [39] and anterior cingulate [40, 41]. Studies of stimulants effects on the brain using fMRI have been very limited to date but are progressing. Initially, Vaidya et al. [42] showed that MPH, relative to placebo, increased frontal activation in both ADHD patients and controls. Striatal activation was increased on MPH relative to placebo in children with ADHD, but controls showed the opposite pattern, even though both groups improved in the cognitive task performance. A group of concordantly diagnosed ADHD parent-child dyads from the National Institute of Mental Health Multimodal Treatment of ADHD study (MTA) was compared with a matched sample of normal parent-child dyads [43]. The ADHD dyads were administered double-blind MPH and placebo in a counterbalanced fashion over two consecutive days of testing. In both groups, frontostriatal function was measured using functional magnetic resonance imaging (fMRI) during performance of a Go/No-Go task. Parents with ADHD showed greater activation of left caudate nucleus on MPH relative to placebo, while youth showed greater activation on medication in the anterior cingulate, bilateral caudate, and the right inferior parietal lobule. Adults with ADHD showed increased activation of the anterior cingulate on MPH relative to placebo while performing a difficult interference task; and an increase in cingulate activity predicted response to medication [44].

Rubia et al. [45] compared 13 boys with ADHD and matched controls during fMRI while they performed a rewarded continuous performance test; the boys with ADHD preformed the task twice, once on placebo and again on MPH, in a double blind counterbalanced design. MPH, compared to placebo, significantly increased brain activation in cerebellum, precuneus and posterior cingulate gyrus; MPH also enhanced right hemisphere activity in inferior prefrontal, premotor and parietal cortices. In the condition where the subjects were rewarded for task performance, MPH further enhanced activity in the anterior cingulate, the caudate and the right ventromedial frontal cortex. When children with ADHD on placebo were compared to controls, there were numerous differences in brain activity across multiple areas, but these differences were no longer significant when the children with ADHD were on MPH, suggesting a normalizing effect of the stimulant.

Recent work has distinguished between an active and "default" mode state in brain activity. The default or resting mode consists of activity in the precuneus and ventral medical prefrontal cortex, while the active mode is represented by dorsal anterior cingulate and inferior frontal cortex. These groups of regions (active and default) are anticorrelated in their levels of brain activity and this anticorrelation is decreased in subjects with ADHD relative to controls [46]. Peterson et al. [47] compared the default mode activity of youth with ADHD to controls; subjects with ADHD were studied both on and off stimulant medication. Results showed that on medication, those with ADHD were more able to suppress default mode activity during the Stroop Task. Functional magnetic resonance imaging can also be used to study cerebral perfusion through the continuous arterial spin labeling (CASL) technique. After withdrawing MPH, cerebral perfusion was found to be increased in adults with ADHD in the left caudate, as well as in frontal and parietal regions relative to controls [48]. Thus the fMRI data to date is consistent with a picture of activation of MPH for brain regions involved in attention (anterior cingulate, frontal regions and caudate), and reassuringly, this appears to represent normalization of brain function in MPH.

Increasingly, data is emerging showing the long-term impact of stimulant treatment on neuroanatomy. Relative to controls, children with ADHD have about a 3% reduction in brain volume but this reduction is less pronounced in children with ADHD who have a history of stimulant treatment [49]. Anterior cingulate and cerebellar vermis volume was found to be reduced in children with ADHD relative to controls but only in those who were treatment-naïve [50, 51]. Change in cortical thickness was estimated from two neuroanatomic MRI scans at different time points in 43 youths with ADHD. The mean age at the first scan was 12.5 years and at the second scan, 16.4 years [52]. Nineteen patients not treated with stimulants between the scans were compared with an age-matched group of 24 patients who were treated with stimulants. This was a naturalistic follow-up study, so patients were not randomized to treatment. Adolescents who took stimulants showed reduced thinning of cortex relative to those not taking stimulants in the right motor strip, left middle/inferior frontal gyrus, and right parieto-occipital region. There was no difference in clinical outcome between the groups and those who had taken stimulants, however those who had taken stimulants showed rates of cortical thinning similar to control subjects. Normalizing effects of stimulants in patients with ADHD have also been shown in the basal ganglia [53] and thalamus [54]. This is reassuring evidence to provide to parents worried about long term effects of stimulants on brain development, although more definitive long-term studies on this subject are needed.

Studies of short-term efficacy

Stimulants have consistently shown robust behavioral efficacy in hundreds of randomized controlled trials conducted since the 1960s. By 1993, Swanson's "Review of reviews" reported over 3000 citations and 250 reviews of stimulant treatment [55]. Robust short-term stimulant-related improvements in ADHD symptoms were found in 161 studies encompassing five preschool, 140 school age, seven adolescent and nine adult RCTs [56]. Improvement was noted for 65–75% of the 5899 patients assigned to stimulant treatment versus only 4–30% of those assigned to placebo for

MPH (n = 133 trials), (DEX) (n = 22 trials), and pemoline (n = 6 trials). (Pemoline was removed from the market as a result of hepatotoxicity and will not be discussed further.) In the mid-1990s the short-acting mixed salts of AMP (MSA) were introduced [57]. Methylphenidate has both a dextro (d) and levo (l) isomer; the d-MPH isomer alone shows efficacy equal to that of the d, 1-MPH form, with some evidence that the d-isomer administered alone has a slightly longer duration of action than d, l-MPH [58]. Short-acting stimulants rarely have duration of action longer than six hours, requiring multiple doses per day. In recent years, long-acting forms have been developed for d, l MPH (Concerta, Daytrana Transdermal System, Metadate CD, Ritalin LA), AMP (Adderall XR, Vyvanse) and d-MPH (Focalin XR). Studies documenting the efficacy of these agents relative to placebo are listed in Table 6.1. All of these studies are characterized by large samples, rigorous diagnostic criteria for ADHD, use of standardized rating scales for assessing symptoms of ADHD and double blind, controlled designs. Results showed long acting agents to have a response rate similar to that shown by short acting stimulants in the earlier studies. Furthermore, they show that adults respond in a manner similar to school age children.

In the National Institute of Mental Health (NIMH)—Preschool ADHD Treatment Study (PATS), 183 children aged 3 to 5 years underwent an open-label trial of MPH; subsequently, 165 of these subjects were randomized into a double-blind, placebo-controlled crossover trial of MPH lasting 6 weeks [59]. One-hundred-and-forty subjects who completed this second phase went on to enter a long-term maintenance study of MPH. Parents of subjects in this study were required to complete a ten-week course of parent training before their child was treated with medication. Of note, only 37 of 279 enrolled parents felt that the behavior training resulted in significant or satisfactory improvement.

Results from the short-term, open-label run-in and double-blind crossover studies do show that MPH is effective in preschoolers with ADHD [60]. The mean optimal dose of MPH was found to be 0.7 + 0.4 mg/kg/day, which is lower than the mean of 1.0 mg/kg/day found to be optimal in the studies with school-age children [61]. Eleven percent of subjects discontinued MPH because of adverse events [60]. The preschool group showed a higher rate of emotional adverse events, including crabbiness, irritability, and proneness to crying than older children. The conclusion was that the dose of MPH (or any stimulant) should be titrated more conservatively in preschoolers than in school-age patients, and lower mean doses may be effective. A pharmacokinetic study done as part of the PATS protocol showed that preschoolers metabolized MPH more slowly than did school-age children, perhaps explaining these results [62].

Table 6.1 Summary of recent studies of the use of stimulants in the treatment of ADHD

Generic name	Brand	N, age group	Design	Efficacy data	Safety	Author
MSA	Adderall XR	509 children, aged 6–12 years	4 week, DBPC parallel groups	a.m. and p.m. teacher and behavior rating scales improved relative to placebo	Decreased appetite—22%, Headache—14%, Insomina—16%, Abdominal pain—14%, Moodiness—9%	Biederman et al. [94]
OROS-MPH	Concerta	282 children aged 6–12 years	MPH responders randomized to placebo, MPH or OROS MPH	Response rates: OROS MPH: 47%, MPH—47%, Placebo—17%	Decreased appetite, headache and insomnia	Wolraich et al. [92]
MPH	Metadate CD	321 children aged 6–16 years	3 week DBPC parallel groups	Response rates: MPH—64%, Placebo—27%	Headache—15%, Decreased appetite—10%, Abdominal pain—10%, Insomnia—7%	Greenhill et al. [93]
MPH	Ritalin LA	134 children aged 6–12	2 week DBPC parallel groups	Teacher ratings significantly improved over placebo	Decreased appetite and insomnia	Package Insert
d-MPH	Focalin XR	97 children aged 6–17 years	7 week, DBPC parallel groups	Response rates: d-MPH—67%, Placebo—13%		Greenhill et al. [148]
OROS-MPH	Concerta	141 adults	6 weeks, DBPC parallel groups	66% response to MPH, 39% to placebo	Small but clinically insignificant effects on blood pressure	Biederman et al. [149]
MSA	Adderall XR	278 adolescents aged 10–17 years	4 weeks, DBPC parallel groups	Response rates: Placebo—27%, 10 mg—52%, 20 mg 66%, 30 mg 71%, 40 mg 64%	Decreased appetite—36%, Headache—16%, Weight loss—9%, Insomnia—12%	Spencer et al. [150]

MSA	Adderall XR	223 adults	4-week, DBPC parallel group, placebo vs. 4 doses of MSA (20, 40 or 60 mg)	Significant improvement of ADHD symptoms relative to baseline	Insomnia—33% Decreased appetite—32% Headache—30% Nervousness—26%	Weisler et al. [151]
OROS MPH	Concerta	220 adolescents	Open titration to efficacious dose of OROS MPH, then randomized for two weeks to OROS MPH or placebo	Response rates: OROS MPH—52% Placebo—31% 37% of subjects required 72 mg of OROS MPH a day	Headache—7% Decreased appetite—2% Insomnia—4% (only MPH responders in study)	Wilens et al. [152]
MPH transdermal system (MTS)	Daytrana	270 children aged 6–12	5-week DBPC parallel groups, 4 dose levels of MTS	Response rate: MPH MTS—72% Placebo—24%	Decreased appetite—25% Insomnia—10% Nausea—10% Decreased weight—10% Tic—5% Moodiness—5%	Findling et al. [153]
LDX	Vyvanse	290 children aged 6–12	4-week DBPC parallel group, 30, 50 and 70 mg doses of drug	Response rate: Placebo—18% All three drug groups: >70%	Decreased appetite—39% Irritability—10% Insomnia—10% Nausea—6% Weight loss—9%	Biederman et al. [154]
LDX	Vyvanse	420 adults	4-week DBPC parallel group, 30, 50 and 70 mg doses of drug	Response rate: Placebo—29% 30 mg: 57% 50 mg: 62% 70 mg: 61%	Decreased appetite—22% Dry mouth—18% Headache—12% Insomnia—14%	Alder et al. [155]

ADHD = attention-deficit/hyperactivity disorder; CD = conduct disorder; DBPC = Double blind placebo controlled; d-MPH = dextro-methylphenidate; LA = Long acting; MPH = methylphenidate; MSA = mixed salts of AMP; MTS = MPH transdermal system; OROS = Osmotic Release Oral System; OROS-MPH = OROS methylphenidate; XR = extended release.

Studies of long-term efficacy

The Multimodality Treatment of ADHD (MTA) is a major long-term study of the treatment outcome of ADHD. Subjects underwent a year of active treatment [63, 64] then had follow up assessments two [65, 66], three [67–70], and most recently, 6–8 years [71] after the formal research treatment ended. Subjects will most likely be followed into adulthood. A large number of children with ADHD aged 7–10 years of age (n = 579) were randomized to one of four groups for 13 months of active intervention: (1) Medication Management (Med-Mgt), wherein children first underwent a 28-day double-blind placebo-controlled, MPH trial to determine the best dose of stimulant for symptom reduction and then received 13 months of regular medication follow up. Pharmacotherapists had regular access to parent and teacher behavior rating scales. (2) Intensive behavior therapy (Beh), consisting of 35 parent- training sessions, biweekly consultation with the child's teacher, an eight-week summer camp program designed for children with ADHD and three months of classroom aide support. (3) Combined treatment (Comb) consisting of Med-Mgt and Beh together or (4) community comparison (CC). It would not be ethical to deprive children with ADHD of all treatments for a year, so the "control" group was referred to standard treatment in the community. About two-thirds of these children received medication treatment, primarily with stimulants.

The MTA findings address several major areas: (1) how comorbidity affects symptoms at entry to the study, (2) outcome of acute treatment at the end of the year, and (3) outcome at future time points *after active treatment had ended*. This latter point is particularly important in understanding the results of the MTA. After the first year of the study, families chose whichever standard treatment they wished, or they could also drop out of treatment. Children who were in the behavior group could begin medication, while children in the medication group could stop pharmacologic intervention. For the purposes of the analyses in years 2, 3 and 6–8, children were still classified according to the group in which they were originally randomized.

Figure 6.3 shows how the children undergoing different treatments in the first year of the MTA fared over time. All of the children met DSM-IV criteria at study entry; at 14 months, all four groups showed improvement in symptoms such that many children no longer met criteria for ADHD [63]. As shown, the two groups that were treated with rigorous medication management were significantly better than the CC and Beh groups, which were not different from each other. Beh appeared to do as well as the "standard" CC group in reducing symptoms, so it might be claimed that behavior therapy works as well as medication and is an alternative to medication. However, when children who had not received

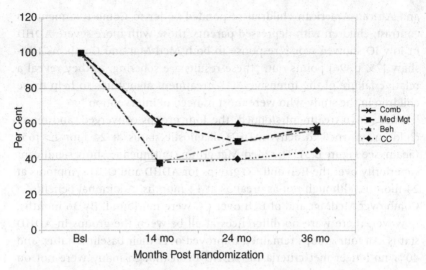

Figure 6.3 Attention-deficit hyperactivity disorder diagnostic status. (Reprinted from the Journal of the American Academy of Child and Adolescent Psychiatry, Vol 46/8, Jensen PS, Arnold LE, Swanson JM, et al, '3-Year Follow-up of the NIMH MTA Study' Pages no. 989–1002, Copyright 2007, with permission from Elsevier.)

any medication were excluded from the CC group, the CC group in fact did better than the Beh group. Thus, behavior therapy is not as effective as medication treatment. The American Academy of Child and Adolescent Psychiatry practice parameters regard pharmacological intervention as the first-line treatment for ADHD [72]. While combined treatment did not show superiority over Med-Mgt in the initial intention-to-treat analysis, a secondary analysis suggested there might be a higher proportion of "excellent responders," that is children whose ADHD rating scale scores fell into the normative range [73].

Before moving to the long-term outcome, it is critical to look at moderators that affected the response of subgroups in the sample. Not surprisingly, comorbidity was a key factor [64,74]. For children with ADHD alone, Beh did not have any effect greater than CC, whereas, there was a significantly larger effect size for Med-Mgt and Comb over CC (though not different from each other). The comorbidity of ODD/CD did not moderate treatment, as can be seen that the lines for ADHD plus ODD/CD essentially overlap with the ADHD group. This means that the ODD/CD comorbid children responded to treatment just like the ADHD group. The pattern was quite different for comorbid anxiety, however. Note that children with comorbid anxiety were much more responsive to all treatments, with a large effect size over the CC group. Comb was more effective than Med-Mgt. This was particularly true for the group with dual comorbidity, that is, children with ADHD, ODD/CD and anxiety. Hinshaw [75] described other moderators of outcome in the MTA. Children on public assistance and African-American children responded better to Comb treatment. In contrast, children with depressed parents, those with more severe ADHD or low IQ showed worse response to both Med-Mgt and Comb. As Hinshaw [75, p. 96] points out, "these results are sobering, as they reveal a relative failure of the intensive MTA treatment algorithms to help those children in the study who were most in need of intervention."

Once active treatment stopped, the four groups converged, and many children returned to active ADHD diagnostic status at 24 months [65] (again, see Figure 6.3). The Med-Mgt group continued to show significant superiority over the Beh and CC groups for ADHD and ODD symptoms at 24 months, although not as great as at 14 months. Additional benefits of Comb over MedMgt and of Beh over CC were not found. By 36 months, however, there were no differences at all between the groups in ADHD status. All four groups remained improved over their baseline status, and 40% no longer met criteria for ADHD even though many were not on medication [67], At 36 months, 70% of the Med-Mgt and Comb groups were still taking medication, compared to 60% of the CC group and 45% of the Beh group. While there were differences in outcome between those taking and not taking medication at 24 months, there was no such difference at 36 months [70]. The 6–8 year follow up of the MTA subjects has been published [71]. Overall, the patients continued on the course noted in the 36-month follow up. There was no difference in outcome among the originally assigned treatment groups. Only one-third of the subjects were still taking medication at the 6–8 year follow up, "taking medication" being defined very liberally as on medication 50% of the time in the last year. There was no difference in outcome between those who remained on medication and those who did not. It is possible that the lack of effect was due to the fact that even when subjects did take medication; it was not taken consistently enough to have an impact. The study did find a positive relationship between taking medication and mathematics achievement, consistent with gains in academic achievement found in another long term follow up study of youth with ADHD [76]. Nonetheless, the results were surprising. Does this suggest medication treatment of ADHD "is not worth it" in the long run?

First, it is important to note that none of the 36-month data takes away from the fact that medication showed strong effects in the 14- and 24-month follow up, far superior to the only alternative to medication, that is, behavior therapy. Secondly, psychiatry is not alone in having treatments that are highly effective in the short term but do not seem to alter the underlying disease process. Indeed, a recent review of treatments in childhood asthma shows that inhaled corticosteroids and long-acting beta agonists clearly improve acute symptoms of asthma but do not "alter the natural progression of the childhood asthma nor halt progressive airway damage" [77, p. 1528]. Yet, no one would suggest not using inhalers during acute asthmatic attacks. We should continue our acute management of ADHD with medication, but research on other interventions to improve long-term outcomes are needed.

Clinical use

Table 6.2 shows the wide variety of stimulant preparations that are currently available for clinical use. Reviews of stimulant trials suggest that both AMP and MPH are equally efficacious, typically about 50–60% of patients with ADHD will respond to whichever stimulant is tried first. The response rate will rise to 70–90% if two different stimulant classes are tried in succession [78, 79]. It is estimated that approximately 40% of patients will have a preferential response to one of the stimulant classes but there are no aspects of the patient (gender, age, ADHD subtype, etc.) or laboratory measures that distinguish who will respond to which stimulant. Thus the choice of agent depends on family and physician preference. Clinical experience suggests that families prefer long-acting agents because school dosing is more easily avoided. Table 6.3 shows the dosing schedule for the stimulant preparations as well as the equivalent dosing across agents. Immediate release (IR) D-MPH and AMP preparations have equal potency, which is twice that of d,l MPH. Potency should never be confused with efficacy; on average, a given dose of AMP or d-MPH will yield the same effect as double that dose of d,l MPH.

Stimulants have a rapid onset of action (often on the first day of dosing). Some early work suggested stimulants have a "therapeutic window" in which MPH dosages of 0.3 mg/kg/dose are optimal for enhancing cognition while dosages of 0.6 mg/kg/day resulted in greater improvements in behavior [80]. Extensive work with analog classroom studies in which children with ADHD perform arithmetic problems every hour over the course of a day has shown that on *average*, all stimulants have linear effects on both behavior and cognition [81–83]. Figure 6.4 shows hypothetical data from individual subjects exposed to different doses of MPH. Note that while the average of the subjects shows a linear effect, there are wide individual differences. Subject 1 follows the group mean and has clear linear effects of MPH, whereas subject 2's response hits a plateau at 10 mg with no further improvement as the dose increases. Subject 3 shows a curvilinear response with decline to baseline at higher doses, whereas subject 4 is a complete non-responder. Thus each child's dosing needs to be individualized. Typically, textbooks and guidelines have expressed the dose range for stimulants as 0.3–1.0 mg/kg/dose for MPH and 0.15–0.5 mg/kg/dose for AMP [7]. Several points of confusion about this dosing principle need to be

Table 6.2 Available preparations and cost of psychostimulants

	Commercially available preparations	Dosage form	Mechanism
DextroAMP	Generic (dextroAMP sulfate)	5, 10 mg tablets	IR
	Dexedrine	5, 10 mg tablets; 5 mg / 5 ml elixir	IR
	Dexedrine spansules (sustained release)	5 mg, 10 mg, 15 mg capsules	Not clearly documented
	Vyvanse (lisdexamfetamine lystate)	10, 20, 30, 40, 50, 60, 70 mg	d-AMP is covalently bonded to the amino acid L-lysine, after oral administration, it is converted to active d-AMP
	Procentra (liquid)	5 mg/5 ml solution	IR
Dextro and Levo AMP	Adderall	5, 10, 20 mg (scored)	IR
	Adderall XR	5, 10, 15, 20, 25, 30 mg capsules	50:50% ratio of IR to delayed release beads designed to simulate bid AMP administration
MPH	Generic	5, 10, 20 mg tablets	IR
	Ritalin	5, 10, 20 mg tablets	IR
	Ritalin LA	10, 20, 30, 40 mg capsules	50:50% ratio of IR to delayed release beads
	Ritalin—SR (sustained release)	20 mg tablet	MPH embedded in waxy cellulose compounds, The time to peak rate in children was 4.7 hours for the SR tablets compared to 1.9 hours for the tablets
	Metadate—ER (extended release)	10, 20 mg tablets	MPH embedded in wax matrix, allowing slow release as the table passes through GI tract
	Metadate CD	10, 20, 30, 40, 50, 60 mg capsules	Mixture of IR and delayed released beads, 30% released in a.m., 70% delayed
	Methylin (pill, chewable and liquid)	5 mg (unscored), 10 mg (scored), 20 mg (scored) tablets	IR
	Concerta (extended release)	18, 27, 36, and 54 mg tablets	22% of MPH dose released immediately, the remaining is released via an osmotic pump to create an ascending blood level of MPH
	Focalin (d-MPH)	2.5, 5 and 10 mg tablets	IR
	Focalin XR (d-MPH)	5, 10, 15, 20, 30 mg capsule	50:50% mixture of IR and delayed release beads
	Daytrana Transdermal System	10, 20, 30 mg patch	MPH is contained within a multipolymeric adhesive layer attached to a transparent backing. Avoids first pass metabolism

AMP = amphetamine; IR—immediate release; MPH = methylphenidate.

Table 6.3 Comparative dosing of stimulants. (Reprinted from the Journal of the American Academy of Child and Adolescent Psychiatry, Vol 46/8, Jensen PS, Arnold LE, Swanson JM, et al, '3-Year Follow-up of the NIMH MTA Study' Pages no. 989–1002, Copyright 2007, with permission from Elsevier.)

	MPH (bid)	Concerta (q am)*	Daytrana (q am)	Metadate CD (q am)	Focalin (bid)	Focalin XR (q am)	AMP given (bid)	Adderall XR (q am)	Vyvanse (q am)
Preschool to early school age range (<25 kg)	2.5				1.25		1.25		
	5	18	10	10	2.5	5	2.5	5	20
	7.5	27			3.75				
Later school age and early adolescent (25–40 kg)	10	36	20	20	5	10	5	10	30
	15	54	30	30	7.5	15	7.5	15	40
	20	72		40	10	20	10	20	50
Later adolescent and adults (>40 kg)	25	90		50	12.5		12.5	25	60
	30	108		60	15	30	15	30	70
		126					20	40	
		144					30	60	

AMP = Amphetamine; bid = twice per day; MPH = methylphenidate; q am = every morning.
*a.m. doses equivalent; Concerta simulates tid (three times per day) dosing of MPH.

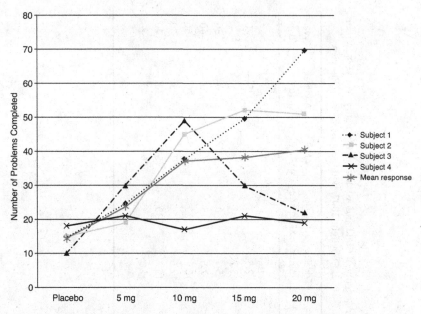

Figure 6.4 Hypothetical data from individual subjects exposed to different doses of Methylphenidate MPH.

cleared up. First, this dosing regimen was designed with regard to school age children and does not apply for adolescents, adults or heavy children. For instance a 70 kg 17 year old would never be given 70 mg of MPH three times a day! Secondly, it does not imply a "target dose" but a range. As shown in Table 6.3, the starting and ending doses are determined by the patient's weight. For any given patient, one selects the starting dose, then administers it for at least a period of one week. If response is not optimal (and side-effects are not impairing), the physician should advance the dose to the next level and repeat the process.

What is the best way to assess response? A wide variety of behavior rating scales are available, which the parent can fill out during the session to quantify the child's response (see Table 6.4). For assessing the child's behavior at home and school repeatedly over several weeks, the short 10-item versions of these scales are preferable. Ideally, one should continue to titrate the stimulant until scores on the ADHD rating scale fall into the "normative" range (T-Score below 60, which is one standard deviation above the mean). Teacher ratings can be examined as well, but some parents may not want to have the school informed that the child is on medication. In other cases obtaining teacher input is difficult to com-munication issues (i.e. getting someone to fax the rating scale to the doctor's office). Parents are generally good reporters of their child's behav-ior at school [84], so obtaining teacher ratings is not mandatory, but when they are not available, the physician should consider examining samples of school work or report cards. Dosing for older adolescents and adults

Table 6.4 Widely used rating scales for assessing stimulant response in ADHD

Scale	Reference
Academic Performance Rating Scale (APRS)	The APRS is a 19-item scale for determining a child's academic productivity and accuracy in grades 1–6 that has six scale points; construct, concurrent, and discriminant validity data, as well as norms (n = 247), available [156] http://www.guilford.com
ADHD Rating Scale-IV	The ADHD Rating Scale-IV is an 18-item scale using *DSM-IV* criteria [157] http://www.guilford.com
Brown ADD Rating Scales for Children, Adolescents and Adults	Psychological Corporation, San Antonio, TX (2001) http://www.drthomasebrown.com/assess_tools/index.html [158]
Conners 3	The parent form includes 110 items, the teacher form includes 115 items, and the self-report form includes 99 items. The short form, consisting of 43 items on the parent form, 39 on the teacher form, and 39 on the self-report form can be used for screening. ADHD and Global Indexes are included http://www.mhs.com
Swanson, Nolan, and Pelham (SNAP-IV) and SWANP	The SNAP-IV [159] is a 26-item scale that contains *DSM-IV* criteria for ADHD and screens for other *DSM* diagnoses; the SWANP is a 30-item scale that measures impairment of functioning at home and at school http://www.adhd.net
Vanderbilt ADHD Diagnostic Parent and Teacher Scales	Teachers rate 35 symptoms and eight performance items measuring ADHD symptoms and common comorbid conditions [160] The parent version contains all 18 ADHD symptoms with items assessing comorbid conditions and performance [161]

can lead to difficulties in determining the "maximum" dose. The Food and Drug Administration has approved a dose of Adderall XR up to 60 mg a day for adults. What is the equivalent dose of this in immediate release MPH or Concerta? Using the rule that MPH is half as potent as AMP, this would suggest the maximum dose of Concerta is 144 mg day or 120 mg a day of immediate-release MPH [85]. In general most physicians are uncomfortable with such doses, and 108 mg a day of Concerta or 90 mg a day of MPH have been a more commonly used maximum dose. Despite these data, physicians must beware of the dangers of tolerance and toxicity (psychosis, severe anorexia and perseveration) at very high doses and monitor carefully. Diversion of stimulants is covered in the section on substance abuse below.

Even long-acting stimulants can be noted to wear off in the late evening. This effect, commonly referred to as "rebound," may often cause caretakers to report that the child is "worse" on the medication because the parent may only observe the effect of the medication after school. It is important for the physician to inquire about the child's behavior on weekends and distinguish the period 8 AM to 4 PM (when most long-acting medications are at peak action) and the late afternoon period. It is clear that the long-acting stimulants are equally effective as their short acting equivalents, though direct comparisons to short acting are limited to Concerta [86] and Adderall XR [83]. In a comparison study in the laboratory setting, effects of Concerta were equivalent to three-times-a day MPH and lasted at least through 12 hours after dosing. Parents preferred Concerta more than tid IR MPH or placebo. This adds empirical weight to the widespread clinical impression that the long-acting agents are more beneficial, in addition to providing enhanced convenience and privacy.

Once a therapeutic dose is established, long-term treatment is generally required. Parents commonly ask, "How long must my child remain on the medication?" Review of the long-term outcome of children with ADHD is beyond the scope of this chapter, but only about a third of children with ADHD experience complete remission of symptoms by young adulthood [87]. To determine if an individual patient is ready to discontinue stimulant medication, parents can stop the medication on the weekend or the summer and observe their child or adolescent's behavior during a cognitively stressful task. If they note marked improvements relative to the child's behavior at the time of diagnosis, then a medication-free period may be advisable. Generally, this should not be at the start of school, but at a mid-point in the fall or spring semester. If grades or behavior in school deteriorate quickly, the stimulant can be restarted. If a patient still has impairing symptoms by age 25, will those symptoms be life long? This has not yet been established, but clinically, many physicians are treating their patients with ADHD into their 40s and 50s.

Common side-effects

The acute side-effects of stimulants, both common and rare, are:

Common:
Insomnia
Decreased appetite
Gastrointestinal pain
Irritability (primarily when medication wears off)
Increased heart rate (clinically insignificant)

Uncommon or idiosyncratic:
Psychosis at therapeutic dose
Excitement/agitation
Sadness/isolation
Preservation ("zombie" effect)

Growth suppression
Tics/skin picking/finger nail biting
Increased heart rate (clinically significant)
Increased blood pressure (clinically significant)
Nausea, constipation
Rash/hives (may be related to tablet/capsule material)

Longer term, open-label studies of these agents, often lasting up to 2 years [88–90] have also been performed, giving the field more data about efficacy and safety after prolonged use. These studies do not show the presence of any major medical adverse events, with no abnormalities of hematological or chemical measures [83, 91–94]. Management of common side-effects is a critical skill for physicians managing ADHD. Appetite that is clearly reduced by medication (and not an expression of baseline "pickiness" about eating) can be managed by being sure the child eats a large breakfast before the stimulant is administered in the morning or by providing snacks in the evening when the child's appetite returns. An alternative stimulant could be tried, but if appetite is reduced on all stimulants, cyproheptadine may be added in the evening to stimulate the child's appetite [95]. Many children with ADHD have sleep issues before beginning treatment. If a child experiences insomnia (or a worsening of baseline sleep problems) with stimulants, then behavioral counseling about avoiding caffeine and removing distractions (computer, TV) from the child's room is often helpful. If this fails, then a trial of over-the-counter melatonin should be tried first. After this, a dose of clonidine (0.05 to 0.10 mg) can be administered about an hour before bedtime. The problem of irritability with stimulants is a vexing one, as many children with ADHD (particularly those with comorbid oppositional defiant disorder), are already irritable before treatment. Indeed, controlled trials of stimulant medications show that they often reduce irritability, on average, relative to baseline. The physician should inquire if the irritability occurs when the medication is peaking in the bloodstream (a direct drug effect) or in the evening when the medication wears off (rebound). Changing to a different stimulant or a nonstimulant will be necessary for the former situation while the latter can be dealt with by adding a low dose of a stimulant in the evening, adding a low dose of atomoxetine [72] or by adding an alpha agonist [96].

Post-marketing safety data for stimulants has also been reviewed by the FDA for reports of mania/psychotic symptoms, aggression and suicidality [97]. Such reports have many limitations as information about dosage, comorbid diagnoses, and concomitant medications is often not available. Nonetheless, for each of the stimulants, there occurred very rare events of psychotic symptoms, specifically involving visual and tactile hallucinations of insects. Symptoms of aggression and suicidality (but no completed suicides) were also reported. The FDA ordered changes to stimulant medication labeling, which more prominently discusses these risks. While such labeling changes will encourage families and clinicians to more closely monitor patients for these rare events, the new label does not require a change in the clinical use of stimulant medications.

Cardiovascular safety issues

In 2005, Health Canada briefly suspended the sale of Adderall XR due to concerns regarding a small number of cases of sudden death in both children and adolescents. A review by the U.S. Food and Drug Administration (FDA) [98] estimated the rate of sudden death in stimulant-treated ADHD children for the exposure period January 1, 1992 to December 31, 2004 to be 0.2/100 000 patient years for MPH, and 0.3/100 000 patient-years for AMP (the differences between the agents are not clinically meaningful). Thus the rate of sudden death of children on ADHD medications *does not* exceed the base rate of sudden death in the general population. Nonetheless, controversy over this subject continues. A retrospective cohort study used ten years of Florida Medicaid claims data cross-linked to Vital Statistics Death Registry data [99]. All youth 3 to 20 years old who were newly diagnosed with attention-deficit/hyperactivity disorder were classified at follow up according to stimulant claims (MPH, AMPs, and pemoline) as current use (on stimulant), former use, or nonuse (time preceding the first stimulant claim, including follow-up of youth who were never exposed to stimulants). The study's end points were cardiac death, first hospital admission for cardiac causes or first emergency department visit for cardiac causes. During 124 932 person-years of observation (n = 55 383), 73 youth died, five because of cardiac causes. No cardiac death occurred during 42 612 person-years of stimulant use. Hospital admissions for cardiac cause occurred for 27 children (eight during stimulant use, 11 during 35 671 person-years of former use, and eight during 46 649 person-years of nonuse); and 1091 children visited the emergency department for cardiac causes (8.7 per 1000 person-years). Current stimulant use was associated with a 20% increase in the hazard for emergency department visits when compared with nonuse. Use of multiple medications, particularly combinations of stimulants and bronchodilators, was associated with ER visits for cardiac reasons. No increased risk was found for periods of former use when compared with nonuse, suggesting any risk is associated only to current use, not to past effects of stimulants.

Gould et al. [100] performed a matched case-control design examining mortality data from 1985–96 state vital statistics. They identified 564 cases of sudden death occurring at ages seven through 19 years across the United States along with a matched group of 564 young people who died as passengers in motor vehicle traffic accidents. Exposure to AMP, dextroAMP, methAMP, or MPH (according to informant reports or as noted in medical examiner records, toxicology results, or death certificates) was examined in the two groups. In ten (1.8%) of the sudden unexplained deaths the youths were taking stimulants, specifically MPH; in contrast, use of stimulants was found in only two subjects in the motor vehicle accident comparison group (0.4%), with only one involving MPH use. A significant association of stimulant use with sudden unexplained death emerged, based on exact conditional logistic regression (odds ratio = 7.4, 95% CI = 1.4 to 74.9). While the study raises concerns, it is of note that the rate of stimulant use in the sudden death group was typical of the rate of use in the general population at the time. Indeed, statistical significance was achieved only because the rate of reported stimulant use in the accident population was *lower* than that in the general population. The FDA did not alter any of the stimulant package labeling regarding cardiovascular risk or screening as a result of this study.

Just prior to the publication of the above results, the American Heart Association (AHA) published a statement widely interpreted as indicating that an electrocardiogram (EKG) should always be done prior to starting a child on any medication for ADHD, based on the reasoning that all current ADHD medications affect the cardiovascular system in some manner [101]. The concept was based on the idea that children may have rare occult heart defects that could be identified by EKG, thus abnormal EKG findings would be followed up for more in-depth cardiovascular work up. Children with fully identified heart disease would then either never be treated with stimulants or only be treated if they had ongoing cardiovascular follow up, though this was never clearly specified. Once the statement was issued, there were major discussions between the AHA, the American Academy of Pediatrics (AAP), and the American Academy of Child and Adolescent Psychiatry (AACAP) regarding this issue, resulting in major revision of the statement on May 16, 2008 [102]. In particular, the AHA clarified that,

- Acquiring an ECG is a Class IIa recommendation. This means that it is reasonable for a physician to consider obtaining an ECG as part of the evaluation of children being considered for stimulant drug therapy, but this should be at the physician's judgment, and it is not mandatory to obtain one.
- Treatment of a patient with ADHD should not be withheld because an ECG is not done. The child's physician is the best person to make the assessment about whether there is a need for an ECG.

Cardiology evaluation should be sought only if the history and physical examination raise suspicion of cardiovascular disease [72].

Growth suppression

Whether stimulants effect the growth of children with ADHD has been controversial for many years. Recently, two major reviews [103,104] have examined all of the available data and concluded that stimulant treatment may be associated with a reduction in expected height gain, at least in the first one to three years of treatment. The Multi-modality Treatment of ADHD study showed reduced growth in ADHD patients after two years of stimulant treatment compared with those patients who received no medication [66] and these deficits persisted at 36 months [69]. Interestingly, the children with ADHD in the MTA study were taller and heavier than average at the start of the study; those treated continuously with medication tended to approach the mean of the population for height and weight by year three of follow up. Charach et al. [105] found higher doses of stimulant correlated with reduced gains in height and weight; indeed the effect did not become significant until the dose in MPH equivalents was >2.5 mg/kg/day for four years. In her review, Poulton [103] raised concern that children with ADHD treated with stimulants might show a reduced height gain of about 1 cm/year and called for more long-term studies. Children with ADHD treated with stimulants should have height and weight measured at least semi-annually. Children whose height or weight percentile drops across two major lines (fifth, tenth, 25th, 50th, 75th, 90th, and 95th) should be considered for treatment with a nonstimulant. Drug holidays should be considered if the child's symptoms of ADHD are not causing severe impairment on weekends and during the summer.

Substance use and diversion

Do children with ADHD treated with stimulants show a greater propensity to abuse illicit substances (particularly stimulants or cocaine) as adults? Wilens and colleagues [106] performed a meta-analysis of six follow- up studies that tracked stimulant treatment and substance-use problems; two of these studies followed subjects into adolescence while four continued follow-up into adulthood. Altogether 674 medicated and 360 unmedicated subjects were followed for at least four years. The pooled estimate of the odds ratio indicated a 1.9-fold *reduction* in risk for SUD in youths who were treated with stimulants compared with youths who did not receive pharmacotherapy for ADHD, with similar reductions in risk for later drug and alcohol use disorders. Furthermore, there was no predilection for patients with ADHD to specifically abuse stimulants or cocaine. More recent studies published since this review have not shown this protective effect of stimulants. The MTA study did not find any association with original assignment to either of the medication or nonmedication groups to future substance abuse, nor was there any relationship of substance-use disorder to ongoing use of stimulant [68,71]. There was no relationship between treatment with stimulants and future substance abuse (positive or negative) in 112 adults with ADHD followed up ten years after diagnosis as children [107]. It should be noted, however, that 75% of the sample has been treated at some point in their lives. A retrospective study of 206 adults with ADHD also did not find that stimulant treatment either increased or decreased substance use disorder risk [108]. Certainly it is well established that stimulant treatment of ADHD does not *increase* the risk of future substance abuse but whether stimulant treatment *protects* against the development of adult substance use disorders remains to be established.

Given that substance-use disorders in adolescence are highly comorbid with ADHD [109] it would be valuable to know what the impact of stimulant treatment would be in those with ADHD who have a *concurrent* substance use disorder. Riggs and colleagues [110] randomized 318 adolescents aged 13–17 years with ADHD and comorbid substance use disorder to either placebo or OROS MPH (Concerta) for 16 weeks. Both groups received cognitive behavioral therapy focusing on their substance-use issues. While both groups improved both in terms of ADHD and substance use, the MPH and placebo groups did not differ from each other in either self-report or laboratory measures of substance use. More detailed results of the study are yet to be published but it appears that treatment of ADHD does not accelerate recovery from substance abuse.

Diversion of stimulant is a growing concern. Wilens et al. [111] reviewed 21 studies representing 113 104 subjects. The studies reported rates of past-year nonprescribed stimulant use ranging from 5–9% in adolescents and 5–35% in college-age individuals. Lifetime rates of diversion of students with stimulant prescriptions asked to give, sell, or trade their medications ranged from 16–29%. Those at higher risk for diversion were whites, members of fraternities and sororities, and individuals with lower grade point averages. Immediate-release preparations were also more likely to be diverted. Reported reasons for use, misuse, and diversion of stimulants included need to concentrate, improve alertness, "get high," or experimentation. Physicians need to be aware of this phenomenon and be cautious about replacing "lost" refills or prescribing to adults without adequate documentation of the diagnosis of ADHD.

Comparison with nonstimulant treatment

Given the fact that 20–25% of children with ADHD fail to respond to a single trial of a stimulant medication, there has always been a need for nonstimulant alternatives. Furthermore, it would be useful to have an agent for ADHD that was not a controlled substance and did not have the stimulants' aforementioned effects on appetite, growth and mood. For many years, tricyclic antidepressants (TCAs), particularly desipramine, filled this role [112]. Desipramine was subsequently associated with a number of cases of sudden death [113]; this, coupled with the TCAs' unfavorable side-effect profile and their lesser efficacy compared to stimulants [114] led to a search for an alternative. Atomoxetine is a selective NE reuptake blocker, though it has indirect effects on DA in the frontal lobe [115]. It is free of effects at noradrenergic, cholinergic and histaminic receptors [116]. Numerous double-blind placebo-controlled trials have demonstrated its efficacy in the treatment of ADHD in children, adolescents, and adults [117–119]. In analog classroom settings, however, stimulants proved superior to atomoxetine in improving behavior and number of arithmetic problems completed [120]. Newcorn et al. [121] directly compared the efficacy of OROS MPH and atomoxetine in a double blind, placebo-controlled parallel groups study. Children and adolescents aged 6–16 with ADHD (N = 222) were randomly assigned to receive 0.8–1.8 mg/kg per day of atomoxetine, 18–54 mg/day of osmotically released MPH, or placebo for six weeks. After six weeks, patients treated with MPH were switched to atomoxetine under double-blind conditions. The response rates for both atomoxetine (45%) and MPH (56%) were superior to that for placebo (24%), but the response to OROS MPH was superior to that for atomoxetine. Of the 70 subjects who did not respond to MPH, 30 (43%) subsequently responded to atomoxetine. Likewise, 29 (42%) of the 69 patients who did not respond to atomoxetine had previously responded to osmotically released MPH.

Thus while atomoxetine is an acceptable first-line agent for the treatment of ADHD [72], most physicians view it as second line if a patient has failed two stimulants or has intolerable side-effects to stimulants [122]. Stimulants can also be combined with atomoxetine to treat partial responders; when MPH was added to atomoxetine, there was a further mean reduction of 40% in ADHD rating [123], but increased rates of insomnia, irritability, and loss of appetite compared to atomoxetine alone [124]. When combined with stimulants, atomoxetine is often dosed lower (~0.5 mg/kg/day) than when used as a monotherapy and may be more often used as a single afternoon dose. Atomoxetine does carry a warning regarding possible suicidal ideation. In a meta-analysis of atomoxetine studies, the frequency of suicidal ideation was 0.37% (5/1357) in pediatric patients taking atomoxetine versus 0% (0/851) for the placebo group [125]. There were no completed suicides. While rare, physicians should warn families about the possibility of suicidal ideation.

Alpha agonists such as clonidine and guanfacine have had a long history of use in the treatment of ADHD, dating back to the 1980s [126]. Recently, an extended release form of guanfacine (GXR, Intuniv) has been approved by the FDA for the treatment of ADHD after showing efficacy in controlled trials [127, 128] and lack of serious adverse events in safety trials [129–131]. The dose of GXR ranges from 1–4 mg a day with the principal side-effect being sedation. It should be noted that 77% of subjects discontinued treatment in the Sallee et al. study [130]. While only 12.5% of these subjects cited lack of efficacy, 13.5% of subjects were "lost to follow up" and 28% "withdrew" consent. Recently Wilens et al. [96] enrolled 461 stimulant partial responders in a double-blind placebo-controlled trial of GXR. Suboptimal response to stimulants was defined as an ADHD rating scale greater than 24 after 4 weeks of stimulant treatment. After nine weeks of treatment, 61% of subjects on stimulant plus GXR met criteria for remission (ADHD rating scale < 18) compared to only 46% meeting remission criteria on stimulant plus placebo. There were no additional side-effects in the combination groups relative to the stimulant only group. Thus it appears that co-administration of GXR to stimulants can result in further improvement in ADHD symptoms without added adverse events.

Despite many years of use, there have been few studies directly comparing clonidine to stimulants in the treatment of ADHD. Palumbo et al. [132] conducted a 16-week, randomized, double-blind, placebo-controlled clinical trial in 122 children aged 7 to 12 with ADHD. They were randomly assigned to clonidine, MPH, clonidine in combination with MPH, or placebo. In two successive four-week titration periods, clonidine (or matching placebo) and added MPH (or matching placebo)were adjusted to optimal doses and then continued for eight weeks. On the Conners Teachers Abbreviated Symptom Questionnaire, monotherapy with clonidine was not found to improve ADHD symptoms, whereas subjects treated with MPH showed significant improvement compared to those not treated with MPH. Subjects treated with clonidine had greater improvements on the Conners Abbreviated Symptom Questionnaire for Parents and Children's Global Assessment Scale, but also a higher rate of sedation compared with subjects not treated with clonidine. While there was a trend for the combination group to have better results than either MPH or clonidine alone, this difference did not reach statistical significance. The study suggested that parents perceived greater benefit to clonidine due to its evening sedative effect, but it should be borne in mind that this study did not administer an evening dose of MPH. An extended release version of clonidine has shown superiority to placebo in the treatment of ADHD in youth aged 6–17 [133]. Thus the alpha-agonists may soon play a larger role in the treatment of ADHD, particularly in combination with stimulants for partial responders or those with tic disorders (see below).

Since the mid-1990s there has been concern as to whether the combination of clonidine and stimulant creates a greater risk for cardiovascular side-effects relative to the use of either medication alone [134, 135]. The above study examined blood pressure, pulse and electrocardiograms

(EKG) in each of the four medication groups [136]. Increased incidents of bradycardia were found in subjects treated with clonidine compared with those not treated with clonidine (17.5% versus 3.4%) but no increased rate of EKG abnormalities were found whether subjects were treated with clonidine alone or the MPH/clonidine combination. Somnolence was more common in subjects treated with clonidine, but generally resolved after six to eight weeks of treatment.

Treatment of comorbidity

In general, the presence of a significant comorbid illness suggests the need for adjunctive psychosocial intervention. The Texas Children's Medication Algorithm Project (CMAP) algorithm discusses the pharmacologic treatment of ADHD with major depressive disorder (MDD), anxiety disorders, tics disorder and severe aggression [122]. The CMAP recommended that the patient with both ADHD and MDD be assessed for the severity of the two disorders, and the most severe disorder should be treated first. Thus a child whose ADHD is causing more impairment should be treated for ADHD first. If the ADHD and MDD symptoms simultaneously resolve with ADHD treatment, no further pharmacologic intervention is needed. If the MDD symptoms persist despite resolution of the ADHD symptoms, then treatment of depression should be added, this could consist of either an antidepressant or a psychosocial intervention. In contrast, if the MDD symptoms are more severe (pervasive depression, weight loss, loss of functioning) than the ADHD symptoms, then treatment for MDD should be initiated (usually a serotonin reuptake inhibitor). If the ADHD symptoms persist after remission of the depression, than an ADHD treatment should be added for treatment of the depression (see above).

Children with tic disorders can be treated safely with stimulants without increasing tics [137] and the CMAP algorithm suggests beginning with stimulant medications for this subgroup. If stimulants worsen tics, then the clinician should utilize a nonstimulant medication such as atomoxetine [138]. Some children with ADHD and comorbid tics respond only to stimulants in terms of their ADHD, yet the stimulant worsens their tics. In such cases, alpha-agonist medications should be added to the stimulant so classes of symptoms are reduced [139].

Severe aggressive behavior occurs in substantial numbers of children with ADHD, particularly in those with comorbid oppositional defiant, conduct disorder or bipolar disorder [140]. Stimulant or atomoxetine treatment of children with ADHD often reduces comorbid oppositional or aggressive behavior [141, 142]. Thus aggressive and conduct disorders symptoms will resolve in the comorbid child when the ADHD is robustly treated [143]. If treatment of ADHD is not sufficient to eliminate the aggressive behavior, then a behavioral treatment should be added to the ADHD treatment. It is prudent to address any psychosocial or parent management problems contributing to the aggression [144, 145].

Pharmacogenetics

The heritability of ADHD approaches 80% and over the last decade a number of candidate genes have been associated with ADHD, though their impact on the risk for ADHD is quite low [146]. Nonetheless, those genes thought to be relevant to the catecholamine action of the stimulant medications have been examined to determine if they can predict response to stimulants, either in terms of symptom reduction or emergence of adverse events [147]. The results of these studies in children are summarized in Table 6.5. The most widely studied polymorphism are those for the DA transporter and the DA D4 receptor, but results are inconsistent in terms

Table 6.5 Pharmacogenetic studies of stimulant response in children with ADHD [147]

Gene	Number of studies/design	Results
Adrengeric α-2 receptor (ADRA2A)	2 open label, n = 165	Improved response on inattention symptoms with G allele
Catechol-O-methyltransferase (COMT)	1 open label, n = 122	Improved hyperactive/impulsive symptoms with homozygous valine allele (fast metabolism of dopamine DA)
DA Transporter (SLC6A3)	3 double blind, n = 287	Decreased response with 9-repeat allele (3 double blind studies
	11 open label or retrospective studies, n = 1016	Decreased response with 10-repeat allele in 5 open label studies
		No effect of transporter allelle in remaining 6 open label studies
DA 4 -receptor (DRD4)	1 double-blind study, n = 81	In double-blind study, no effect of 7 or 4 repeat allele on response to MPH, but modest relationship to side effects
	9 open-label studies, n = 779	In open-label, 7 repeat related to better response in two studies, worse response in two studies and no relationship to response in other studies
Serotonin(5-HT) receptors and transporters	4 open-label studies, n = 317	No relationship of any allele for 5-HT receptors or the transporter related to stimulant response
Synaptosomal-associated protein 25 kDa (SNAP25)	1 double-blind study, n = 81	Association of T1065G G homozygotes and T1069C C homozygotes with side effects to methylphenidate (MPH)

of which, if any of the alleles for these entities predict response. A similar picture emerges for the other candidate genes studied. Four studies of the relationship of DA and NE genes to stimulant response in adults yielded only one study that showed a positive response between the 10-repeat DA transporter allele and MPH response of ADHD symptoms. Thus genotyping of patients with ADHD does not, at this point, yield clinically useful information.

Conclusions

Stimulants are the most effective agents available for the treatment of ADHD. Despite their high success rate in reducing acute symptoms, it is difficult to judge their impact on longer term outcome of patients with ADHD. They are very safe medications, but children must be monitored for growth suppression. Routine cardiovascular assessment is not necessary for every patient undergoing stimulant treatment, but those whose history suggests possible cardiac disease should be referred to a cardiologist prior to beginning treatment. Many children will need to continue ADHD treatment as adults, and physicians should be alert to signs of diversion as patients enter adolescence. Adjunctive psychosocial interventions are important for those who have only a partial response to medication or who have significant comorbidity. Neuroimaging studies may begin to unlock the mechanisms of actions of these agents and genetic studies may identify subtypes that are clinically indistinguishable but respond preferentially to certain agents. Understanding of the pathophysiology of ADHD will hopefully lead to the development of new and more effective agents, particularly to improve long-term outcome.

References

1 Barkley RA: Comorbid disorders, social and family adjustment, and subtyping. In: Barkley RA (ed.). *Attention Deficit Hyperactivity Disorder*. New York, NY: Guilford Press, 2006, pp. 184–218.
2 Bradley C: The behavior of children receiving benzedrine. *Am J Psychiatry* 1937; **94:** 577–85.
3 Swanson JM, Volkow ND: Psychopharmacology: concepts and opinions about the use of stimulant medications. *J Child Psychol Psychiatry* 2009; **50:** 180–93.
4 Centers for Disease Control and Prevention: Prevalence of diagnosis and medication treatment for attention deficit/hyperactivity disorder—United States 2003. *MMWR* **2005:** 842–7.
5 Kuczenski R: Biochemical actions of amphetamine and other stimulants. In: Creese I (ed.). *Stimulants: Neurochemical, Behavioral, and Clinical Perspectives*. New York, NY: Raven Press, 1983, pp. 31–62.

6 Berridge CW: Arousal and attention-related actions of the locus coeruleus-noradrenergic system: potential target in the therapuetic actions of amphetamine-like stimulants. In: Solant MV, Arnsten AFT, Castellanos FX (eds). *Stimulant Drugs and ADHD: Basic and Clinical Neuroscience.* New York, NY: Oxford University Press, 2001, pp. 158–84.

7 Connor DF, Meltzer BM: *Pediatric Psychopharmacology: Fast Facts.* New York, NY: W.W. Norton & Company, 2008.

8 Aston-Jones G, Chiang C, Alexinsky T: Discharge of noradrenergic locus coeruleus neurons in behaving rats and monkeys suggests a role in vigilance. *Prog Brain Res* 1991; **88:** 501–20.

9 Gamo NJ, Wang M, Arnsten AF: Methylphenidate and atomoxetine enhance prefrontal function through alpha2-adrenergic and dopamine D1 receptors. *J Am Acad Child Adolesc Psychiatry* 2010; **49:** 1011–23.

10 Arnsten AF, Li BM: Neurobiology of executive functions: catecholamine influences on prefrontal cortical functions. *Biol Psychiatry* 2005; **57:** 1377–84.

11 Arnsten AF: Stimulants: therapeutic actions in ADHD. *Neuropsychopharmacology* 2006; **31:** 2376–83.

12 Arnsten AFT: Dopaminergic and Noradrenergic influences on cognitive functions mediated by prefrontal cortex. In: Solanto MV, Arnsten AFT, Castellanos FX (eds) *Stimulant Drugs and ADHD: Basic and Clinical Neuroscience.* New York: Oxford University Press, NY, 2001, pp. 185–208.

13 Spencer TJ, Biederman J, Madras BK et al.: In vivo neuroreceptor imaging in attention-deficit/hyperactivity disorder: a focus on the dopamine transporter. *Biol Psychiatry* 2005; **57:** 1293–300.

14 Volkow ND, Wang GJ, Fowler JS et al.: Imaging the effects of methylphenidate on brain dopamine: new model on its therapeutic actions for attention-deficit/hyperactivity disorder. *Biol Psychiatry* 2005; **57:** 1410–15.

15 Volkow ND, Wang G, Fowler JS et al.: Therapeutic doses of oral methylphenidate significantly increase extracellular dopamine in the human brain. *J Neurosci* 2001; **21:** RC121.

16 Rosa-Neto P, Lou HC, Cumming P et al.: Methylphenidate-evoked changes in striatal dopamine correlate with inattention and impulsivity in adolescents with attention deficit hyperactivity disorder. *Neuroimage* 2005; **25:** 868–76.

17 Jucaite A, Fernell E, Halldin C et al.: Reduced midbrain dopamine transporter binding in male adolescents with attention-deficit/hyperactivity disorder: association between striatal dopamine markers and motor hyperactivity. *Biol Psychiatry* 2005; **57:** 229–38.

18 Volkow ND, Wang GJ, Kollins SH et al.: Evaluating dopamine reward pathway in ADHD: clinical implications. *JAMA* 2009; **302:** 1084–91.

19 Krause KH, Dresel SH, Krause J et al.: The dopamine transporter and neuroimaging in attention deficit hyperactivity disorder. *Neurosci Biobehav Rev* 2003; **27:** 605–13.

20 Vles JS, Feron FJ, Hendriksen JG et al.: Methylphenidate down-regulates the dopamine receptor and transporter system in children with attention deficit hyperkinetic disorder (ADHD). *Neuropediatrics* 2003; **34:** 77–80.

21 Feron FJ, Hendriksen JG, van Kroonenburgh MJ et al.: Dopamine transporter in attention-deficit hyperactivity disorder normalizes after cessation of methylphenidate. *Pediatr Neurol* 2005; **33:** 179–83.

22 Barry RJ, Clarke AR, Johnstone SJ: A review of electrophysiology in attention-deficit/hyperactivity disorder: I. Qualitative and quantitative electroencephalography. *Clin Neurophysiol* 2003; **114:** 171–83.

23 Loo SK, Barkley RA: Clinical utility of EEG in attention deficit hyperactivity disorder. *Appl Neuropsychol* 2005; **12:** 64–76.

24 Clarke AR, Barry RJ, McCarthy R et al.: Electroencephalogram differences in two subtypes of attention-deficit/hyperactivity disorder. *Psychophysiology* 2001; **38:** 212–21.

25 Clarke AR, Barry RJ, Bond D et al.: Effects of stimulant medications on the EEG of children with attention-deficit/hyperactivity disorder. *Psychopharmacology (Berl)* 2002; **164:** 277–84.

26 Clarke AR, Barry RJ, McCarthy R et al.: EEG differences between good and poor responders to methylphenidate and dexamphetamine in children with attention-deficit/hyperactivity disorder. *Clin Neurophysiol* 2002; **113:** 194–205.

27 Loo SK, Hopfer C, Teale PD et al.: EEG correlates of methylphenidate response in ADHD: association with cognitive and behavioral measures. *J Clin Neurophysiol* 2004; **21:** 457–64.

28 Loo SK, Specter E, Smolen A et al.: Functional effects of the DAT1 polymorphism on EEG measures in ADHD. *J Am Acad Child Adolesc Psychiatry* 2003; **42:** 986–93.

29 Barry RJ, Johnstone SJ, Clarke AR: A review of electrophysiology in attention-deficit/hyperactivity disorder: II. Event-related potentials. *Clin Neurophysiol* 2003; **114:** 184–98.

30 Kok A: Event-related-potential (ERP) reflections of mental resources: a review and synthesis. *Biol Psychol* 1997; **45:** 19–56.

31 Klorman R: Cognitive event-related potentials in attention deficit disorder. *J Learn Disabil* 1991; **24:** 130–40.

32 Barkley RA: *ADHD and the Nature of Self Control*. New York, NY: Guilford Press, 1997.

33 Kok A: Effects of degradation of visual stimuli on components of the event-related potential (ERP) in go/nogo reaction tasks. *Biol Psychol* 1986; **23:** 21–38.

34 Pliszka SR, Liotti M, Woldorff MG: Inhibitory control in children with attention deficit/hyperactivity disorder: event related potentials identify the processing component and timing of an impaired right-frontal response-inhibition mechanism. *Biol Psychiatry* 2000; **48:** 238–46.

35 Broyd SJ, Johnstone SJ, Barry RJ et al.: The effect of methylphenidate on response inhibition and the event-related potential of children with attention deficit/hyperactivity disorder. *Int J Psychophysiol* 2005; **58:** 47–58.

36 Schmajuk M, Liotti M, Busse L et al.: Electrophysiological activity underlying inhibitory control processes in normal adults. *Neuropsychologia* 2006; **44:** 384–95.

37 Seifert J, Scheuerpflug P, Zillessen KE et al.: Electrophysiological investigation of the effectiveness of methylphenidate in children with and without ADHD. *J Neural Transm* 2003; **110:** 821–9.

38 Pliszka SR, Liotti M, Bailey BY et al.: Electrophysiological effects of stimulant treatment in children with attention deficit hyperactivity disorder (ADHD). *J Child Adolesc Psychopharmacol* 2007; **17:** 356–66.

39 Rubia K, Smith AB, Brammer MJ et al.: Abnormal brain activation during inhibition and error detection in medication-naive adolescents with ADHD. *Am J Psychiatry* 2005; **162:** 1067–75.

40 Bush G, Frazier JA, Rauch SL et al.: Anterior cingulate cortex dysfunction in attention-deficit/hyperactivity disorder revealed by fMRI and the Counting Stroop. *Biol Psychiatry* 1999; **45:** 1542–52.

41 Pliszka SR, Glahn DC, Semrud-Clikeman M et al.: Neuroimaging of inhibitory control areas in children with attention deficit hyperactivity disorder who were treatment naive or in long term treatment. *Am J Psychiatry* 2006; **163**: 1052–60.

42 Vaidya CJ, Austin G, Kirkorian G et al.: Selective effects of methylphenidate in attention deficit hyperactivity disorder: a functional magnetic resonance study. *PNAS* 1998; **95**: 14494–9.

43 Epstein JN, Casey BJ, Tonev ST et al.: ADHD- and medication-related brain activation effects in concordantly affected parent-child dyads with ADHD. *Journal of Child Psychology and Psychiatry and Allied Disciplines* 2007; **48**: 899–913.

44 Bush G, Spencer TJ, Holmes J et al.: Functional magnetic resonance imaging of methylphenidate and placebo in attention-deficit/hyperactivity disorder during the multi-source interference task. *Arch Gen Psychiatry* 2008; **65**: 102–14.

45 Rubia K, Halari R, Cubillo A et al.: Methylphenidate normalises activation and functional connectivity deficits in attention and motivation networks in medication-naive children with ADHD during a rewarded continuous performance task. *Neuropharmacology* 2009; **57**: 640–52.

46 Castellanos FX, Margulies DS, Kelly C et al.: Cingulate-precuneus interactions: a new locus of dysfunction in adult attention-deficit/hyperactivity disorder. *Biol Psychiatry* 2008; **63**: 332–7.

47 Peterson BS, Potenza MN, Wang Z et al.: An FMRI study of the effects of psychostimulants on default-mode processing during Stroop task performance in youths with ADHD. *Am J Psychiatry* 2009; **166**: 1286–94.

48 O'Gorman RL, Mehta MA, Asherson P et al.: Increased cerebral perfusion in adult attention deficit hyperactivity disorder is normalised by stimulant treatment: a non-invasive MRI pilot study. *Neuroimage* 2008; **42**: 36–41.

49 Castellanos FX, Lee PP, Sharp W et al.: Developmental trajectories of brain volume abnormalities in children and adolescents with attention-deficit/hyperactivity disorder. *JAMA* 2002; **288**: 1740–8.

50 Bledsoe J, Semrud-Clikeman M, Pliszka SR: A magnetic resonance imaging study of the cerebellar vermis in chronically treated and treatment-naive children with attention-deficit/hyperactivity disorder combined type. *Biol Psychiatry* 2009; **65**: 620–4.

51 Semrud-Clikeman M, Pliszka SR, Lancaster J et al.: Volumetric MRI differences in treatment-naive vs. chronically treated children with ADHD. *Neurology* 2006; **67**: 1023–7.

52 Shaw P, Sharp WS, Morrison M et al.: Psychostimulant treatment and the developing cortex in attention deficit hyperactivity disorder. *Am J Psychiatry* 2009; **166**: 58–63.

53 Sobel LJ, Bansal R, Maia TV et al.: Basal ganglia surface morphology and the effects of stimulant medications in youth with attention deficit hyperactivity disorder. *Am J Psychiatry* 2010; **167**: 977–86.

54 Ivanov I, Bansal R, Hao X et al.: Morphological abnormalities of the thalamus in youths with attention deficit hyperactivity disorder. *Am J Psychiatry* 2010; **167**: 397–408.

55 Swanson JM, McBurnett K, Wigal T et al.: Effect of stimulant medication on children with attention deficit disorder: a "review of reviews". *Exceptional Child* 1993; **60**: 154–62.

56 Spencer T, Biederman J, Wilens T et al.: Pharmacotherapy of attention-deficit hyperactivity disorder across the life cycle. *J Am Acad Child Adolesc Psychiatry* 1996; **35**: 409–32.

57 Pliszka SR, Browne R, Olvera RL et al.: A double-blind placebo controlled trial of Adderall and methylphendiate in the treatment of Attention deficit hyperactivity disorder. *J Am Acad Child Adolesc Psychiatry* 2000; **39:** 619–26.

58 Weiss M, Wasdell M, Patin J: A post hoc analysis of d-threo-methylphenidate hydrochloride (focalin) versus d,l-threo-methylphenidate hydrochloride (ritalin). *J Am Acad Child Adolesc Psychiatry* 2004; **43:** 1415–21.

59 Greenhill LL, Kollins S, Abikoff H et al.: Efficacy and safety of immediate-release methylphenidate treatment for preschoolers with ADHD. *J Am Acad Child Adolesc Psychiatry* 2006; **45:** 1284–93.

60 Wigal T, Greenhill LL, Chuang S et al.: Safety and tolerability of methylphenidate in preschool children with ADHD. *J Am Acad Child Adolesc Psychiatry* 2006; **45:** 1294–303.

61 Boyle MH, Jadad AR: Lessons from large trials: the MTA study as a model for evaluating the treatment of childhood psychiatric disorder. (Review) (21 refs). *Canadian Journal of Psychiatry—Revue Canadienne de Psychiatrie* 1999; **44:** 991–8.

62 McGough J, McCracken J, Swanson J et al.: Pharmacogenetics of methylphenidate response in preschoolers with ADHD. *J Am Acad Child Adolesc Psychiatry* 2006; **45:** 1314–22.

63 MTA Cooperative Group: 14 month randomized clinical trial of treatment strategies for children with attention deficit hyperactivity disorder. *Arch Gen Psychiatry* 1999; **56:** 1073–86.

64 MTA Cooperative Group: Moderators and mediators of treatment response for children with attention deficit hyperactivity disorder: The MTA study. *Arch Gen Psychiatry* 1999; **56:** 1088–96.

65 MTA Cooperative Group: National Institute of Mental Health Multimodal Treatment Study of ADHD Follow-up: 24-Month Outcomes of Treatment Strategies for Attention-Deficit/Hyperactivity Disorder. *Pediatrics* 2004; **113:** 754–61.

66 MTA Cooperative Group: National Institute of Mental Health Multimodal Treatment Study of ADHD Follow-up: Changes in Effectiveness and Growth After the End of Treatment. *Pediatrics* 2004; **113:** 762–9.

67 Jensen PS, Arnold LE, Swanson JM et al.: 3-Year Follow-up of the NIMH MTA Study. *J Am Acad Child Adolesc Psychiatry* 2007; **46:** 989–1002.

68 Molina BS, Flory K, Hinshaw SP et al.: Delinquent behavior and emerging substance use in the MTA at 36 Months: prevalence, course, and treatment effects. *J Am Acad Child Adolesc Psychiatry* 2007; **46:** 1028–40.

69 Swanson JM, Elliott GR, Greenhill LL et al.: Effects of stimulant medication on growth rates across 3 Years in the MTA follow-up. *J Am Acad Child Adolesc Psychiatry* 2007; **46:** 1015–27.

70 Swanson JM, Hinshaw SP, Arnold LE et al.: Secondary evaluations of MTA 36-Month outcomes: propensity score and growth mixture model analyses. *J Am Acad Child Adolesc Psychiatry* 2007; **46:** 1003–14.

71 Molina BS, Hinshaw SP, Swanson JM et al.: MTA at 8 years: prospective follow-up of children treated for combined-type ADHD in a multisite study. *J Am Acad Child Adolesc Psychiatry* 2009; **48:** 484–500.

72 American Academy of Child and Adolescent Psychiatry: Practice parameter for the assessment and treatment of children and adolescents with attention-deficit/hyperactivity disorder. *J Am Acad Child Adolesc Psychiatry* 2007; **46:** 894–921.

73 Conners CK, Epstein JN, March JS et al.: Multimodal treatment of ADHD in the MTA: an alternative outcome analysis. *J Am Acad Child Adolesc Psychiatry* 2001; **40:** 159–67.

74 Jensen PS, Hinshaw SP, Kraemer HC et al.: ADHD comorbidity findings from the MTA study: comparing comorbid subgroups. *J Am Acad Child Adolesc Psychiatry* 2001; **40:** 147–58.

75 Hinshaw SP: Moderators and mediators of treatment outcome for youth with ADHD: understanding for whom and how interventions work. *Ambul Pediatr* 2007; **7:** 91–100.

76 Scheffler RM, Brown TT, Fulton BD et al.: Positive association between attention-deficit/hyperactivity disorder medication use and academic achievement during elementary school. *Pediatrics* 2009; **123:** 1273–9.

77 Tamesis GP, Covar RA: Long-term effects of asthma medications in children. *Curr Opin Allergy Clin Immunol* 2008; **8:** 163–7.

78 Arnold LE: Methylphenidate vs. amphetamine: comparative review. *J Atten Disord* 2000; **3:** 200–11.

79 Elia J, Borcherding BG, Rapoport JL et al.: Methylphenidate and dextroam-phetamine treatments of hyperactivity: are there true nonresponders? *Psychiatry Res* 1991; **36:** 141–55.

80 Sprague RL, Sleator EK: Methylphenidate in hyperkinetic children: differences in dose effects on learning and social behavior. *Science* 1977; **198:** 1274–6.

81 Biederman J, Boellner SW, Childress A et al.: Lisdexamfetamine dimesylate and mixed amphetamine salts extended-release in children with ADHD: A double-blind, placebo-controlled, crossover analog Classroom Study. *Biol Psychiatry* 2007; **62:** 970–6.

82 Swanson JM, Gupta S, Williams L et al.: Efficacy of a new pattern of delivery of methylphenidate for the treatment of ADHD: effects on activity level in the classroom and on the playground. *J Am Acad Child Adolesc Psychiatry* 2002; **41:** 1306–14.

83 McCracken JT, Biederman J, Greenhill LL et al.: Analog classroom assessment of a once-daily mixed amphetamine formulation, SLI381 (Adderall XR), in children with ADHD. *J Am Acad Child Adolesc Psychiatry* 2003; **42:** 673–83.

84 Biederman J, Keenan K, Faraone SV: Parent-based diagnosis of attention deficit disorder predicts a diagnosis based on teacher report. *J Am Acad Child Adolesc Psychiatry* 1990; **29:** 698–701.

85 Biederman J: Practical considerations in stimulant drug selection for the attention-deficit/hyperactivity disorder patient-efficacy, potency and titration. *Today's Therapeutic Trends* 2002; **20:** 311–28.

86 Pelham WE, Gnagy EM, Burrows-MacLean L et al.: Once-a-day Concerta methylphenidate versus three-times-daily methylphenidate in laboratory and natural settings. *Pediatrics* 2001; **107:** E105.

87 Biederman J, Monuteaux MC, Mick E et al.: Young adult outcome of attention deficit hyperactivity disorder: a controlled 10-year follow-up study. *Psychol Med* 2006; **36:** 167–79.

88 Wilens T, Pelham W, Stein M et al.: ADHD treatment with once-daily OROS methylphenidate: interim 12-month results from a long-term open-label study. *J Am Acad Child Adolesc Psychiatry* 2003; **42:** 424–33.

89 Wilens T, McBurnett K, Stein M et al.: ADHD treatment with once daily OROS methylphendiate treatment: final results from a long term open-label study. *J Am Acad Child Adolesc Psychiatry* 2005; **44:** 1015–23.

90 McGough JJ, Biederman J, Wigal SB et al.: Long-term tolerability and effectiveness of once-daily mixed amphetamine salts (Adderall XR) in children with ADHD. *J Am Acad Child Adolesc Psychiatry* 2005; **44:** 530–8.

91 Wolraich ML: Evaluation of efficacy and safety or OROS methylphenidate HCl (MPH) extended release tablets, methylphenidate tid, and placebo in children with ADHD. *Pediatr Res* 2000; **47**: 36A.

92 Wolraich ML, Greenhill LL, Pelham W et al.: Randomized, controlled trial of oros methylphenidate once a day in children with attention-deficit/hyperactivity disorder. *Pediatrics* 2001; **108**: 883–92.

93 Greenhill LL, Findling RL, Swanson JM: A double-blind, placebo-controlled study of modified-release methylphenidate in children with attention-deficit/hyperactivity disorder. *Pediatrics* 2002; **109**: E39.

94 Biederman J, Lopez FA, Boellner SW et al.: A randomized, double-blind, placebo-controlled, parallel-group study of SLI381 (Adderall XR) in children with attention-deficit/hyperactivity disorder. *Pediatrics* 2002; **110**: 258–66.

95 Daviss WB, Scott J: A chart review of cyproheptadine for stimulant-induced weight loss. *J Child Adolesc Psychopharmacol* 2004; **14**: 65–73.

96 Wilens TE, Bukstein OG, Cutler AJ et al.: A multicenter placebo-controlled study of extended release guanfacine coadministered with psychostimulants in the treatment of attention-deficit /hyperactivity disorder: effects on overall, morning, and evening ADHD assessments. Presented at the Annual Meeting of the American Academy of Child and Adolescent Psychiatry, New York, October 25–31, 2010.

97 Gelperin K: Psychiatric adverse events associated with drug treatment of ADHD: review of post marketing safety data. Available at: Food and Drug Administration Website 2006 (cited 2006 Apr 1); Available from http://www.fda.gov/ohrms/dockets/ac/06/briefing/2006-4210B-Index.htm.

98 Villalaba L: Follow up review of AERS search identifying cases of sudden death occurring with drugs used for the treatment of attention deficit hyperactivity disorder (ADHD). Available from http://www.fda.gov/ohrms/dockets/ac/06/briefing/2006-4210B-Index.htm.

99 Winterstein AG, Gerhard T, Shuster J et al.: Cardiac safety of central nervous system stimulants in children and adolescents with attention-deficit/hyperactivity disorder. *Pediatrics* 2007; **120**: e1494–e1501.

100 Gould MS, Walsh BT, Munfakh JL et al.: Sudden death and use of stimulant medications in youths. *Am J Psychiatry* 2009; **166**: 992–1001.

101 Vetter VL, Elia J, Erickson C et al.: Cardiovascular monitoring of children and adolescents with heart disease receiving stimulant drugs: a scientific statement from the American Heart Association Council on Cardiovascular Disease in the Young Congenital Cardiac Defects Committee and the Council on Cardiovascular Nursing. *Circulation* 2008; **117**: 2407–23.

102 American Heart Association. American Academy of Pediatrics/American Heart Association clarification of statement on cardiovascular evaluation and monitoring of children and adolescents with heart disease receiving medications for ADHD. Circulation 2008 (cited 2010 Nov 19). Available from http://www.newsroom.heart.org/index.php?s=43&item=398.

103 Poulton A: Growth on stimulant medication; clarifying the confusion: a review. *Arch Dis Child* 2005; **90**: 801–6.

104 Faraone SV, Biederman J, Morley CP et al.: Effect of stimulants on height and weight: a review of the literature. *J Am Acad Child Adolesc Psychiatry* 2008; **47**: 994–1009.

105 Charach A, Figueroa M, Chen S et al.: Stimulant treatment over 5 years: effects on growth. *J Am Acad Child Adolesc Psychiatry* 2006; **45**: 415–21.

106 Wilens TE, Faraone SV, Biederman J et al.: Does stimulant therapy of attention-deficit/hyperactivity disorder beget later substance abuse? A meta-analytic review of the literature. *Pediatrics* 2003; **111**: 179–85.

107 Biederman J, Monuteaux MC, Spencer T et al.: Stimulant therapy and risk for subsequent substance use disorders in male adults with ADHD: a naturalistic controlled 10-year follow-up study. *Am J Psychiatry* 2008; **165**: 597–603.

108 Faraone SV, Biederman J, Wilens TE et al.: A naturalistic study of the effects of pharmacotherapy on substance use disorders among ADHD adults. *Psychol Med* 2007; **37**: 1743–52.

109 Wilens TE, Fusillo S: When ADHD and substance use disorders intersect: relationship and treatment implications. *Current Psychiatry Reports* 2007; **9**: 408–14.

110 Riggs PD: Treatment of co-occurring substance use and attention deficit hyperactivity disorder: New findings from the NIDA Clinical Trials Network. Presented at the 20th Annual Meeting of the American Academy of Addiction Psychiatry, Los Angeles, CA (December 2–6), 2009.

111 Wilens TE, Adler LA, Adams J et al.: Misuse and diversion of stimulants prescribed for ADHD: a systematic review of the literature. *J Am Acad Child Adolesc Psychiatry* 2008; **47**: 21–31.

112 Daly JM, Wilens T: The use of tricyclics antidepressants in children and adolescents. *Pediatr Clin North Am* 1998; **45**: 1123–35.

113 Riddle MA, Nelson JC, Kleinman CS et al.: Sudden death in children receiving Norpramin: a review of three reported cases and commentary. *J Am Acad Child Adolesc Psychiatry* 1991; **30**: 104–8.

114 Pliszka SR: Tricyclic antidepressants in the treatment of children with attention deficit disorder. *J Am Acad Child Adolesc Psychiatry* 1987; **26**: 127–32.

115 Bymaster FP, Katner JS, Nelson DL et al.: Atomoxetine increases extracellular levels of norepinephrine and dopamine in prefrontal cortex of rat: a potential mechanism for efficacy in attention deficit/hyperactivity disorder. *Neuropsychopharmacology* 2002; **27**: 699–711.

116 Fuller RW, Wong DT: Effects of antidepressants on uptake and receptor systems in the brain. *Prog Neuropsychopharmacol Biol Psychiatry* 1985; **9**: 485–90.

117 Michelson D, Adler L, Spencer T et al.: Atomoxetine in adults with ADHD: two randomized, placebo-controlled studies. *Biol Psychiatry* 2003; **53**: 112–20.

118 Michelson D, Faries D, Wernicke J et al.: Atomoxetine in the treatment of children and adolescents with attention-deficit/hyperactivity disorder: a randomized, placebo-controlled, dose-response study. *Pediatrics* 2001; **108**: 1–9.

119 Michelson D, Allen AJ, Busner J et al.: Once-daily atomoxetine treatment for children and adolescents with attention deficit hyperactivity disorder: a randomized, placebo-controlled study. *Am J Psychiatry* 2002; **159**: 1896–901.

120 Wigal SB, McGough JJ, McCracken JT et al.: A laboratory school comparison of mixed amphetamine salts extended release (Adderall XR) and atomoxetine (Strattera) in school-aged children with attention deficit/hyperactivity disorder. *J Atten Disord* 2005; **9**: 275–89.

121 Newcorn JH, Kratochvil CJ, Allen AJ et al.: Atomoxetine and osmotically released methylphenidate for the treatment of attention deficit hyperactivity disorder: acute comparison and differential response. *Am J Psychiatry* 2008; **165**: 721–30.

122 Pliszka SR, Crismon ML, Hughes CW et al.: The Texas Children's Medication Algorithm Project: revision of the algorithm for pharmacotherapy of attention-deficit/hyperactivity disorder. *J Am Acad Child Adolesc Psychiatry* 2006; **45**: 642–57.

123 Wilens TE, Hammerness P, Utzinger L et al.: An open study of adjunct OROS-methylphenidate in children and adolescents who are atomoxetine partial responders: I. Effectiveness. *J Child Adolesc Psychopharmacol* 2009; **19**: 485–92.

124 Hammerness P, Georgiopoulos A, Doyle RL et al.: An open study of adjunct OROS-methylphenidate in children who are atomoxetine partial responders: II. Tolerability and pharmacokinetics. *Journal of Child and Adolescent Psychopharmacology* 2009; **19**: 493–9.

125 Bangs ME, Tauscher-Wisniewski S, Polzer J et al.: Meta-analysis of suicide-related behavior events in patients treated with atomoxetine. *J Am Acad Child Adolesc Psychiatry* 2008; **47**: 209–18.

126 Connor DF, Fletcher KE, Swanson JM: A meta-analysis of clonidine for symptoms of attention-deficit hyperactivity disorder. *J Am Acad Child Adolesc Psychiatry* 1999; **38**: 1551–9.

127 Sallee FR, McGough J, Wigal T et al.: Guanfacine extended release in children and adolescents with attention-deficit/hyperactivity disorder: a placebo-controlled trial. *J Am Acad Child Adolesc Psychiatry* 2009; **48**: 155–65.

128 Biederman J, Melmed RD, Patel A et al.: A randomized, double-blind, placebo-controlled study of guanfacine extended release in children and adolescents with attention-deficit/hyperactivity disorder. *Pediatrics* 2008; **121**: e73–e84.

129 Faraone SV, Glatt SJ: Effects of Extended-Release Guanfacine on ADHD Symptoms and Sedation-Related Adverse Events in Children with ADHD. *J Atten Disord* 2009; **13**: 532–8.

130 Sallee FR, Lyne A, Wigal T et al.: Long-term safety and efficacy of guanfacine extended release in children and adolescents with attention-deficit/hyperactivity disorder. *J Child Adolesc Psychopharmacol* 2009; **19**: 215–26.

131 Biederman J, Melmed RD, Patel A et al.: Long-term, open-label extension study of guanfacine extended release in children and adolescents with ADHD. *CNS Spectr* 2008; **13**: 1047–55.

132 Palumbo DR, Sallee FR, Pelham WE, Jr. et al.: Clonidine for attention-deficit/hyperactivity disorder: I. efficacy and tolerability outcomes. *J Am Acad Child Adolesc Psychiatry* 2008; **47**: 180–8.

133 Kollins S, Findling RL, Wigal SB et al.: Modified-release clonidine for the treatment of children/adolescents with ADHD. Presented at the 56th Annual Meeting of the American Academy of Child and Adolescent Psychiatry, October 27–November 1, Honolulu, HI. 2009.

134 Swanson JM, Flockhart D, Udrea D et al.: Clonidine in the treatment of ADHD: questions about safety and efficacy. *J Child Adolesc Psychopharmacol* 1995; **5**: 301–4.

135 Swanson JM, Connor DF, Cantwell D: Combining methylphenidate and clonidine: ill-advised. *J Am Acad Child Adolesc Psychiatry* 1999; **38**: 614–22.

136 Daviss WB, Patel NC, Robb AS et al.: Clonidine for attention-deficit/hyperactivity disorder: II. ECG changes and adverse events analysis. *J Am Acad Child Adolesc Psychiatry* 2008; **47**: 189–98.

137 Gadow KD, Sverd J, Sprafkin J et al.: Long-term methylphenidate therapy in children with comorbid attention-deficit/hyperactivity disorder and chronic multiple tic disorder (see comments). *Arch Gen Psychiatry* 1999; **56**: 330–6.

138 Allen AJ, Kurlan RM, Gilbert DL et al.: Atomoxetine treatment in children and adolescents with ADHD and comorbid tic disorders. *Neurology* 2005; **65**: 1941–9.

139 Tourette's Syndrome Study Group: Treatment of ADHD in children with tics: a randomized controlled trial. *Neurology* 2002; **58**: 527–36.

140 Jensen PS, Youngstrom Y, Steiner H et al.: Consensus report: Impulsive aggression as a symptom across diagnostic categories in child psychiatry. *J Am Acad Child Adolesc Psychiatry* 2007; **46:** 309–22.

141 Connor DF, Glatt SJ, Lopez ID et al.: Psychopharmacology and aggression. I: A meta-analysis of stimulant effects on overt/covert aggression-related behaviors in ADHD. *J Am Acad Child Adolesc Psychiatry* 2002; **41:** 253–61.

142 Newcorn JH, Spencer TJ, Biederman J et al.: Atomoxetine treatment in children and adolescents with attention-deficit/hyperactivity disorder and comorbid oppositional defiant disorder. *J Am Acad Child Adolesc Psychiatry* 2005; **44:** 240–48.

143 Klein RG, Abikoff H, Klass E et al.: Clinical efficacy of methylphenidate in conduct disorder with and without attention deficit hyperactivity disorder. *Arch Gen Psychiatry* 1997; **54:** 1073–80.

144 Pappadopulos E, Macintyre Ii JC, Crismon ML et al.: Treatment recommendations for the use of antipsychotics for aggressive youth (TRAAY). Part II. *J Am Acad Child Adolesc Psychiatry* 2003; **42:** 145–61.

145 Schur SB, Sikich L, Findling RL et al.: Treatment recommendations for the use of antipsychotics for aggressive youth (TRAAY). Part I: a review. *J Am Acad Child Adolesc Psychiatry* 2003; **42:** 132–44.

146 Mick E, Faraone SV: Genetics of attention deficit hyperactivity disorder. *Child Adolesc Psychiatr Clin N Am* 2008; **17:** 261–84.

147 Froehlich TE, McGough JJ, Stein MA: Progress and promise of attention-deficit hyperactivity disorder pharmacogenetics. *CNS Drugs* 2010; **24:** 99–117.

148 Greenhill LL, Muniz R, Ball RR et al.: Efficacy and safety of dexmethylphenidate extended-release capsules in children with attention-deficit/hyperactivity disorder. *J Am Acad Child Adolesc Psychiatry* 2006; **45:** 817–23.

149 Biederman J, Mick E, Surman C et al.: A randomized, placebo-controlled trial of OROS methylphenidate in adults with attention-deficit/hyperactivity disorder. *Biol Psychiatry* 2006; **59:** 829–35.

150 Spencer TJ, Wilens TE, Biederman J et al.: Efficacy and safety of mixed amphetamine salts extended release (Adderall XR) in the management of attention-deficit/hyperactivity disorder in adolescent patients: a 4-week, randomized, double-blind, placebo-controlled, parallel-group study. *Clin Ther* 2006; **28:** 266–79.

151 Weisler RH, Biederman J, Spencer TJ et al.: Mixed Amphetamine Salts Extended-Release in the Treatment of Adult ADHD: A Randomized, Controlled Trial. *CNS Spectr* 2006; **11:** 625–39.

152 Wilens TE, McBurnett K, Bukstein O et al.: Multisite controlled study of OROS methylphenidate in the treatment of adolescents with attention-deficit/hyperactivity disorder. *Arch Pediatr Adolesc Med* 2006; **160:** 82–90.

153 Findling RL, Bukstein OG, Melmed RD et al.: A randomized, double-blind, placebo-controlled, parallel-group study of methylphenidate transdermal system in pediatric patients with Attention-Deficit/Hyperactivity Disorder. *J Clin Psychiatry*, 2008: e1–e11.

154 Biederman J, Krishnan S, Zhang Y et al.: Efficacy and tolerability of lisdexamfetamine dimesylate (NRP-104) in children with attention-deficit/hyperactivity disorder: a phase III, multicenter, randomized, double-blind, forced-dose, parallel-group study. *Clin Ther* 2007; **29:** 450–63.

155 Adler LA, Goodman DW, Kollins SH et al.: Double-blind, placebo-controlled study of the efficacy and safety of lisdexamfetamine dimesylate in adults with attention-deficit/hyperactivity disorder. *J Clin Psychiatry* 2008; **69:** 1364–73.

156 Barkley RA: *Attention Deficit Hyperactivity Disorder: A Handbook for Diagnosis and Treatment*. New York, NY: Guilford Press, 1990.

157 DuPaul GJ, Power TJ, Anastopoulos AD, Reid R: *ADHD Rating Scales-IV: Checklists, Norms and Clinical Interpretation*. New York, NY: Guilford Press, 1998.

158 Brown TE: *The Brown Attention Deficit Disorder Scales*. San Antonio, TX: Psychological Corporation, 2001.

159 Swanson JM: *School-based Assessments and Intervention for ADD Students*. Irvine: K.C. Publishing, 1992.

160 Wolraich ML, Lambert EW, Baumgaertel A et al.: Teachers' screening for attention deficit/hyperactivity disorder: comparing multinational samples on teacher ratings of ADHD. *J Abnorm Child Psychol* 2003; **31**: 445–55.

161 Wolraich ML, Lambert W, Doffing MA et al.: Psychometric properties of the Vanderbilt ADHD diagnostic parent rating scale in a referred population. *J Pediatr Psychol* 2003; **28**: 559–67.

CHAPTER 7

Tricyclic Antidepressants and Monoamine Oxidase Inhibitors for the Treatment of Child and Adolescent Psychiatric Disorders

Charlotte M. Heleniak, Tejal Kaur, Kareem D. Ghalib &
Moira A. Rynn
Columbia University/New York State Psychiatric Institute, New York, USA

Tricyclic antidepressants (TCAs)

Overview

In recent years, the serotonin reuptake inhibitors (SRIs) have become the first-line antidepressants used by most clinicians for adults suffering from major depression and anxiety disorders because of their established efficacy, relatively benign side-effects, and ease of administration (See Chapter 8). Tricyclic antidepressants (TCAs), despite their established efficacy in adults for conditions such as major depressive disorder (MDD) and anxiety disorders such as panic disorder, are no longer considered first-line treatment [1].

Historically TCAs were also used with some success in child and adolescent populations, however the evidence base has always been weaker. In meta-analyses of youth with MDD, for example, there is no conclusive evidence that TCAs are superior to placebo [2, 3]. In fact, some assert that noradrenergic and mixed noradrenergic/serotonergic TCAs do not appear to be effective at all in pediatric MDD [2, 4]. Nonetheless, there are other clinical indications for considering the use of TCAs such as enuresis, obsessive compulsive disorder (OCD), and attention-deficit hyperactivity disorder (ADHD), which will be discussed in this chapter.

Chemical properties

The TCAs are dibenzapine derivatives—tricyclic in structure—and block the reuptake of norepinephrine and serotonin in to the presynaptic

Pharmacotherapy of Child and Adolescent Psychiatric Disorders, Third Edition.
Edited by David R. Rosenberg and Samuel Gershon.
© 2012 John Wiley & Sons, Ltd. Published 2012 by John Wiley & Sons, Ltd.

neuron. The TCAs are first absorbed through the gastrointestinal tract. They undergo significant first-pass metabolism by the liver and are less tightly bound to proteins which leads to a rapid metabolism in children and adolescents as compared to adults. Furthermore, the greater liver mass in relation to body size in children and adolescents is also associated with a faster metabolism. Children and adolescents, like adults, can show a more than thirtyfold difference in heterocyclic blood levels at a particular dose [5–7] and steady-state TCA levels can vary widely in children receiving fixed daily doses of medication [8]. Liver biotransformation of TCAs primarily involves oxidation, aromatic hydroxylation, and demethylation.

Indications
See Table 7.1.

Major depressive disorder (MDD)
Controlled studies have failed to demonstrate that TCAs are superior to placebo in the treatment of childhood and adolescent MDD [9–13]. Furthermore, meta-analyses have supported the evidence of lack of efficacy for tricyclic antidepressants in the treatment of child and adolescent MDD [2, 4, 14]. Smith Kline Beecham conducted a multicenter randomized controlled study of pediatric MDD comparing 270 patients treated with paroxetine, imipramine or placebo [15, 16]. Paroxetine was found to be superior to both imipramine and placebo, whereas imipramine was not significantly better than placebo. Furthermore, Attari et al. [12] found that fluoxetine was significantly more effective than nortriptyline in the treatment of child and adolescent major depression. Thus, tricyclic antidepressants do not appear to be effective in child and adolescent MDD [13]. It is worth noting that Sallee et al. [17] found that intravenous clomipramine administration in non-suicidal adolescents with MDD resulted in a significant decrease in depressive symptoms six days after treatment. The intravenous clomipramine led to an 88% response rate compared to a 38% response rate in patients receiving placebo [17]. Further study is warranted before this direct administration can be recommended.

Recently, Braconnier et al. [11] found that paroxetine and clomipramine demonstrated similar efficacy in adolescent severe major depression. This finding is consistent with a recent meta-analysis of SRI and TCA trials in youth under the age of 20, in which the meta-analytically pooled difference between these antidepressant groups was not statistically significant [18].

While it is clear that tricyclic antidepressants are not superior to placebo in the treatment of pediatric depression, it is not clear when or why young adults begin to respond to TCAs. A study comparing noradrenergic vs.

Table 7.1 U.S. FDA approved uses of TCAs in children and adolescents

Generic	Adult dose	Pediatric dose	FDA Indication	FDA Approved for children?
Amitriptyline	50–100 mg/day	>12 yrs 10 mg tid and 20 mg qhs	MDD	No
Clomipramine	25–250 mg/day	>10 yrs 25–200 mg/day, Max: 3 mg/kg/day	OCD	Yes
Desipramine	100–200 mg/day	25–100 mg/day	MDD	No
Doxepin	25–300 mg/day	N/A	MDD and/or anxiety	No
Imipramine	75–300 mg/day	MDD: Adolescents: 30–40 mg/day Enuresis: ≥6 yrs 25–50 mg qhs, Max: 2.5 mg/kg/day	MDD and enuresis	Yes
Nortriptyline	25–150 mg/day	Adolescents 30–50 mg/day	MDD	No
Protriptyline	15–60 mg/day	Adolescents 5 mg tid	MDD	No
Trimipramine	50–200 mg/day	Adolescents 50–100 mg/day	MDD	No

MDD = major depressive disorder; OCD = obsessive compulsive disorder; tid = three times per day; qhs = at each bedtime.
Adapted from the Physicians Desk Reference (2010).

serotonergic antidepressant treatment response in young adults (18–24) to adults (25 and older) demonstrated a relatively lower response rate to noradrenergic TCAs in young adults, whereas there was no difference in treatment response in the older cohort [19]. This maturational difference in response has led to the hypothesis that the slower maturation of the noradrenergic system is a likely explanation for the poor response rate of children and adolescents to tricyclic antidepressants [20,21]. Animal studies, where serotonergic systems have been shown to mature earlier than dopaminergic and noradrenergic systems, are consistent with this [22–24].

In recent rodent studies, TCA effect on the forced swim test has been inconclusive. Reed et al. [25] found that juvenile rats model adolescent human response to antidepressant treatment in depression, however both Pechnick et al. [26] and Mason et al. [27] found no difference in adult and juvenile efficacy of the TCAs desmethylimipramine and imipramine respectively in the forced swim test. It has been suggested that the earlier maturation of serotonergic systems and the later maturation of noradrenergic systems allow for effective intervention with SRIs in child and adolescent MDD, but preclude intervention with noradrenergic and mixed serotonergic/noradrenergic TCAs [15].

Given the safety profile and recent data suggesting the efficacy of SRIs in child and adolescent MDD (see Chapter 8), these medications are now first-line treatment. Although SRIs are first line psychopharmacological treatment for pediatric MDD, and fluoxetine and escitalopram are the only medications approved by the FDA in the treatment of pediatric MDD, it is worth noting that one recent review failed to find the superiority of SRIs over TCAs [18]. Because TCAs have not been demonstrated to be superior to placebo in the treatment of pediatric MDD, and given their side-effect profile and potential for toxicity in overdose, we do not recommend their use for child and adolescent MDD.

Anxiety disorders

School refusal and separation anxiety disorder

To date, two studies have shown the efficacy of imipramine in reducing school refusal. Gittelman-Klein and Klein [28] found that imipramine was superior to placebo in treating children with school refusal, and Bernstein et al. [29] found that CBT augmented by imipramine significantly increased school attendance in adolescents with comorbid anxiety and depressive disorders as compared to those with CBT and placebo [28, 29]. However, other studies have failed to show the efficacy of tricyclic antidepressants in the treatment of school refusal [29–31]. These inconsistencies in response to tricyclic antidepressants are probably due to many factors such as different diagnoses, comorbidities, small sample sizes, and differing doses [32]. Because of the mixed data and side-effect profile of TCAs, they are not recommended as a first-line treatment for school refusal.

Obsessive-compulsive disorder

Clomipramine is a TCA that has been found to be effective in the treatment of adult OCD, and it has also been FDA-approved for the treatment of pediatric OCD. Clomipramine inhibits serotonin reuptake, thereby potentiating its effects, and its primary metabolite, desmethylclomipramine, inhibits norepinephrine reuptake [33]. Blocking serotonin reuptake is believed to be crucial to its anti-obsessive-compulsive actions. In a double-blind, placebo-controlled study of 19 OCD children and adolescents 10 to 18 years of age, clomipramine was shown to be superior to placebo [34]. In a follow-up study, Flament et al. [35] showed the continued superiority of clomipramine over placebo. In another study, children and adolescents with OCD were studied in an eight-week multicenter, double-blind, parallel group trial of clomipramine versus placebo [36]. After eight weeks, clomipramine-treated patients showed a mean reduction in OCD symptoms of 37% versus 8% treated with placebo [36]. In a one-year open-label treatment, clomipramine therapy continued to be effective and well tolerated.

Clomipramine has been shown to be superior to other TCAs in the treatment of OCD. In a 10-week crossover design, Leonard et al. [37] found clomipramine to be superior to desipramine in the treatment of 49 children and adolescents with severe OCD. In addition, several studies have shown the success of maximizing the therapeutic effects and minimizing adverse effects of clomipramine treatment by augmenting clomipramine with low doses of fluoxetine and fluvoxamine [38, 39]. In 1999, Fitzgerald et al. [40] published results from an open label study demonstrating that risperidone augmentation of clomipramine (or paroxetine or fluoxetine) resulted in marked improvement in patients who had not responded sufficiently to SRI treatment or other monodrug therapy.

Trichotillomania

While not classified in the DSM-IV as an anxiety disorder but under impulse-control disorders, given its common comorbidity with OCD, trichotillomania will also be considered here. Swedo et al. [41] performed a double-blind comparison of clomipramine and desipramine in the treatment of trichotillomania and found clomipramine to be effective. In fact, a recent review of the adult trichotillomania treatment literature found that while habit reversal therapy is the most effective in the treatment of trichotillomania, clomipramine is also superior not only to placebo

but even to SRIs [42]. Currently, there is no consensus for what constitutes the best treatment of trichotillomania in children and adolescents.
Further study of clomipramine in pediatric patients with this condition
is warranted.

Attention-deficit hyperactivity disorder

Although not first-line treatments, imipramine, desipramine,
nortriptyline, amitriptyline and clomipramine have all been shown
to be superior to placebo in the treatment of ADHD [43–51]. However,
stimulants have been established as most effective and first line treatment
of pediatric ADHD [52,53]. In a double-blind, placebo-controlled crossover
study of 12 prepubertal male children with ADHD comparing the efficacy
of methylphenidate, desipramine and clomipramine, it was seen that
while methylphenidate was significantly better than desipramine and
clomipramine in improving classroom functioning, clomipramine was
more effective than desipramine in decreasing aggressive, impulsive,
and depressive/mood symptoms [46]. Desipramine is still considered the
first-line TCA to treat ADHD because it is the most studied of the antidepressants, and it has a relatively favorable anticholinergic and sedating
side-effect profile as compared with other TCAs, including clomipramine.
TCAs are not recommended in ADD without hyperactivity [54]. It is
important to point out that the long-term efficacy of the TCAs for ADHD
has not been established [44, 55].

Attention-deficit hyperactivity disorder and comorbid disorders

ADHD is often comorbid with several disorders, some of which may
strengthen the indication for treating with a TCA. In individuals with
a history of tics and for whom stimulants have exacerbated tic
symptoms, a TCA trial should be considered, as these agents have
demonstrated efficacy in the treatment of ADHD but do not typically
exacerbate tics [56, 57]. Literature suggests the efficacy of the TCA
nortriptyline in reducing both symptoms of ADHD and oppositionality
in children and adolescents [58]. A recent meta-analysis confirmed the
efficacy of atomoxetine and desipramine in the treatment of children with
ADHD and comorbid tics, but also demonstrated that methylphenidate
is the fastest and most effective treatment for these co-occurring
disorders [59].

Enuresis

Enuresis (involuntary urination—bedwetting—in children over five to six
years old) has several established treatments. Behavioral approaches are

recommended as a first-line treatment for nocturnal enuresis, and desmopressin should be considered first-line pharmacotherapy for enuresis [60]. Enuresis remains one of the only FDA-established indications for the use of TCAs in children and adolescents; their efficacy in treating this disorder have been demonstrated in over 40 double-blind studies [61]. An antienuretic effect can be seen without delay once treatment is initiated. Patients may become tolerant to the antienuretic effect, which may wear off after several weeks. Additionally, many patients relapse once the medication is withdrawn. The only antidepressants that have been approved by the FDA for the treatment of enuresis are desipramine and imipramine [62]. Recent literature suggests that imipramine may be more efficacious than both placebo and other anticholinergic medications in treating refractory enuresis [62–64]. Imipramine has more side-effects (such as sedation and anticholinergic effects) but is less expensive [62]. Desipramine should be reserved for patients who have both diurnal and nocturnal enuresis, or for those whose nocturnal enuresis has not responded to conservative behavioral measures or 1-Deamino-8-d-Arginine-Vasopressin (DDAVP) [65]. Clomipramine has also been used to treat enuresis, with a therapeutic effect observed at plasma concentrations of 20–60 ng/ml [66,67]. While TCAs have been proven effective in the treatment of nocturnal enuresis, most children relapse after treatment is withdrawn, whereas half of the children who complete behavioral treatment do not relapse [61]. Tricyclic antidepressants are recommended as second-line only after behavioral approaches have failed.

Pain

Headache/migraine prophylaxis
Two studies have examined amitriptyline in the prophylaxis of migraines or headaches in children and adolescents. Lewis et al. [68] found amitriptyline to be the most commonly prescribed treatment for the prevention of pediatric migraines and that it was 89% effective. Hershey et al. [69] also found amitriptyline to be effective in headache prevention in children and adolescents. Furthermore, many adult reviews have established the use of tricyclic antidepressants as effective, and more so than SRIs, in the treatment of headaches and neuropathic pain [70–72].

Irritable bowel syndrome
In a review of the adult irritable bowel syndrome (IBS) literature, Brandt et al. [73] found that tricyclic antidepressants are not superior to placebo in the reduction of global IBS symptoms. However, they have been established as effective in treating abdominal pain associated with IBS. Recently,

Bahar et al. [74] found amitriptyline to be significantly more effective than placebo in the treatment of irritable bowel syndrome in adolescents.

Initiating, maintaining and withdrawing treatment

Before starting medication

Tricyclic antidepressants are not considered first-line pharmacologic intervention for any pediatric neuropsychiatric disorder [75]. Careful weighing of the risks, particularly potential cardiac side-effects, versus potential benefits must always be considered and communicated to the parents/legal guardians and the child.

Prior to initiating a TCA trial, children and adolescents should have a physical examination, with special attention paid to heart rate, blood pressure, weight, and height. It is also important to elicit any family history of cardiac disease, require a pregnancy test, complete a thorough evaluation of substance abuse and nicotine history, and to check liver function. It should be noted that oral contraceptives containing estrogen can interfere with the metabolism of TCAs. To increase the chances of detecting a preexisting cardiac conduction defect, a baseline ECG is required [62]. Thereafter, an ECG rhythm strip should be obtained in children and adolescents at frequent intervals during the period of dose elevation [62].

Treatment initiation

In an attempt to minimize cardiac side-effects associated with peak TCA plasma levels in children, Dugas et al. [66] recommended giving divided doses-b.i.d. or t.i.d. dosages for total daily doses of over 1 mg/kg. Administering the total daily dose at one time, as at bedtime, is not recommended for children. Ryan et al. [62] did, however, observe that, once the dosage was stabilized, the total daily dose of imipramine could be safely given to adolescents at bedtime without increasing the risk of cardiac side-effects [62].

When children and adolescents are treated with TCAs, it is important to check blood pressure, pulse, and ECG rhythm strip at each dose increase. Plasma TCA levels should be drawn five to seven days after the last dose increase, and 12 hours after the most recently administered dose. Children and adolescents should have an annual physical examination by their pediatrician or family practitioner.

Interference with diagnostic blood tests

These agents can interfere with a number of diagnostic tests, such as increasing the blood levels of cholesterol, aspartate transaminase (SGOT), alkaline transaminase (SGPT), bilirubin, lactate dehydrogenase (LDH), alkaline phosphatase, eosinophils, catecholamines, and glucose. They can also decrease blood glucose levels, granulocytes, and platelets.

Dispensing TCAs

Given the toxicity of TCAs in overdose, we recommend that parents dispense medications and keep the medications in child-protective containers. When potential for overdose is a clinical concern, we also advocate prescribing no more than a two-week supply of medication at one time, with refills if necessary.

Maintaining treatment

There are no firm guidelines as to how long to continue treatment with TCAs for children and adolescents with psychiatric disorders. Since they are not considered first-line medication for any psychiatric conditions in childhood and adolescence, it is difficult to offer definitive guidelines on the use of these agents. Our recommendations are based on a review of the available literature and on clinical experience. For the dosing and administration of specific agents, see Table 7.1.

Withdrawal of medication

Children are at higher risk than adults for experiencing withdrawal symptoms when TCAs are discontinued because they metabolize these medications more rapidly than do adults [62]. Withdrawal symptoms of TCAs are similar in children and adults, including anxiety, agitation, disrupted sleep, behavioral activation, and somatic or GI distress [76]. The symptoms often give the overall impression of a flu-like syndrome and are largely related to the anticholinergic effects [62]. On withdrawal of TCAs, the anticholinergic effects are responsible for the resultant withdrawal effects. These can be avoided or minimized by gradually tapering the medication over a period of two weeks. If withdrawal symptoms do occur, they can be treated by restarting the medication and/or tapering it more gradually [62].

Side-effect profile

Common

Anticholinergic

Dry mouth and constipation are frequently seen in both children/adolescents and adults; these side-effects are usually dose dependent and often dissipate with time. Blurred vision and urinary retention are believed to be less common in children and adolescents than in adults [62]. Sedation as a result of anticholinergic and antihistaminergic effects is also common [77].

Dry mouth may be ameliorated by reducing the dose, or by using sugar-free gum or candy. Rarely, bethanechol, a cholinergic agonist, can be used in doses of 10 mg q.i.d. to 50 mg q.i.d. to reduce this symptom when conservative measures are unsuccessful. The only common side-effect of bethanechol therapy is stomach cramps, which necessitates lowering the dose [62]. Constipation, another commonly encountered anticholinergic side-effect of TCA therapy, can often be managed with colace or metamucil. Laxatives should not be used. When the more serious anticholinergic complication of delayed urination occurs (which is rare in children and adolescents), dose reduction and/or bethanechol treatment is warranted. Discontinuation of the medication is advised in the case of seizure, allergic reaction, or confusion—a sign of anticholinergic toxicity.

Antihistamine
Weight gain and somnolence are common but less severe side-effects of TCAs.

Cardiac
Tricyclic antidepressants may slow cardiac conduction [78]. Mild increases in the PR interval (5–10%), QRS duration (7–25%) and prolongation of the QT interval (3–10%) are common in children and adolescents [62,79]. A corrected QT interval (QTc) of >460 ms has been reported in 8% of patients treated with TCAs, but mean QTc intervals remained within the normal range in pediatric patients treated with TCAs [80–84]. A mild increase in the pulse rate of up to 120 beats per minute with sinus tachycardia is common, and is frequently asymptomatic [62,79]. Large increases in cardiac conduction slowing (i.e., PR >0.21 and QRS >0.12) can be dangerous, and can result in arrhythmias and/or heart block. By prospectively looking at the records of 14 784 patients over eight years and comparing risk of cardiovascular disease against antidepressant users and nonusers, a recent epidemiological study showed that the use of tricyclic antidepressants in adults increases the risk of cardiovascular disease [85].

While a case of ventricular fibrillation resulting in sudden cardiac death was reported in a patient who had a family history of sudden death [79, 86], torsade de pointes and other malignant arrhythmias have not been reported in children and adolescents treated with TCAs.

Cardiovascular side-effects are of particular concern in children and younger adolescents because of the efficiency with which they convert TCAs to potentially toxic 2-hydroxy metabolites [7,87]. These patients appear to be more sensitive to cardiac toxicity than are older adolescents and adults [87] and there is greater variability in heart rate in children than in adults [75]. Interestingly, desipramine treatment has been found to significantly decrease variability of heart rate [88, 89]. Increased risk for cardiovascular side-effects may also be associated with concomitant use of other medications including methylphenidate, cimetidine, and sympathomimetic agents [79]. Further study of the risk of developing cardiovascular disease from using TCAs during childhood is warranted.

Uncommon

Sudden cardiac death

There may be a relationship between sudden cardiac death and tricyclic antidepressants in children and adolescents, although this is not a well-established fact [90]. At least eight deaths in pediatric patients have been associated with the TCAs imipramine and desipramine [90]. Amitai and Frischer [91] found excess case fatality rate from desipramine in children and adolescents. It is worth noting that sudden cardiac death and syncope have been associated with family history of prolonged QT intervals and torsade de pointes [79, 86]. Therefore, drugs including TCAs that can prolong the QT interval should be avoided in children and adolescents with familial prolongation of the QT interval and torsade de pointes.

It is not known how many children have been treated with TCAs, although the number is believed to be quite large. This suggests that if such a risk exists, it most likely is small [80, 92]. Nonetheless, this potential risk and other side-effects need to be taken into account when TCA therapy is considered. The American Heart Association [79] specifically recommends a comprehensive baseline history and physical examination, detailed delineation of current medication history, family history assessment for cardiac disease, baseline ECG and follow-up ECG and history after achieving steady state level of the TCA on 3–5 mg/kg for desipramine or imipramine.

Other uncommon side-effects

Ryan et al. [62] noted the following uncommon side-effects of tricyclic antidepressants: psychosis, seizures, hypertension, nightmares and insomnia, rash, tics, and sexual dysfunction [62]. Mania is another established uncommon side-effect [93, 94], as is confusion [6, 95].

Overdose

The TCAs have a very high potential for causing death when taken in overdose even if the child is taken to the hospital immediately after the event [96]. When a patient overdoses on more than 1 g of a TCA, toxicity often results and death can occur [93]. Heart arrhythmias, seizures, hypotension, respiratory arrest and other medically emergent conditions can result in death [93]. It should be noted that, as in adults, plasma TCA levels often do not reflect the severity of the overdose [96]. Almost all symptoms develop within 24 hours of the overdose [93].

Central-nervous system side-effects ranging from drowsiness to coma are common [93]. These side-effects can be exacerbated and potentiated if the patient has also ingested other CNS depressants, such as benzodiazepines, alcohol, or barbiturates [93]. Antimuscarinic side-effects are frequent and often pronounced, and include dry mucous membranes, warm dry skin, blurred vision, and mydriasis [93]. Cardiovascular toxicity may also occur. Respiratory arrest and uncontrolled seizures can result from a severe overdose [93]. If any of the above symptoms are noted, or if there is any reason to believe someone has overdosed on these medications, emesis should be induced and the person should be transported to the ER immediately. Gastric lavage and administration of activated charcoal may be indicated to reduce the absorption of residual drug and intensive care interventions may be necessary [93].

Abuse

TCAs have a low risk for abuse. Anticholinergic side-effects are very rarely used to induce an altered mind state [62].

Drug interactions, contraindications

Please see Box 7.1.

Box 7.1   Contraindications to tricyclic antidepressant (TCA) use

Concomitant illness or state: pregnancy, prior hypersensitivity reaction, prior cardiac problems (especially recovery from myocardial infarction), family history of cardiac disease, thyroid, epilepsy, psychosis, cardiac problems

Drug interactions: may increase effect of: central nervous system (CNS) stimulants, CNS depressants, MAOIs[a], sympathominetics (ephedrine), alcohol, antipsychotics, benzodiazepines, barbiturates, anticholinergic agents, thyroid medications (cardiac effects), seizure-potentiating drugs, phenytoin may decrease effects of: clonidine, guanethidine

Effects may be increased by: phenothiazines, methylphenidate, oral contraceptives (estrogen), marijuana (tachycardia)

Effects may be decreased by: lithium, barbiturates, chloral hydrate, smoking

---

MAOI = monoamine oxidase inhibitor; SRIs = serotonin reuptake inhibitors; TCAs = tricyclic antidepressant.

[a]It is now understood that the only TCAs that are unsafe to combine with MAOIs are those with the potency of SRIs – clomipramine and imipramine. Other TCAs are safe to combine with the MAOIs [132].

Monoamine oxidase inhibitors (MAOIs)

Overview

Monoamine oxidase inhibitors (MAOIs) are a class of antidepressant defined by function rather than structure, such that all drugs in this class either reversibly or irreversibly inhibit the enzyme monoamine oxidase (MAO). Monoamine oxidase inhibitors have restricted applications in child psychiatry due to both their potential adverse effects related to dietary non-compliance and as studies displaying efficacy in this population are also limited. Currently, no MAOI compound is FDA approved for psychiatric indications in children under 16 years of age. Despite their decline in clinical use, MAOIs remain important investigative tools due to efficacy in treating atypical and treatment resistant depression and anxiety in adults. However, before recommending use in children and adolescents, further treatment trials assessing both safety and efficacy are necessary.

Chemical properties

Monoamine oxidase inhibitors (MAOIs) are compounds which inhibit the enzyme monoamine oxidase (MAO). Monoamine oxidase is a mitochondrial, flavin- adenosine-dinucleotide containing enzyme found in the brain, intestines and liver which converts biogenic amines, such as norepinephrine, dopamine and serotonin, to aldehydes [94]. The antidepressant properties of MAOIs are hypothesized to be related to receptor mediated pre-synaptic and post-synaptic events or to the function of MAOIs in inactivating the enzyme MAO, reducing the breakdown of monoamines and therefore increasing the concentration of monoamines, such as norepinephrine, dopamine and serotonin [97, 98].

Monoamine oxidases can be subdivided into categories based on which isomer, MAO-A or MAO-B, they selectively inhibit, or based on whether they reversibly or irreversibly bind to monoamine oxidase [99]. MAO-A, whose inhibition is most closely linked to antidepressant activity, is found primarily in the brain and intestine, with primary substrates being epinephrine, norepinephrine, dopamine and serotonin in the brain, and tyramine in the intestine. MAO-B is found primarily in the brain, platelets, and other tissues, with preferred substances being beta-phenylethylamine, dopamine and tyramine. While MAO-A inhibition is most closely linked to antidepressant effect, it is also most linked to accumulation of tyramine, leading to adverse effects, as tyramine causes the release of stored catecholamines from nerve terminals, leading to hypertension, headache, tachycardia, nausea, cardiac arrhythmias and stroke. In contrast to oral MAOIs, the transdermal delivery of selegiline (Emsam) bypasses enzyme inhibition in the intestines and first pass metabolism in the liver, improving safety by decreasing risk of tyramine reactions. As all FDA approved MAOIs are irreversible inhibitors, these MAOIs bind to the MAO enzyme for the lifetime of the molecule so that tyramine cannot displace the MAOI from the MAO, leading to potential tyramine accumulation, and requiring a washout period of 7–10 days for the MAO enzyme to be regenerated [100].

Indications
See Table 7.2.

There are currently five U.S. Food and Drug Administration (FDA)-approved MAOIs. In adult populations, studies have shown MAOIs to be effective in treating "atypical depression" [101–105] and treatment-resistant depression [101, 104, 106, 107]. The American Psychiatric Association Practice Guidelines for the Treatment of Patients with Major Depressive Disorder (MDD) [108] recommends MAOI therapy particularly in MDD with atypical features and in treatment resistant depression. However, traditionally, the adverse effect profile of MAOIs, in comparison to the less risky profiles of other antidepressants, such as (SRIs), have led to the relatively low use of MAOIs in adult populations, with even fewer use, and no FDA indications, for children and adolescents.

After MAOIs fell out of favor in the 1960s, some of the few persistent indications were social phobia, panic disorder and "atypical depression" [109, 110]. Frommer [111] conducted a double blind, placebo controlled study of phenelzine combined with chlordiazepoxide in 16 depressed, and 15 "phobic" children aged 9–15 years. The clinical descriptions appear to meet criteria for major depression in the first group and separation anxiety/school phobia in the second although the presence and nature

Table 7.2 U.S. FDA approved uses of MAOIs in adults

Generic	Starting dose	Usual dose	FDA indication
Selegiline transdermal patch	6 mg	6–12 mg	Major depressive disorder
Selegiline	5 mg	5–10 mg	Parkinsonism
Phenelzine	15 mg	45–90 mg	Depression
Tranylcypromine	10 mg	30–60 mg	Depression without melancholia
Isocarboxazid[a]	10–20 mg	30–60 mg	Depression

[a] Approved in adolescents ≥16.

Adapted from American Psychiatric Association Practice Guideline for Treatment of Patients with Major Depressive Disorder (2010).

of neurovegetative signs was not mentioned. Although the groups were merged for analysis, the phenelzine-chlordiazepoxide combination was superior to placebo-chlordiazepoxide overall [111].

The more persisting indication for MAOIs, particularly in the adult literature, remains atypical depression, defined as a subtype of major depression with "reversed" neurovegetative signs: weight gain rather than loss, hypersomnia rather than insomnia, mood reactivity, and mood worsening in the evening rather than morning [109]. This subtype is not included in DSM-IV, but is the only approved indication for MAOI therapy in adults (Parnate[tm]) or adolescents older than 16 years of age (Nardil[tm]; Marplan[tm]). The frequency of atypical depressive symptoms in adolescents and young adults has led to the proposal that "atypical" depression may, in fact, be the primary manifestation of major depression in young people [62, 112, 113].

Yet, no controlled trials exist that compare MAOIs to SRIs or bupropion, both of which have seen use for atypical depression (see Chapter 8). The only two studies of MAOIs in child and adolescent depression are favorable, albeit inconclusive. In the only other published series, Ryan et al. [3] conducted a retrospective study of 23 cases of adolescent major depression treated with MAOI. In each case the child had failed a trial of a tricyclic compound and was subsequently treated with either phenelzine or tranylcypromine. If the tricyclic had shown no benefit a MAOI was used alone. If there had been incomplete response, a MAOI was prescribed in combination with the TCA. When used in this manner, 74% of children responded to treatment, but only 57% both responded and maintained dietary restrictions. Of the seven adolescents who became noncompliant with dietary restrictions, one experienced a pressor response described as blood pressure of 162/104 and headache after eating one sausage, which resolved after treatment with chlorpromazine, with no further sequelae. Another adolescent described myoclonic jerks after a cheese sandwich, which also resolved without sequelae. While no patients in the study had serious consequences, two other patients described brief periods of hypomania with subsequent clinical improvement on MAOI, and one other was noted to have a suicide attempt by taking a "handful of pills" but with no medical sequelae. Generally, the authors found MAOIs to be well tolerated in the study when patients were compliant with dietary restrictions.

In adult populations 18 years and older, randomized controlled, double blind placebo controlled trials of selegiline transdermal demonstrated efficacy in treating major depressive disorder and in preventing relapse at 52 weeks [114–117]. Significantly, in these trials selegiline transdermal displayed a similar safety profile to placebo despite absence of dietary tyramine restrictions at doses of 6 mg/24 h [115–117] or flexible dosing of 6 mg/24 h–12 mg/24 h [117].

With the development of the transdermal selegiline patch and with ongoing studies in children and adolescents, MAOI prescription in children and adolescents may become a viable alternative in the treatment of psychiatric illness. Currently, a multisite clinical trial evaluating the efficacy of the selegiline patch in adolescents is ongoing but preliminary data are not yet available [118].

Initiating, maintaining, and withdrawing treatment

As guidelines for MAOI use are not established in children and adolescents, this section will briefly review strategies in adults. Clinicians should note that there is currently no evidence base to suggest that adult guidelines may be translated into the treatment of children and adolescents. Only isocarboxazid is approved for use in adolescents of age 16 and older.

Education about and adherence to dietary and medication restrictions is necessary before starting MAOI therapy, particularly by providing well-organized and simply written handouts that may be posted at home and referred to frequently (see Rappaport [119] for additional information on dietary restrictions in adults). Since a washout period of 7–14 days or more is required when changing from most other antidepressant agents to a MAOI, this time may be used to ensure the absence of contraindications to treatment (see Box 7.2) and to evaluate the patient's ability to comply with dietary restrictions by keeping a detailed log of all foods and beverages ingested. The physician may then review the log for compliance and counsel the family on any misinterpretations of the guidelines before prescribing a MAOI. If a MAOI is initiated after fluoxetine, the washout period should be 5–6 weeks due to the long half-life of fluoxetine and its metabolites [120].

After initiating MAOI treatment (see Table 7.2), dose increases should not be more frequent than every 14 days, since maximal MAO inhibition is achieved 7–14 days after the last change. Upon abrupt discontinuation, monoamine oxidase activity returns to normal gradually over two weeks, suggesting that any withdrawal is related to non-MAOI properties of the compound itself. Nevertheless, symptoms have ranged from anxiety and agitation to psychosis and have been compared to stimulant withdrawal [121]. Gradual discontinuation of the medication is recommended. Regardless of how the medication is discontinued, MAO activity is suppressed for up to two weeks after the last dose, necessitating full compliance to dietary and medication restrictions for that period of time.

> ## Box 7.2   Contraindications to monoamine oxidase inhibitor (MAOI) use: [119, 130, 131]
>
> **Concomitant illness:** cerebrovascular disease, which increases risk of hypertensive consequences; pre-existing hepatic disease or abnormal liver function; pheochromocytoma, which causes high levels of endogenous sympathomimetic amines, and pending surgical procedures that will require anesthesia
>
> **Drug interactions:** serotonin reuptake inhibitors, tricyclic antidepressants, trazodone, nefazodone, venlafaxine, duloxetine, or narcotics (especially meperidine), general anesthesia, or local anesthesia containing sympathomimetic vasoconstrictors, guanethidine; over-the-counter cold and weight loss products
>
> **Dietary:** foods with increased amounts of tyramine such as aged cheeses or meats, fermented products, yeast extracts, fava or broad beans, red wine, draft beers, and over-ripe or spoiled foods (of note, dietary restrictions have not been found necessary at 6 mg/24 h dose of selegiline transdermal patch)

Side-effects

Adverse effects are largely from the adult literature as studies of MAOIs in children and adolescents are limited.

Tyramine pressor effect/hypertensive crisis

Dietary tyramine in high doses acts as a pseudotransmitter, with stimulant and depressor effects. Since tyramine is a substrate of MAO, MAOI therapy is associated with a tenfold to thirtyfold increase in sensitivity to these effects [122]. While unmedicated volunteers can tolerate 200–400 mg of oral tyramine before blood pressure increases [123], as little as 6–10 mg of dietary tyramine in a subject taking MAOIs can result in a significant rise in blood pressure, and 20–25 mg may induce a hypertensive crisis [124]. Violation of dietary guidelines or concurrent use of any sympathomimetic agent may result in a hypertensive crisis, including occipital headache, palpitation, neck stiffness, nausea, vomiting, diaphoresis, pupillary dilation, photophobia and chest pain, and can be lethal [125].

The serotonergic syndrome

Occurring in combination with MAOIs and either agents that inhibit serotonin reuptake or tryptophan (serotonin precursor), the clinical features of serotonin syndrome include mental status changes (confusion, agitation, hypomania), myoclonus, hyperreflexia, tremor, ataxia, diaphoresis, fever, and autonomic dysregulation [126,127]. This syndrome may be difficult to distinguish from neuroleptic malignant syndrome (NMS) (see Chapter 8); however, unlike NMS, serotonergic syndrome does not commonly produce pronounced rigidity, CPK levels over 1000 U/L, or leukocytosis.

Cardiovascular effects

MAOI therapy is associated with both decreased and increased resting blood pressure (RBP), with decrease in RBP being most notable in subjects who were hypertensive at baseline [128] and making orthostatic hypotension a common side-effect due to the alpha adrenergic agonist properties of norepinephrine. Hypertension as a consequence of MAOI therapy is most often part of the tyramine reaction or a result of concurrent sympathomimetic use (see discussion above).

General effects

The most common side-effect of MAOI use is hypotension (discussed above) and dizziness. Much less common, but established adverse effects include insomnia, overstimulation (jitteriness; tremors; twitching), impotence, edema, weight gain, and elevated hepatic enzymes [94].

Overdose

Toxic symptoms reported by manufacturers and clinicians include drowsiness, dizziness, mental status changes (including agitation, hyperactivity, confusion or psychosis), headache, seizures and coma [94, 129, 130]. Hypotension or hypertension may develop along with hyperreflexia and general autonomic dysregulation (tachycardia, hyperthermia, tachypnea, pupillary dilation) [94, 129, 130]. Toxic blood levels are not established in humans. If the patient has also ingested a source of tyramine or sympathomimetics then an overdosage is treated much like a hypertensive crisis [131]. It is of note that MAOIs have not been known to have abuse potential.

General summary

Given the very limited evidence for safety and efficacy of MAOIs in the treatment of childhood disorders, this chapter has incorporated evidence and dosing from the adult psychiatric literature. Considering the lack of pediatric studies, it is unclear whether adult guidelines and responses can be, or should be, translated into pediatric practice. Further studies, potentially studying transdermal preparations of MAOIs, which may have fewer adverse effects, are needed before clinical guidelines can be established in pediatric populations.

On the other hand, many studies have evaluated the safety and efficacy of TCAs in treating many indications in children and adolescents. Although TCAs have been approved by the FDA to treat child and adolescent enuresis and OCD, their side-effect profile precludes us from recommending TCAs as first line treatments in any pediatric illness. Only after other approved and established medications and behavioral treatments have failed should TCAs be considered.

References

1 Glassman A, Roose S: Tricyclic treatment: What is adequate and who is refractory? In: Tasman A, Goldfinger SM, Kaufmann CA (eds) *Review of Psychiatry.* Washington DC: American Psychiatric Press, 1990, vol. 9, pp. 60–73.
2 Hazell P: Depression in children and adolescents. Clin Evid (Online), 2009. Available at http://www.consumerreports.org/health/resources/pdf/clinical-guidelines/sr-depression–children-and-adolescents-1008.pdf, accessed July 29, 2011.
3 Ryan ND, Puig-Antich J, Rabinovich H et al.: MAOIs in adolescent major depression unresponsive to tricyclic antidepressants. *J Am Acad Child Adolesc Psychiatry* 1998; **27:** 755–58.
4 Papanikolaou K, Richardson C, Pehlivanidis A et al.: Efficacy of antidepressants in child and adolescent depression: a meta-analytic study. *J Neural Transm* 2006; **113:** 399–415.
5 Sjoqvist F, Bertilsson L: Clinical pharmacology of antidepressant drugs: pharmacogenetics. *Adv Biochem Psychopharmacol* 1984; **39:** 359–72.
6 Preskorn S, Weller E, Weller R et al.: Plasma levels of imipramine and adverse effects in children. *Am J Psychiatry* 1983; **140:** 1332–5.
7 Ryan ND, Puig-Antich J, Cooper TB et al.: Relative safety of single versus divided dose imipramine in adolescent major depression. *J Am Acad Child Adolesc Psychiatry* 1987a: **26:** 400–6.
8 Preskorn SH, Jerkovich GS, Beber JH et al.: Therapeutic drug monitoring of tricyclic antidepressants: a standard of care issue. *Psychopharmacol Bull* 1989; **25:** 281–4.
9 Puig-Antich J, Perel JM, Lupatkin W et al.: Imipramine in prepubertal major depressive disorders. *Arch Gen Psychiatry* 1987; **44:** 81–9.
10 Birmaher B, Waterman GS, Ryan ND et al.: Randomized, controlled trial of amitriptyline versus placebo for adolescents with "treatment-resistant" major depression. *J Am Acad Child Adolesc Psychiatry* 1989; **37:** 527–35.
11 Braconnier A, Le Coent R, Cohen D: Paroxetine versus clomipramine in adolescents with severe major depression: a double-blind, randomized, multicenter trial. *J Am Acad Child Adolesc Psychiatry* 2003; **42:** 22–9.
12 Attari A, Yadollah F, Hansanzadeh A et al.: Comparison of efficacy of fluoxetine with nortriptyline in treatment of major depression in children and adolescents: a double-blind study. *J Res Med Sci* 2006; **11:** 24–30.
13 Hazell P, O'Connell D, Heathcote D et al.: Tricyclic drugs for depression in children and adolescents. *Cochrane Database Syst Rev* 2002; **2:** CD002317.
14 Hazell P, O'Connell D, Heathcote D et al.: Efficacy of tricyclic drugs in treating child and adolescent depression: a meta-analysis. *BMJ* 1995; **310:** 897–901.
15 Ryan ND, Varma D: Child and adolescent mood disorders—experience with serotonin-based therapies. *Biol Psychiatr* 1998; **44:** 336–40.
16 Beecham S: data cited in Ryan ND, Varma D: Child and adolescent mood disorders—experience with serotonin-based therapies. *Biol Psychiatry* 1998; **44**(5): 336–40.
17 Sallee FR, Vrindavanam NS, Deas-Nesmith D et al.: Pulse intravenous clomipramine for depressed adolescents: double-blind, controlled trial. *Am J Psychiatry* 1997; **154:** 668–73.

18 Tsapakis EM, Soldani F, Tondo L et al.: Efficacy of antidepressants in juvenile depression: meta-analysis. *Br J Psychiatry* 2008; **193:** 10–17.

19 Mulder RT, Watkins WG, Joyce PR et al.: Age may affect response to antidepressants with serotonergic and noradrenergic actions. *J Affect Disord* 2003; **76:** 143–9.

20 Murrin LC, Sanders JD, Bylund DB: Comparison of the maturation of the adrenergic and serotonergic neurotransmitter systems in the brain: implications for differential drug effects on juveniles and adults. *Biochem Pharmacol* 2007; **73:** 1225–36.

21 Bylund DB, Reed AL: Childhood and adolescent depression: why do children and adults respond differently to antidepressant drugs? *Neurochem Int* 2007; **51:** 246–53.

22 Goldman-Rakic PS, Brown RM: Postnatal development of monoamine content and synthesis in the cerebral cortex of rhesus monkeys. *Brain Res* 1982; **256:** 339–49.

23 Rosenberg DR, Lewis DA: Changes in the dopaminergic innervation of monkey prefrontal cortex during late postnatal development: a tyrosine hydroxylase immunohistochemical study. *Biol Psychiatry* 1994; **36:** 272–7.

24 Rosenberg DR, Lewis DA: Postnatal maturation of the dopaminergic innervation of monkey prefrontal and motor cortices: a tyrosine hydroxylase immunohistochemical analysis. *J Comp Neurol* 1995; **358:** 383–400.

25 Reed AL, Happe HK, Petty F et al.: Juvenile rats in the forced-swim test model the human response to antidepressant treatment for pediatric depression. *Psychopharmacology (Berl)* 2008; **197:** 433–41.

26 Pechnick RN, Bresee CJ, Manalo CM et al.: Comparison of the effects of desmethylimipramine on behavior in the forced swim test in peripubertal and adult rats. *Behav Pharmacol* 2008; **19:** 81–4.

27 Mason SS, Baker KB, Davis KW et al.: Differential sensitivity to SSRI and tricyclic antidepressants in juvenile and adult mice of three strains. *Eur J Pharmacol* 2009; **602:** 306–15.

28 Gittelman-Klein R, Klein DF: Controlled Imipramine Treatment of School Phobia. *Arch Gen Psychiatry* 1971; **25:** 204–7.

29 Bernstein GA, Garfinkel BD, Borchardt CM: Comparative studies of pharmacotherapy for school refusal. *J Am Acad Child Adolesc Psychiatry* 1990; **29:** 773–81.

30 Berney T, Kolvin I, Bhate S et al.: School phobia: a therapeutic trial with clomipramine and short-term outcome. *Br J Psychiatry* 1981; **138:** 110–18.

31 Klein RG: Pharmacotherapy of adolescent depression. *Clin Neuropharmacol* 1992; (**15** Suppl 1): A:227A–228A.

32 King NJ, Bernstein GA: School refusal in children and adolescents: a review of the past 10 years. *J Am Acad Child Adolesc Psychiatry* 2001; **40:** 197–205.

33 Davis J, Glassman A: *A Comprehensive Textbook of Psychiatry*, 5th edn. Baltimore: Williams & Wilkens, 1991.

34 Flament MF, Rapoport JL, Berg CJ et al.: Clomipramine treatment of childhood obsessive-compulsive disorder. A double-blind controlled study. *Arch Gen Psychiatry* 1985; **42:** 977–83.

35 Flament MF, Rapoport JL, Murphy DL et al.: Biochemical changes during clomipramine treatment of childhood obsessive-compulsive disorder. *Arch Gen Psychiatry* 1987; **44:** 219–25.

36 DeVeaugh-Geiss J, Moroz G, Biederman J et al.: Clomipramine hydrochloride in childhood and adolescent obsessive-compulsive disorder—a multicenter trial. *J Am Acad Child Adolesc Psychiatry* 1992; **31:** 45–9.

37 Leonard HL, Swedo SE, Rapoport JL et al.: Treatment of obsessive-compulsive disorder with clomipramine and desipramine in children and adolescents. A double-blind crossover comparison. *Arch Gen Psychiatry* 1989; **46:** 1088–2.

38 Simeon JG, Thatte S, Wiggins D: Treatment of adolescent obsessive-compulsive disorder with a clomipramine-fluoxetine combination. *Psychopharmacol Bull* 1990; **26:** 285–90.

39 Figueroa Y, Rosenberg DR, Birmaher B et al.: Combination treatment with clomipramine and selective serotonin reuptake inhibitors for obsessive-compulsive disorder in children and adolescents. *J Child Adolesc Psychopharmacol* 1998; **8:** 61–7.

40 Fitzgerald KD, Stewart CM, Tawile V et al.: Risperidone augmentation of serotonin reuptake inhibitor treatment of pediatric obsessive compulsive disorder. *J Child Adolesc Psychopharmacol* 1999; **9:** 115–23.

41 Swedo SE, Leonard HL, Rapoport JL,et al.: A double-blind comparison of clomipramine and desipramine in the treatment of trichotillomania (hair pulling). *N Engl J Med* 1989; **321:** 497–501.

42 Bloch MH, Landeros-Weisenberger A, Dombrowski P et al.: Systematic review: pharmacological and behavioral treatment for trichotillomania. *Biological Psychiatry* 2007; **62:** 839–46.

43 Winsberg BG, Goldstein S, Yepes LE et al.: Imipramine and electrocardiographic abnormalities in hyperactive children. *Am J Psychiatry* 1975; **132:** 542–5.

44 Quinn PO, Rapoport JL: One-year follow-up of hyperactive boys treated with imipramine or methylphenidate. *Am J Psychiatry* 1975; **132:** 241–5.

45 Werry JS, Aman MG, Diamond E: Imipramine and methylphenidate in hyperactive children. *J Child Psychol Psychiatry* 1980; **21:** 27–35.

46 Garfinkel BD, Wender PH, Sloman L et al.: Tricyclic antidepressant and methylphenidate treatment of attention deficit disorder in children. *J Am Acad Child Psychiatry* 1983; **22:** 343–8.

47 Biederman J, Baldessarini RJ, Wright V et al.: A double-blind placebo controlled study of desipramine in the treatment of ADD: I. Efficacy. *J Am Acad Child Adolesc Psychiatry* 1989; **28:** 777–84.

48 Donnelly M, Zametkin AJ, Rapoport JL et al.: Treatment of childhood hyperactivity with desipramine: Plasma drug concentration, cardiovascular effects, plasma and urinary catecholamine levels, and clinical response. *Clin Pharm Ther* 1986; **39:** 72–81.

49 Gittleman-Klein R: Pharmacotherapy of childhood hyperactivity: an update. In: Meltzer HY (ed.) Psychopharmacology: The Third Generation of Progress. New York: Raven Press. 1987, pp. 1215–24.

50 Prince JB, Wilens TE, Biederman J et al.: A controlled study of nortriptyline in children and adolescents with attention deficit hyperactivity disorder. *J Child Adolesc Psychopharmacol* 2000; **10:** 193–204.

51 Overtoom CC, Verbaten MN, Kemner C et al.: Effects of methylphenidate, desipramine, and L-dopa on attention and inhibition in children with attention deficit hyperactivity disorder. *Behav Brain Res* 2003; **145:** 7–15.

52 Brown RT, Amler RW, Freeman WS et al.: Treatment of attention-deficit/hyperactivity disorder: overview of the evidence. *Pediatrics* 2005; **115:** e749–57.

53 Yildiz O, Sismanlar S, Memik N et al.: Atomoxetine and Methylphenidate Treatment in Children with ADHD: The Efficacy, Tolerability and Effects on Executive Functions. *Child Psychiatry Hum Dev* 2010; **42:** 257–69.

54 Wender P: *The Hyperactive Child, Adolescent, and Adult: Attention Deficit Disorder through the Lifespan.* New York, NY: Oxford University Press, 1987.

55 Yepes LE, Balka EB, Winsberg BG et al.: Amitriptyline and methylphenidate treatment of behaviorally disordered children. *J Child Psychol Psychiatry* 1977; **18:** 39–52.

56 Singer HS, Brown J, Quaskey S et al.: The treatment of attention-deficit hyperactivity disorder in Tourette's syndrome: a double-blind placebo-controlled study with clonidine and desipramine. *Pediatrics* 1995; **95**: 74–81.

57 Spencer T, Biederman J, Coffey B et al.: A double-blind comparison of desipramine and placebo in children and adolescents with chronic tic disorder and comorbid attention-deficit/hyperactivity disorder. *Arch Gen Psychiatry* 2002; **59**, 649–56.

58 Prince JB, Wilens TE, Biederman J et al.: A controlled study of nortriptyline in children and adolescents with attention deficit hyperactivity disorder. *J Child Adolesc Psychopharmacol* 2000; **10**: 193–204.

59 Bloch MH, Panza KE, Landeros-Weisenberger A et al.: Meta-analysis: treatment of attention-deficit/hyperactivity disorder in children with comorbid tic disorders. *J Am Acad Child Adolesc Psychiatry* 2009; **48**: 884–93.

60 Darling JC: Management of nocturnal enuresis. Trends in urology, *Gynaecology and Sexual Health* 2010; **15**: 18–22.

61 Glazener CM, Evans JH, Peto RE: Tricyclic and related drugs for nocturnal enuresis in children. *Cochrane Database Syst Rev* 2002; **3**: CD002117.

62 Ryan ND: Heterocyclic antidepressants in children and adolescents. *J Child Adolesc Psychopharmacol* 1990; **1**: 21–31.

63 Neveus T, Tullus K: Tolterodine and imipramine in refractory enuresis; a placebo-controlled crossover study. *Pediatr Nephrol* 2008; **23**: 263–7.

64 Gepertz S, Neveus T: Imipramine for therapy resistant enuresis: a retrospective evaluation. *J Urol* 2004; **171**: 2607–10; discussion 9–10.

65 Rapoport JL, Mikkelsen EJ, Zavadil A et al.: Childhood enuresis. II. Psychopathology, tricyclic concentration in plasma, and antienuretic effect. *Arch Gen Psychiatry* 1980; **37**: 1146–52.

66 Dugas M, Zarifian E, Leheuzey M-Fo et al.: Preliminary observations of the significance of monitoring tricyclic antidepressant plasma levels in the pediatric patient. *Therapeutic Drug Monitoring* 1980; **2**: 307–14.

67 Morselli PL, Bianchetti G, Dugas M: Therapeutic drug monitoring of psychotropic drugs in children. *Pediatr Pharmacol* (New York) 1983; **3**: 149–56.

68 Lewis DW, Diamond S, Scott D et al.: Prophylactic treatment of pediatric migraine. headache: *The Journal of Head and Face Pain* 2004; **44**: 230–37.

69 Hershey AD, Powers SW, Bentti A-L et al.: Effectiveness of amitriptyline in the prophylactic management of childhood headaches. *Headache: The Journal of Head and Face Pain* 2000; **40**: 539–49.

70 Jackson JL, Shimeall W, Sessums L et al.: Tricyclic antidepressants and headaches: systematic review and meta-analysis. *BMJ* 2010; **341**: c5222.

71 McMahon S, Koltzenburg M: *Wall and Melzack's Textbook of Pain*, 5th edn. Philadelphia, PA: Churchill Livingstone, 2006.

72 Finnerup NB, Otto M, McQuay HJ et al.: Algorithm for neuropathic pain treatment: an evidence based proposal. *Pain* 2005; **118**: 289–305.

73 Brandt LJ, Bjorkman D, Fennerty MB et al.: Systematic review on the management of irritable bowel syndrome in North America. *Am J Gastroenterol* 2002; **97**(11 Suppl): S7–26.

74 Bahar RJ, Collins BS, Steinmetz B et al.: Double-blind placebo-controlled trial of amitriptyline for the treatment of irritable bowel syndrome in adolescents. *J Pediatr* 2008; **152**: 685–9.

75 Geller B, Reising D, Leonard HL et al.: Critical Review of Tricyclic Antidepressant Use in Children and Adolescents. *J Am Acad Child Adolesc Psychiatry* 1999; **38**: 513–16.

76 Dilsaver S, Greden J: Antidepressant withdrawal phenomena. *Biological Psychiatry* 1984; **19**: 237–56.

77 Zajecka J, Tummala R: Tricyclics: still solid performers for the savvy psychiatrist. *The Journal of Family Practice* 2002; **1**(6). Available at http://www.jfponline.com/Pages.asp?AID=520, accessed July 27, 2011.

78 Roose SP, Glassman AH, Giardina EG et al.: Tricyclic antidepressants in depressed patients with cardiac conduction disease. *Arch Gen Psychiatry* 1987; **44**:, 273–5.

79 Gutgesell H, Atkins D, Barst R et al.: Cardiovascular monitoring of children and adolescents receiving psychotropic drugs : a statement for healthcare professionals from the committee on congenital cardiac defects, Council on Cardiovascular Disease in the Young, American Heart Association. *Circulation* 1999; **99**: 979–82.

80 Biederman J, Baldessarini RJ, Wright V et al.: A double-blind placebo controlled study of desipramine in the treatment of ADD: II. Serum drug levels and cardiovascular findings. *J Am Acad Child Adolesc Psychiatry* 1989a; **28**: 903–11.

81 Fletcher SE, Case CL, Sallee FR et al.: Prospective study of the electrocardiographic effects of imipramine in children. *J Pediatr* 1993; **122**: 652–4.

82 Schroeder JS, Mullin AV, Elliott GR et al.: Cardiovascular effects of desipramine in children. *J Am Acad Child Adolesc Psychiatry* 1989; **28**: 376–79.

83 Wilens TE, Biederman J, Baldessarini RJ et al.: Electrocardiographic effects of desipramine and 2-hydroxydesipramine in children, adolescents, and adults treated with desipramine. *J Am Acad Child Adolesc Psychiatry* 1993; **32**: 798–804.

84 Wilens TE, Biederman J, Baldessarini RJ et al.: Cardiovascular effects of therapeutic doses of tricyclic antidepressants in children and adolescents. *J Am Acad Child Adolesc Psychiatry* 1996; **35**: 1491–501.

85 Kemp AH, Quintana DS, Gray MA et al.: Impact of depression and antidepressant treatment on heart rate variability: a review and meta-analysis. *Biological Psychiatry* 2010; **67**: 1067–74.

86 Vieweg WV, Wood MA: Tricyclic antidepressants, QT interval prolongation, and torsade de pointes. *Psychosomatics* 2004; **45**: 371–7.

87 Baldessarini R: *Goodman and Gilman's The Pharmacological Basis of Therapeutics*, 8th edn. New York, NY: Pergamon Press, 1990.

88 Mezzacappa E, Steingard R, Kindlon D et al.: Tricyclic antidepressants and cardiac autonomic control in children and adolescents. *J Am Acad Child Adolesc Psychiatry* 1998; **37**: 52–9.

89 Walsh BT, Giardina EG, Sloan RP et al.: Effects of desipramine on autonomic control of the heart. J Am Acad Child Adolesc *Psychiatry* 1994; **33**: 191–7.

90 Varley CK: Sudden death related to selected tricyclic antidepressants in children: epidemiology, mechanisms and clinical implications. *Paediatr Drugs* 2001; **3**: 613–27.

91 Amitai Y, Frischer H: Excess fatality from desipramine in children and adolescents. *J Am Acad Child Adolesc Psychiatry* 2006; **45**: 54–60.

92 Biederman J: Sudden death in children treated with a tricyclic antidepressant. *J Am Acad Child Adolesc Psychiatry* 1991; **30**: 495–8.

93 Arana G: Hyman S: *Handbook of Psychiatric Drug Therapy*, 2nd edn. Boston: Little Brown, 1991.

94 Sadock BJ, Sadock VA, Kaplan HI: *Kaplan and Sadock's Concise Textbook of Child and Adolescent Psychiatry*. Philadelphia, PA: Wolters Kluwer/Lippincott Williams & Wilkins, 2009.

95 Preskorn SH, Weller E, Jerkovich G et al.: Depression in children: concentration-dependent CNS toxicity of tricyclic antidepressants. *Psychopharmacol Bull* 1998; **24**: 140–2.

96 Woolf AD, Erdman AR, Nelson LS et al.: Tricyclic antidepressant poisoning: an evidence-based consensus guideline for out-of-hospital management. *Clin Toxicol (Phila)* 2007; **45**: 203–33.

97 Baker GB, Coutts RT, McKenna KF et al.: Insights into the mechanisms of action of the MAO inhibitors phenelzine and tranylcypromine: a review. *J Psychiatry Neurosci* 1992; **17**: 206–14.

98 Fiedorowicz JG, Swartz KL: The role of monoamine oxidase inhibitors in current psychiatric practice. *J Psychiatr Pract* 2004; **10**: 239–48.

99 Robinson DS: Monoamine oxidase inhibitors: a new generation. *Psychopharmacol Bull* 2002; **36**: 124–38.

100 Lotufo-Neto F, Trivedi M, Thase ME: Meta-analysis of the reversible inhibitors of monoamine oxidase type A moclobemide and brofaromine for the treatment of depression. *Neuropsychopharmacology* 1999; **20**: 226–47.

101 Quitkin F, Rifkin A, Klein DF: Monoamine oxidase inhibitors. A review of antidepressant effectiveness. *Arch Gen Psychiatry* 1979; **36**: 749–60.

102 Liebowitz MR, Quitkin FM, Stewart JW et al.: Antidepressant specificity in atypical depression. *Arch Gen Psychiatry* 1988; **45**: 129–37.

103 Stewart JW, McGrath PJ, Quitkin FM et al.: Relevance of DMS-III depressive subtype and chronicity of antidepressant efficacy in atypical depression. Differential response to phenelzine, imipramine, and placebo. *Arch Gen Psychiatry* 1989; **46**: 1080–7.

104 Thase ME, Trivedi MH, Rush AJ: MAOIs in the contemporary treatment of depression. *Neuropsychopharmacology* 1995; **12**: 185–219.

105 Henkel V, Mergl R, Allgaier AK et al.: Treatment of depression with atypical features: a meta-analytic approach. *Psychiatry Res* 2006; **141**: 89–101.

106 Amsterdam JD, Hornig-Rohan M.: Treatment algorithms in treatment-resistant depression. *Psychiatr Clin North Am* 2005; **19**: 371–86.

107 Amsterdam JD, Shults J: MAOI efficacy and safety in advanced stage treatment-resistant depression—a retrospective study. *J Affect Disord* 2005; **89**: 183–8.

108 Gelenberg A, Freeman M, Markowitz J, Rosenbaum J et al.: *Practice Guideline for the Treatment of Patients with Major Depressive Disorder*, 3rd edition. Arlington, VA: American Psychiatric Association, 2010.

109 West ED, Dally PJ: Effects of iproniazid in depressive syndromes. *Br Med J* 1959; **1**: 1491–4.

110 Liebowitz MR, Schneier F, Gitow A, Feerick J: Reversible monoamine oxidase-A inhibitors in social phobia. *Clin Neuropharmacol* 1993; **16**(Suppl 2): S83–S888.

111 Frommer EA: Treatment of childhood depression with antidepressant drugs. *Br Med J* 1967; **1**: 729–32.

112 Casper RC, Redmond DE, Jr., Katz MM et al.: Somatic symptoms in primary affective disorder. Presence and relationship to the classification of depression. *Arch Gen Psychiatry* 1985; **42**: 1098–104.

113 Ryan ND, Puig-Antich J, Cooper T et al.: Imipramine in adolescent major depression: plasma level and clinical response. *Acta Psychiatr Scand* 1986; **73**: 275–88.

114 Bodkin JA, Amsterdam JD: Transdermal selegiline in major depression: a double-blind, placebo-controlled, parallel-group study in outpatients. *Am J Psychiatry* 2002; **159**: 1869–75.

115 Amsterdam JD: A double-blind, placebo-controlled trial of the safety and efficacy of selegiline transdermal system without dietary restrictions in patients with major depressive disorder. *J Clin Psychiatry* 2003; **64**: 208–14.

116 Amsterdam JD, Bodkin JA: Selegiline transdermal system in the prevention of relapse of major depressive disorder: a 52-week, double-blind, placebo-substitution, parallel-group clinical trial. *J Clin Psychopharmacol* 2006; **26:** 579–86.

117 Feiger AD, Rickels K, Rynn MA et al.: Selegiline transdermal system for the treatment of major depressive disorder: an 8-week, double-blind, placebo-controlled, flexible-dose titration trial. *J Clin Psychiatry* 2006; **67:** 1354–61.

118 Phase IV:Safety and Efficacy of EMSAM in Adolescents With Major Depression. Available from: http://clinicaltrials.gov/ct2/show/NCT00531947?term=NCT00531 947&rank=1.

119 Rapaport MH: Dietary restrictions and drug interactions with monoamine oxidase inhibitors: the state of the art. *J Clin Psychiatry* 2007; **68**(Suppl 8): 42–6.

120 Beasley CM, Jr., Masica DN, Heiligenstein JH et al.: Possible monoamine oxidase inhibitor-serotonin uptake inhibitor interaction: fluoxetine clinical data and preclinical findings. *J Clin Psychopharmacol* 1993; **13:** 312–20.

121 Joyce PR, Paykel ES: Predictors of drug response in depression. *Arch Gen Psychiatry* 1989; **46:** 89–99.

122 Murphy DL, Sunderland T, Cohen RM: Monoamine oxidase-inhibiting antidepressants. a clinical update. *Psychiatr Clin North Am* 1984; **7:** 549–62.

123 Simpson GM, de Leon J: Tyramine and new monoamine oxidase inhibitor drugs. *Br J Psychiatry* 1989; (Suppl 6): 32–7.

124 Brown C, Taniguchi G, Yip K: The monoamine oxidase inhibitor-tyramine interaction. *J Clin Pharmacol* 1989; **29**(6): 529–32.

125 Blackwell B, Marley E, Price J et al.: Hypertensive interactions between monoamine oxidase inhibitors and foodstuffs. *Br J Psychiatry* 1967; **113:** 349–65.

126 Boyer EW, Shannon M: The serotonin syndrome. *N Engl J Med* 2005; **352:** 1112–20.

127 Sternbach H: The serotonin syndrome. *Am J Psychiatry* 1991; **148:** 705–13.

128 Goldman LS, Alexander RC, Luchins DJ: Monoamine oxidase inhibitors and tricyclic antidepressants: comparison of their cardiovascular effects. *J Clin Psychiatry* 1986; **47:** 225–9.

129 Sadock BJ, Kaplan HI, Sadock VA: *Kaplan and Sadock's Synopsis of Psychiatry: Behavioral Sciences/Clinical Psychiatry*, 10th edn. Philadelphia, PA: Wolter Kluwer/ Lippincott Williams & Wilkins, 2007.

130 Krishnan KR: Revisiting monoamine oxidase inhibitors. *J Clin Psychiatry* 2007; **68**(Suppl 8): 35–41.

131 Gelenberg AJ, Freeman MP, Markowitz JC et al.: Practice Guideline for the Treatment of Patients with Major Depressive Disorder, 3rd edition. Arlington, VA: American Psychiatric Association, 2010.

132 Gillman PK: Tricyclic antidepressant pharmacology and therapeutic drug interactions updated. *Br J Pharmacol* 2007; **151:** 737–48.

CHAPTER 8
Selective Serotonin Reuptake Inhibitors (SSRIs)

Dara Sakolsky & Boris Birmaher
University of Pittsburgh School of Medicine, Western Psychiatric Institute and Clinic, University of Pittsburgh Medical Center

The selective serotonin reuptake inhibitors (SSRIs) have become the first choice medication for many childhood psychiatric conditions including major depressive disorder (MDD), obsessive compulsive disorder (OCD), and other anxiety disorders. This chapter will discuss the pharmacokinetics, dosing, clinical efficacy, and adverse effects of SSRIs. We will focus on evidence based practice. When available data is limited, we have attempted to synthesize the current scientific knowledge and provided our best clinical judgment.

Pharmacokinetics

As youth differ from adults in many ways, pharmacokinetic studies in children and adolescents can provide useful information regarding how to prescribe these medications most effectively for pediatric populations. This is important because medication dosing strategies in several randomized controlled trials (RCTs) may have contributed not only to the failure of these trials to show a difference in efficacy between medication and placebo, but also to our understanding of the safety and tolerability of these medications [1]. Comprehending the pharmacokinetics of SSRIs is of great clinical importance because withdrawal effects (such as irritability) caused by SSRIs with a short half life can not only interfere with a child's daily functioning, but may also be confused with symptoms of psychiatric illness. For example, if a youth becomes more irritable as a consequence of withdrawal effects, the clinician may think that the symptoms are due to the primary psychiatric illness (for example, depression) and modify treatment without taking into the account that the symptoms may be due to the short half life of the medication (see the section on withdrawal below).

Pharmacotherapy of Child and Adolescent Psychiatric Disorders, Third Edition.
Edited by David R. Rosenberg and Samuel Gershon.

Pharmacokinetic properties for fluoxetine were described in a population pharmacokinetic study of children and adolescents [2]. Mean steady-state levels of fluoxetine (127 ng/ml) and its primary metabolite, norfluoxetine (151 ng/ml), were achieved after four weeks of treatment. High intersubject variability was reported. Concentrations of fluoxetine and norfluoxetine were approximately two times higher in children than adolescents. When normalized to body weight, fluoxetine and norfluoxetine concentrations were comparable for both groups. Time to steady-state concentration, plasma level at steady state, and ratio of drug to metabolite were analogous in adolescents when compared to adult studies. Based on these findings, Wilens et al. [2] suggested that children begin fluoxetine at 10 mg/day whereas; adolescents may start at 20 mg per day.

Pharmacokinetic studies of citalopram, escitalopram and sertraline in youth suggest that these medications have shorter half lives at low doses but their half-life becomes equivalent to the half life in adults at a higher dose range. S-citalopram, marketed as escitalopram, is the therapeutically active isomer of racemic citalopram [3]. A pharmacokinetic study of adolescents examined the half-life of R-citalopram and S-citalopram after a single 20 mg dose and after two weeks of 20 mg/day [4]. The single dose and steady state half-life of S-citalopram was found to be significantly shorter than previously reported in adults. Based on these findings, the authors recommended twice daily dosing when prescribing citalopram 20 mg/day. Likewise, a pharmacokinetic study of a single 10 mg dose of escitalopram found the half-life of escitalopram was shorter in adolescents (19.0 hours) than adults (28.9 hours). A pharmacokinetic study of steady-state citalopram (40 mg/day) found pharmacokinetic parameters were similar in adolescents (for example, half life 38 hours) and adults (for example, half life 44 hours). This same pattern is also observed in pharmacokinetics studies of sertraline. Pharmacokinetic studies of sertraline in adolescents have reported the mean steady state half life is 15.3 h at 50 mg/day, 20.4 h at 100 to 150 mg/day, and 27.1 h at 200 mg/day [5, 6]. The steady state half life of sertraline at 200 mg/day was similar to that previously observed in adults. Based on these findings, Axelson et al. [6] suggested an optimal dosing strategy of twice per day at doses of 50 mg/day and once daily at 200 mg/day. In summary, when prescribing citalopram, escitalopram or sertraline in the low dose range, twice-daily dosing should be considered.

The pharmacokinetic properties of fluvoxamine have been investigated in one study with youth. This study evaluated the steady state pharmacokinetic properties of fluvoxamine at 50, 100, and 200 mg/day in children and 50, 100, 200, and 300 mg/day in adolescents [7]. Children demonstrated higher mean peak plasma concentration, higher means area under the curve, and lower apparent clearance compared to adolescents. No pharmacokinetic differences were observed between adolescents and adults prescribed 150 mg twice daily. Nonlinear kinetics of fluvoxamine were observed over the dose range studied. Based on these findings, the authors concluded that children have a higher exposure to fluvoxamine than adolescents, while adolescents and adults appear to have similar drug exposure.

The pharmacokinetic properties of paroxetine have been reported in two studies with youth. The first study reported the half-life of paroxetine after a single 10 mg dose (11.1 hours) was significantly shorter than the half-life previously observed in adult studies [8]. Other pharmacokinetic parameters (for example, time to maximum concentration, intersubject variability, and nonlinear kinetics) were similar to those found in adult studies. For youth who were maintained on 10 mg/day, paroxetine concentrations generally remained stable during treatment; however, an almost sevenfold increase in drug concentration was reported in participants whose dose was raised to 20 mg/day. Based on these findings, Findling et al. [8] concluded that once daily administration of paroxetine was adequate. The second study assessed steady state pharmacokinetic properties after two weeks of 10 mg/day, 20 mg/day, and 30 mg/day [9]. Nonlinear kinetics of paroxetine were established as supraproportional increases in drug concentration were seen with each dose increase. Drug concentration at steady state was higher in children than adolescents at each dose studied. Based on these findings, the authors suggested that when paroxetine is prescribed to prepubertal children clinicians start paroxetine 5 mg/day or use an extended titration schedule such as 10 mg/day for at least four weeks.

In summary, pharmacokinetic studies with SSRIs suggest optimal dosing strategies may be different for children compared to adolescents and in particular for children with low weight. First, fluoxetine, fluvoxamine, and paroxetine need to be initiated at lower doses in low-weight youth. Second, clinicians may start citalopram, escitalopram, or sertraline at once daily dosing and observe closely for withdrawal effects. If withdrawal effects are noted (see the section on withdrawal), then the dosing regimen should be changed to twice-daily dosing.

Initiation and titration

Although there are some differences in pharmacokinetics between youth and adults, dosing regimens of SSRIs for youth are quite similar to adults. It is advisable to start with a low dose but increase weekly until a minimum effective dosage is reached. If persistent side-effects develop during titration, the medication dose should be lowered to the highest tolerable amount. Children and adolescents should receive an adequate and tolerable dosage for a minimum of four-to-six weeks. If a youth has tolerated the SSRI, but remains symptomatic after four-to-six weeks, a dose increase should be considered [10–12]. Clinical response should be reassessed every four-to-six weeks. When a youth shows only partial improvement or fails to show significant improvement after 10–12 weeks, alternative strategies should be considered (see Practice Parameters for the treatment of major depressive disorder, obsessive-compulsive disorder, anxiety disorders and post-traumatic stress disorder from the American Academy of Child and Adolescent Psychiatry).

Indications and efficacy

Major depressive disorder (MDD)

Approximately 20% of adolescents will experience at least one episode of depression by age 18 [13]. If untreated, depression can affect the development of cognitive, emotional, and social skills [14–16]. Youth with depression are also at high risk for suicide, substance abuse, physical illness, legal problems, early pregnancy, as well as poor academic, family, and psychosocial functioning [17]. Judicious identification and successful treatment may diminish the impact of depression on the academic and psychosocial functioning in youth and decrease the risk for suicide, substance abuse, and other sequelae. Evidence-based interventions have emerged in both psychotherapy and pharmacotherapy.

Many interventions (supportive therapy, cognitive behavioral therapy, attachment-based family therapy, interpersonal therapy, and pharmacotherapy) can be helpful for adolescents with major depression [17]. The choice of treatment should be based on a variety of factors including depression severity, duration of illness, prior response to treatment, familial and environmental factors, availability of treatment, comorbid disorders, patient and family preference. For youth with mild or brief depression, little psychosocial impairment, and the absence of suicidality or psychosis, pharmacotherapy is generally not indicated. In these cases, treatment often begins with education and supportive therapy to target stressors in the family or school. If response is not achieved after 2–4 weeks of supportive therapy, a trial with more specific types of psychotherapy (for example, cognitive behavior therapy or interpersonal psychotherapy) should be considered [17]. For youth with moderate, chronic or recurrent depression, and significant psychosocial impairment, the combination of psychotherapy and pharmacotherapy is often indicated [17]. However, a trial of cognitive behavioral therapy (CBT) or interpersonal therapy alone may help. In some cases, the severity of the depressive symptoms (for example, agitation, poor concentration, sleep disturbance, low motivation, or psychosis) can limit participation in psychotherapy, so initial treatment with only an antidepressant may be indicated. For youth with severe depression, psychosis, or treatment resistant depression, pharmacotherapy is usually needed [17]. Treatment often involves the combination of an antidepressant and psychotherapy, although two large studies have demonstrated that for adolescents with severe MDD there were no differences between fluoxetine alone and fluoxetine plus CBT [18, 19]. Youth with depression and psychosis may need treatment with an antipsychotic medication alone or in combination with an antidepressant [17].

One measure of treatment effectiveness is the number needed to treat (NNT) or the number of patients who must receive treatment to get one response that is attributable to active treatment. A meta-analysis of published and unpublished RCTs of antidepressants [20] reported the NNT to benefit from an antidepressant was 10 (95% confidence interval (CI), 7 to 15) for depression in youth. This meta-analysis also assessed the number needed to harm (NNH) or the number of patients who must receive a treatment to get one adverse effect that can be attributed to active treatment. Bridge et al. [20] reported the overall NNH for the spontaneous report of suicidal ideation and suicide attempt was 112 for patients with major depressive disorder who were treated with an antidepressant. These numbers suggest a favorable risk benefit profile for SSRIs in the treatment of childhood and adolescent depression.

Fluoxetine is usually the first choice for pharmacotherapy for depression in youth because three RCTs [21–23] have demonstrated its acute efficacy. In their meta-analysis, Bridge et al. [20] combined the data from all of fluoxetine RCTs for pediatric depression, and found the NNT to benefit from fluoxetine was 6 (95% CI, 4 to 10) while the NNT to benefit from any antidepressant was 10 (95% CI, 7 to 15). It remains unclear if fluoxetine is superior to other SSRIs for the treatment of adolescent depression (for example, long half-life may reduce the effect of poor adherence) or if the fluoxetine studies were better designed and conducted or recruited more severely depressed patients (for reviews of methodological issues see [24, 25]).

Fluoxetine is often the first choice of antidepressants for depression in youth given its effectiveness and low cost. However, there are many situations when choosing a different SSRI makes sense (e.g., lack of response to an adequate trial of fluoxetine, drug interactions, a strong family history of therapeutic response to an alternative SSRI, or family resistance).

Like fluoxetine, escitalopram has received FDA approval for the treatment of depression in youth. The first RCT with escitalopram compared flexible dose medication (10–20 mg/day, mean dose 12 mg/day) and placebo for eight weeks [26]. On the primary outcome measure, change in Children's Depression Rating Scale-Revised (CDRS-R) score from baseline to week 8, there was no significant difference between escitalopram and placebo. In a post hoc analysis of adolescents (aged 12–17 years) who completed the study, those who received escitalopram had significantly improved scores on all efficacy measures. No difference between escitalopram and placebo was demonstrated with children (aged 6–11 years) on any of the outcome measures. A second RCT compared flexible dose escitalopram (10–20 mg/day, mean dose 13 mg/day) with placebo in depressed adolescents for 8 weeks [27]. This study found significant improvement in depressive symptoms in the escitalopram group compared to the placebo on several outcome measures. Thus, two RCTs have demonstrated the efficacy of escitalopram for the treatment of adolescent depression; no RCTs have shown escitalopram to be efficacious for children with MDD.

Both sertraline and citalopram have demonstrated some efficacy for the treatment of depression in youth. Two identical multicenter randomized, double blind, placebo-controlled studies of sertraline were conducted with children and adolescents [28]. Patients received a flexible dose of sertraline (50–200 mg/day, mean dose 131 mg/day) or placebo for 10 weeks. Results from the two trials were combined in a prospectively defined data-analysis plan. Response rates, defined as 40% decrease in adjusted CDRS-R, were 69% for sertraline and 56% for placebo. Based on these studies, Bridge et al. [20] reported the NNT to benefit from sertraline was 10 (95% CI, 6 to 500). For citalopram, there is one positive study [29] and one negative study [30]. In the positive trial, patients were randomized to flexible dose citalopram (20–40 mg/day, mean dose 24 mg/day) or placebo for eight weeks. Response rates, defined as CDRS-R score of less than 28, were 36% for citalopram and 24% for placebo. In the negative trial, adolescents received citalopram (10–40 mg/day) or placebo for 12 weeks. Unlike other RCTs for MDD in youth, participants in this study included both inpatients and outpatients. Some patients received psychotherapy and/or other medications including anticonvulsants, antipsychotics, benzodiazepines, hypnotics, and stimulants. Response rates, defined as two or less on the Schedule for Affective Disorders and Schizophrenia for school-aged children (K-SADS) depression and anhedonia items, were 60% for citalopram and 61% for placebo. When choosing an alternative to fluoxetine or escitalopram, the data from RCTs supports the use of sertraline or citalopram for depression in youth.

The efficacy of paroxetine has been evaluated in three RCTs [31–33] all of which were negative on the primary efficacy measures. In the first trial [33] adolescents received a flexible dose of paroxetine (20–40 mg/day, mean dose 28 mg/day) or placebo for eight weeks. On the two primary outcome measures, Hamilton Rating Scale for Depression (HAM-D) score ≤ 8 or $\geq 50\%$ reduction in baseline HAM-D and change from baseline

HAM-D score, there was no significant difference between paroxetine and placebo. However, four secondary measures of efficacy demonstrated a significant difference between paroxetine and placebo. In the second study [31] adolescents were randomized to receive a flexible dose of paroxetine (20–40 mg/day, mean dose 26 mg/day) or placebo for 12 weeks. On the two primary efficacy measures, ≥ 50% reduction of Montgomery–Asberg Depression Rating Scale (MADRS) and change from baseline on the K-SADS depression subscale, there was no significant difference between paroxetine and placebo. In the third trial [32], children and adolescents were randomized to flexible dose paroxetine (10–50 mg/day, mean dose 28 mg/day) or placebo for eight weeks. On the primary efficacy measure, change from baseline on the CDRS-R and all secondary measures, there were no significant differences between paroxetine and placebo. In their meta-analysis, Bridge et al. [20] were unable to calculate a NNT to benefit from paroxetine as no benefit was demonstrated in these RCTs.

Caution must be used when interpreting the results of RCTs for depression in youth as several factors may moderate the outcomes of these trials. Industry sponsored trials are often conducted at a larger number of sites than studies funded by the National Institute of Mental Health. In Bridge [20] meta-analysis, the number of trial sites was inversely associated with efficacy suggesting a reduction in antidepressant effect as the number of study sites is increased. Patient characteristics can also moderate the outcome of antidepressant response in RCTs. For example, longer duration of illness and younger age are associated with poorer outcomes [20]. Most importantly, the placebo response rate is high in RCTs for pediatric MDD. Bridge [20] observed that the placebo response was higher for youth with MDD (50%) than youth with OCD (32%) or other anxiety disorders (39%). They found the best predictors of a high placebo response in antidepressant trials for pediatric depression were greater number of study sites and lower baseline illness severity[24]. Thus, some RCTs of SSRIs in youth with depression may have failed to show superiority of medication compared to placebo because of study design issues.

To summarize, evidence from RCTs supports the use of the SSRIs, especially fluoxetine for the acute treatment of childhood and adolescent depression, and escitalopram for the acute treatment of adolescent depression. Both fluoxetine and escitalopram have FDA indications for the treatment of MDD in youth (Table 8.1). Existing data also suggests that sertraline and citalopram may be effective for the treatment of MDD in youth.

While many RCTs have assessed the efficacy of SSRIs in the acute treatment (the initial 12 weeks during which the main goal is symptom reduction) of MDD in youth, only a few controlled studies have examined continuation phase (the subsequent 6- to 12- month period for and

Table 8.1 Clinical use of SSRIs in youth

Generic name (brand name)	Typical starting dose*	Initial dose titration	FDA dose range**	Clinical dose range	Formulations
citalopram (Celexa)	10 mg daily	10 mg for 1 week, then 20 mg		10–80 mg	Tablets: 10, 20, 40 mg Solution: 10 mg/5 ml
escitalopram (Lexapro)	5 mg daily	5 mg for 1 week, then 10 mg	10–20 mg	10–40 mg	Tablets: 5, 10, 20 mg Solution: 5 mg/5 ml
fluoxetine (Prozac)	10 mg daily	10 mg for 1 week, then 20 mg	10–20 mg MDD 20–60 mg OCD	10–80 mg	Tablets: 10, 20 mg Capsules: 10, 20, 40 mg Delayed release capsule: 90 mg Solution: 20 mg/5 ml
fluvoxamine (Luvox)	25 mg daily	25 mg for 1 week, then 50 mg	50–200 mg (children) 50–300 mg (adolescents)	50–300 mg	Tablets: 25, 50, 100 mg Extended release capsule: 100, 150 mg
paroxetine (Paxil)	10 mg daily	10 mg for 1 week, then 20 mg	10–60 mg	10–60 mg	Tablets: 10, 20, 30, 40 mg Extended release capsule: 12.5, 25, 37.5 mg Suspension: 10 mg/5 ml
sertraline (Zoloft)	25 mg daily	25 mg for 1 week, then 50 mg	25–200 mg	50–300 mg	Tablets: 25, 50, 100 mg Solution: 20 mg/ml

*Starting doses for children maybe lower (e.g., 5 mg daily for fluoxetine or paroxetine).

**Escitalopram has an FDA indication for major depressive disorder (MDD) in adolescents (12 years and older); fluoxetine has an FDA indication for MDD in youth (8 years and older) and for obsessive compulsive disorder (OCD) in youth (7 years and older); fluvoxamine has an FDA indication for OCD in youth (8 years and older); paroxetine has an FDA indication for OCD in youth (7 years and older); sertraline has an FDA indication for OCD in youth (6 years and older).

colleagues' remission consolidation and relapse prevention) treatment and no controlled studies have examined maintenance (a period of 12 months or longer for youth with recurrent depression during which the goal is to prevent future depressive episodes) treatments. During continuation treatment, SSRIs are continued at the same dose that resulted in clinical response during acute treatment; the SSRI dose may be increased in the absence of side-effects to target residual depressive symptoms. Continuation treatment with fluoxetine was shown to be more efficacious than placebo in preventing relapse of depression in youth [34]. Furthermore, the risk of relapse is much higher in youth who have not attained full remission, the absence of depressive symptoms [34]. For this reason, the addition of cognitive behavioral therapy to fluoxetine treatment results in a higher rate of sustained remission and lower rate of relapse than medication alone [35]. For youth with SSRI-resistant depression, identifying and addressing the cause of nonresponse (for example, inadequate medication dose or duration, poor adherence, lack of treatment for comorbid psychiatric disorders, inaccurate diagnosis, medical illness, or severe psychosocial stressors) is very important. The only RCT of SSRI-resistant depression, Treatment of Resistant Depression in Adolescents (TORDIA), found that switching to either another SSRI or venlafaxine led to a response rate of around 48% [36]. As there were greater rates of adverse effects with venlafaxine, the switch to another SSRI is recommended before trying venlafaxine. Adding CBT to either medication lead to greater improvement than medication alone [36]. Thus, the addition of CBT, if it is not already being utilized, is recommended.

Obsessive compulsive disorder

Obsessive compulsive disorder (OCD) was once thought to be a rare condition, but is now recognized as a severe condition that affects 1–3% of the world's population [37]. As many as 80% of all cases of OCD have their onset in childhood and adolescence [38, 39]. The development of effective treatments for the condition during childhood and adolescence is therefore critical.

Numerous RCTs have established the acute efficacy of SSRIs in the treatment of pediatric OCD [40]. Three SSRIs (fluvoxamine, fluoxetine, and sertraline) have FDA indications for the treatment of OCD in youth (Table 8.1). A meta-analysis of RCTs of antidepressants for pediatric OCD [20] found the NNT to benefit from an SSRI was 6 (95% CI, 4-8) for youth with OCD. Pooled measures of efficacy were comparable in children and adolescents. This meta-analysis also assessed the NNH for the spontaneous report of suicidal ideation and suicide attempt and found an NNH of 200 for children and adolescents with OCD who were treated with an SSRI.

These numbers suggest a very favorable risk-benefit profile for SSRIs in the treatment of childhood and adolescent anxiety disorders.

Fluvoxamine was the first SSRI to be FDA approved for use in children and adolescents with OCD. A large RCT of fluvoxamine (n = 120) compared medication (50–200 mg/day, mean 157 mg/day in children and 170 mg/day in adolescents) and placebo in youth (8–17 years of age) for 10 weeks. Fluvoxamine was superior to placebo in reducing OCD symptom severity [41]. Subsequent investigation to determine the long-term (12-month) efficacy of fluvoxamine in 99 youth with OCD was conducted [42]. After the first three weeks of treatment, the fluvoxamine dose was increased in all patients to 200 mg/day. A significant reduction in OCD symptom severity was seen initially and this improvement was maintained during the follow-up period. Youth with OCD who improved after acute treatment during the RCT demonstrated additional benefit during long-term treatment (mean additional reduction in OCD symptom severity of 31%). Thus, additional improvement with longer term SSRI treatment may be achieved in pediatric OCD patients.

Two large RCT have assessed the efficacy of fluoxetine in the treatment of OCD in youth. The first large RCT compared flexible dose fluoxetine (20–60 mg/day, mean 25 mg/day) and placebo for 13 weeks in 103 youth (7–17 years of age) with OCD [43]. Children and adolescents treated with fluoxetine showed significantly greater improvement in OCD symptoms on multiple outcome measures compared to placebo. The second RCT compared fluoxetine (20–80 mg/day, mean 65 mg/day) and placebo for 8 weeks in 43 youth (6–18 years of age) with OCD [44]. Both groups had lower OCD symptoms at week 8 but there was no difference between fluoxetine and placebo on the primary outcome measure or most secondary measures. Treatment responders (n = 18) were continued on fluoxetine or placebo for an additional eight weeks. After 16 weeks, youth receiving fluoxetine had significantly lower OCD symptoms than youth taking placebo on the primary outcome measure and some secondary measures. Thus, fluoxetine has been shown to be efficacious in the treatment of pediatric OCD, but its effectiveness may take longer than eight weeks to manifest.

The effectiveness of paroxetine for pediatric OCD has been evaluated in one large RCT [45]. In this study, flexible-dose paroxetine (10–50 mg/day, mean dose of 25 mg/day for children and 37 mg/day for adolescents) was compared to placebo in 207 youth (aged 7–17 years) with OCD for 10 weeks. Children and adolescents treated with paroxetine showed significantly greater improvement in symptoms compared to the placebo group on the primary outcome measure and several secondary measures.

Two large RCTs have evaluated the efficacy of sertraline in the treatment of pediatric OCD. The first RCT compared sertraline (maximum 200 mg/day, mean dose 167 mg/day in children and 180 mg/day in adolescents) and placebo for 12 weeks in 187 youth (6–17 years of age) with OCD [46]. Youth treated with sertraline showed significantly greater improvement in OCD symptoms compared to placebo on three out of four primary outcome measures. To evaluate the long-term effectiveness of sertraline for pediatric OCD, youth who participated in the RCT were offered open treatment with sertraline 50–200 mg/day (mean dose 108 mg/day in children and 132 mg/day in adolescents) for 12 months. As with long-term fluvoxamine treatment, continued sertraline treatment resulted in additional improvement in OCD symptom severity. The acute efficacy of sertraline for pediatric OCD was also evaluated in the Pediatric OCD treatment study (POTS) which compared CBT, flexible dose sertraline (25–200 mg/day, mean dose 170 mg/day), their combination (sertraline mean dose 133 mg/day), and pill placebo in 112 youth (7–17 years of age) for 12 weeks [47]. In the POTS, response to CBT, sertraline, and combination treatment was significantly greater than placebo and response to combination treatment was superior to CBT or sertraline alone. In their meta-analysis, Bridge et al. [20] combined the data from these two RCTs of sertraline for pediatric OCD, and found the NNT to benefit from sertraline was 6 (95% CI, 4 to 16), which was consistent with the NNT to benefit from any SSRI.

In the POTS, remission rates were 53.6% (95% CI: 36–70%) for combination treatment, 39.3% (95% CI: 24–58%) for CBT, 21.4% (95% CI: 10–40%) for sertraline and 3.6% (95% CI: 0–19%) for placebo. The remission rate for combination treatment was not different than CBT, but was superior to sertraline and placebo; the remission rate for CBT was not different from sertraline, but was greater than placebo; and the remission rate for sertraline was not different than placebo. Based on these findings, the POTS Study Team recommended that youth with OCD should begin treatment with combination therapy or CBT alone.

The choice of treatment intervention for youth with OCD should be based on a variety of factors including OCD severity, duration of illness, prior response to treatment, familial and environmental factors, availability of treatment, comorbid conditions, patient and family preference. For youth with mild to moderate OCD and little psychosocial impairment, CBT is usually the first-line treatment. For youth with moderate to severe OCD or significant psychosocial impairment, medication and CBT should be considered [40].

Although RCTs have established the short-term efficacy of SSRIs in the treatment of pediatric OCD, controlled studies are needed to determine the optimal length of continuation or maintenance treatment. Until such studies are preformed, we recommend following the same clinical practice as recommended for adult OCD (i.e., medication should be continued at the same dose that resulted in response during acute treatment for 1–2 years). The SSRI dose may be increased during continuation treatment to diminish residual OCD symptoms in the absence of side-effects. A trial off medication during a low-stress period should be considered after 1–2 years of minimal symptoms. A gradual taper of medication by decrements of 10%–25% every 1–2 months while observing for symptom return or exacerbation is recommended [48].

Generalized anxiety disorder, social phobia, and separation anxiety disorder

Anxiety disorders are among the most common conditions affecting children and adolescents [49]. The National Comorbidity Survey Replication-Adolescent Supplement found 31.9% of adolescents to have an anxiety disorder and 8.3% of anxious youth have a severe or impairing disorder [50]. Generalized anxiety disorder, social phobia, and separation anxiety disorder are among the most common pediatric anxiety disorders, have overlapping symptoms, and are often comorbid with each other [51]. Thus, these three anxiety disorders are often studied together. Research demonstrates that anxious children experience difficulties with school performance [52], peer relationships [53], and family functioning [54]. Childhood anxiety disorders are not only associated with impairment in childhood and adolescence but also confer an increased risk of adult anxiety disorders [55], major depressive disorder [56], suicide attempts [57], and substance use disorders [58]. Early identification and successful treatment of childhood anxiety disorders may reduce the impact of childhood anxiety on academic and psychosocial functioning as well as decrease the risk for other psychiatric disorders later in life. Evidence-based treatments have emerged in both psychotherapy and pharmacotherapy.

A variety of interventions (cognitive behavioral therapy, family therapy, psychodynamic psychotherapy, and pharmacotherapy) can be helpful for youth with anxiety disorders [59]. The choice of treatment should be based on a variety of factors including anxiety severity, duration of illness, prior response to intervention, familial and environmental factors, availability of treatment, comorbid disorders, patient and family preference. Cognitive behavioral therapy (CBT) and SSRIs are the best studied therapies for youth with generalized anxiety disorder (GAD), social phobia (SoP) and separation anxiety disorder (SAD). The Child/Adolescent Anxiety Multimodal Treatment Study [60] compared the efficacy of CBT, flexible dose sertraline (25–200 mg/day, mean dose 134 mg/day), their combination, and pill placebo, in 488 youth with GAD, SoP, and SAD. The CAMS found that CBT and sertraline were more effective than placebo on all primary outcome measures and that the combination of these interventions was superior to either treatment alone. In the CAMS, the NNT was 1.7 (95%

CI: 1.7–1.9) for combination therapy, 2.8 (95% CI: 2.7–3.0) for CBT, and 3.2 (95% CI: 3.2–3.5) for sertraline. Future analyses from the CAMS will explore predictors and moderators of intervention response to help identify who will most likely benefit from each of these effective treatments.

Findings from the CAMS are analogous to those reported by a meta-analysis of published and unpublished RCTs of antidepressants for youth with GAD, SoP, or SAD [20]. Bridge et al. [20] found the NNT to benefit from an antidepressant was 3 (95% CI, 2-5) for youth with non-obsessive compulsive anxiety disorders. This meta-analysis also assessed the NNH for the spontaneous report of suicidal ideation and suicide attempt and found an NNH of 143 for anxious youth who were treated with an antidepressant. These numbers suggest a very favorable risk benefit profile for SSRIs in the treatment of childhood and adolescent anxiety disorders.

Although no SSRI has an FDA indication for GAD, SoP, or SAD, many short-term RCTs of SSRIs have demonstrated the benefit of medication compared to placebo. The first RCT compared flexible dose fluvoxamine (25–250 mg/day children 6–12 years old, 25–300 mg/day for adolescents 13–17 years old) and placebo for eight weeks in 128 youth with GAD, SoP or SAD (Research Units of Pediatric Psychopharmacology Anxiety Group, 2001). On both reported outcome measures there was a significant difference between fluvoxamine and placebo. The second RCT compared sertraline (50 mg/day maximum) and placebo for nine weeks in 22 youth (5–17 years old) with GAD [61]. All primary outcome measures showed significant improvement with sertraline treatment compared to placebo. A third RCT compared fluoxetine (20 mg/day) and placebo for 12 weeks in 74 youth (7–17 years old) with GAD, SoP, or SAD [62]. Fluoxetine was effective in reducing anxiety symptoms and improving functioning on all measures. Youth with social phobia and generalized anxiety disorder responded better to fluoxetine than placebo, but only social phobia moderated clinical response. A fourth RCT compared flexible dose paroxetine (10–50 mg/day, mean dose 27 mg/day for children and 35 mg/day for adolescents) and placebo for 16 weeks in 322 youth (8–17 years of age) with social anxiety disorder [63]. All primary and secondary outcome measures showed a significant improvement in anxiety symptoms with paroxetine treatment. A fifth RCT compared fluoxetine (40 mg/day), Social Effectiveness Therapy for Children (SET-C), and placebo for 12 weeks in 122 youth (7–17 years of age) with social phobia [64]. Both fluoxetine and SET-C were more efficacious than placebo in reducing anxiety symptoms and increasing general functioning. As previously discussed, the CAMS [60] reported sertraline and CBT were more effective than placebo in reducing anxiety symptoms in youth. Thus, numerous RCTs have established the efficacy of SSRIs in the treatment of childhood anxiety disorders.

While many RCTs have confirmed the short-term efficacy of SSRIs in treatment of childhood anxiety disorders, only a few open studies have examined the effectiveness of long-term SSRI use. Following the RCT of fluvoxamine and placebo, youth were offered six months of open treatment; fluvoxamine responders were continued on fluvoxamine (n = 35); placebo non-responders were treated with fluvoxamine (n = 14); and fluvoxamine non-responders were switched to fluoxetine (n = 48) [65]. During the six months of open treatment, anxiety symptoms remained low in youth who had initially responded to fluvoxamine and anxiety symptoms improved when placebo nonresponders were treated with fluvoxamine or when fluvoxamine non-responders were switched to fluoxetine. In a second study, youth were offered one year of open treatment with fluoxetine, alternative medication, and/or CBT following the RCT of fluoxetine and placebo [66]. Youth taking fluoxetine (n = 42) showed superior outcomes on most outcome measures compared to those taking no medication (n = 10). A major limitation of both of these studies was the lack of a randomized control design.

Clearly, controlled studies are needed to establish the long-term efficacy of SSRIs in the treatment of childhood anxiety disorders. Until such studies are performed, we recommend following the same clinical practice as continuation treatment for MDD in youth (i.e., SSRI are continued at the same dose that resulted in response during acute treatment for six to 12-months). The SSRI dose may be increased during continuation treatment to diminish residual anxiety symptoms provided that side-effects are not problematic. A trial off medication during a low-stress period (for example, summer vacation) should be considered after six to 12 months of minimal anxiety symptoms. The SSRI should be restarted if anxiety symptoms reoccur.

Panic disorder

While cued panic attacks are common in youth, panic disorder which is characterized by recurrent, *unexpected* panic attacks occurs at a much lower rate. The National Comorbidity Survey Replication-Adolescent Supplement (NCS-A) found 2.3% of adolescents to have panic disorder [50]. The prevalence of this disorder showed a modest increase with age across adolescence. In the NCS-A, all adolescents with panic disorder endorsed "a lot" or "extreme" impairment in daily activities and "severe" or "very severe" distress from their anxiety symptoms.

Despite the impairment and severity of symptoms for youth with panic disorder, no RCTs have evaluated the efficacy of SSRIs for panic disorder in youth. Renaud et al. [67] openly treated 12 youth with panic disorder. Nine youth received fluoxetine (20–60 mg/day, mean 34 mg/day), two were prescribed paroxetine (20 mg/day) and one was treated with sertraline (125 mg/day). In this open trial, SSRIs were effective for panic disorder in youth. Similarly, a chart review of 18 youth (7–16 years of age) with panic disorder showed flexible dose paroxetine (10–40 mg/day, mean 24 mg/day) to be effective for panic disorder in children and adolescents [68]. A recent small RCT (n = 26) of CBT versus self-monitoring control group, has showed CBT to be feasible and a potentially efficacious intervention for youth with panic disorder [69]. In summary, limited data supports the use of SSRIs and CBT in the treatment of panic disorder in children and adolescents. Large RCTs are needed to confirm effective treatment options for panic disorder in youth.

Post-traumatic stress disorder

Most individuals who experience life-threatening events develop post-traumatic symptoms immediately; however, only about 30% report enduring symptoms beyond the first month [70]. The NCS-A found 5.0% of adolescents (13–18 years of age) endorsed symptoms of post-traumatic stress disorder [50]. Post-traumatic stress disorder was more frequent in females and its prevalence increased modestly with age. In the NCS-A, 30% of adolescents with PTSD reported severe anxiety symptoms and significant daily impairment.

Practice guidelines for the treatment of PTSD in children and adolescent recommend trauma-focused psychotherapies as first-line treatments [71]. Two recent RCTs have assessed the efficacy of SSRIs in the treatment of PTSD [72, 73]. Both studies failed to find a difference between SSRI and placebo. The first RCT compared trauma-focused CBT plus flexible dose sertraline (50–200 mg/day, mean 150 mg/day) and trauma-focused CBT plus placebo for 12 weeks in 24 females (10–17 years of age) with PTSD [73]. Significant improvement was seen in both groups from pre- to post-treatment, but no group-by-time differences were observed for PTSD symptoms. The second RCT compared flexible dose sertraline (50–200 mg/day) and placebo for 10 weeks in 129 youth (6–17 years of age) with PTSD [72]. As in the previous study, both groups experienced a significant improvement in PTSD symptoms from pre- to post-treatment, but no difference between the sertraline and placebo group was found. Like the RCTs for SSRIs in pediatric MDD, the high placebo response rate makes detecting an effect of medication difficult. In summary, current data is lacking to support the use of SSRIs in the treatment of childhood PTSD.

Selective serotonin reuptake inhibitors can be considered for youth with PTSD who have comorbid disorders known to be responsive to SSRI treatment (for example, MDD, OCD, GAD, or SoP) or those who do not respond to psychotherapy alone [71].

Adverse effects

Common

In acute RCTs, SSRIs are generally well tolerated. Most side-effects appear to be dose-dependent and often decrease with time [25, 74, 75]. The most common adverse effects include gastrointestinal symptoms (for example, nausea, abdominal pain, and diarrhea), appetite disturbance (increase or decrease), headache, dizziness, sleep changes (for example, insomnia or somnolence, vivid dreams or nightmares), dry mouth, restlessness, akathisia, and sexual dysfunction (Box 8.1).

Impulsivity, silliness, irritability, disinhibition or "behavioral activation" can be seen in 3% to 8% of youth, especially in children, taking SSRIs. This adverse reaction is characterized by goofiness, silliness, increased activity, is usually mild to moderate in severity and has an abrupt onset after starting or changing a medication dose [76]. It can occur with many types of medications (for example, benzodiazepines, antihistamines, or tricyclic antidepressants). We recommend discussing this side-effect with the parents and child being treated beforehand, as this side-effect is transient. Symptoms resolve quickly when the medication dose is lowered or discontinued. Careful differentiation between this phenomena and hypomania or mania is critical. It is also worth pointing out that many patients treated with SSRIs including patients with anxiety disorders, OCD and severe depression may be remarkably inhibited at baseline and it is important not to confuse healthy childhood behavior with a medication side-effect. For example, if parents are concerned about behavior that is not typical of their

---

Box 8.1   Adverse effects of Serotonin Re uptake Inhibitors (SSRIs)

Common
- GI (nausea, diarrhea, dyspepsia)
- Sleep changes (e.g., insomnia, somnolence, vivid dreams)
- Motor restlessness or akathisia
- Appetite changes (increased or decreased)
- Headaches
- Diaphoresis
- Dry mouth
- Sexual dysfunction (e.g., anorgasmia)
- Behavioral activation (e.g., impulsivity, silliness, irritability)

Rare
- Serotonin syndrome
- Predisposition for bleeding
- Hypomania or mania
- Suicidal ideation or behavior

child but is common in their child's peers, this may suggest a decrease in anxiety and not an adverse medication reaction.

Selective serotonin reuptake inhibitors have been associated with hypomania and mania in children and adolescents. This may be a particular concern in youth with depression who may have a higher risk of ultimately developing bipolar disorder. However, it is not clear at present how to discriminate depressed youth who will develop bipolar disorder from those who will not. A family history of bipolar disorder and depression with psychosis carry an increased risk for bipolar disorder in youth, so that caution is indicated when prescribing SSRIs to these youth. Any patient being treated with an antidepressant should be monitored for symptoms of mania/hypomania. As described by Wilens et al. [76] the unmasking of a primary psychiatric disorder (for example, bipolar disorder with a hypmomanic/manic episode) can be distinguished from disinhibition by the onset of symptoms, the offset of symptoms, the severity of symptoms, and the nature of the symptoms. In comparison to disinhibition, a hypomanic or manic episode has a delayed onset; a prolonged offset; and moderate to severe symptomatology including elated mood, grandiosity, decreased need for sleep, talkativeness, flight of ideas, and excessive involvement in pleasurable activities that have a high potential for painful consequences. The reader is strongly encouraged to read the brief review by Wilens et al. [76], which includes very helpful advice in differentiating disinhibition from the unmasking of a primary psychiatric disorder, such as bipolar disorder.

Uncommon and serious

Less common but more severe side-effects include serotonin syndrome [77] and increased risk of bleeding (for example, easy bruising, epistaxis, gastrointestinal bleeding, and perioperative bleeding) [78, 79]. The most publicized and controversial is the increased spontaneous reports of suicidal ideation and behavior.

Given the serious concerns about suicidal ideation and behavior with SSRIs, two meta-analyses have evaluated the risk of suicidal ideation and behavior in children and adolescents taking antidepressants [20, 80]. In collaboration with researchers at Columbia University, the U.S. Food and Drug Administration (FDA) evaluated the effect of nine antidepressants on suicidality in 24 RCTs of pediatric depression, anxiety disorders or attention deficit hyperactivity disorder [80]. The primary outcome measures were *spontaneous* reports of suicidal ideation and suicidal behavior termed "suicidal adverse events." The overall risk ratio (RR) for suicidality for all the trials and indications was 1.95 (95% CI, 1.28–2.98). When analyses were limited to depression trials with SSRIs, the overall RR was 1.66 (95% CI, 1.02–2.68). These results suggest that 1–3 spontaneously reported suicide adverse events occur for every 100 children or adolescents treated with an antidepressant. This meta-analysis [80] also examined worsening or emergence of suicidality using the suicide item scores of depression rating scales from 17 RCTs. These analyses did not reveal any significant RR for worsening of suicidality (0.92; 95% CI, 0.76–1.1) or for emergence of suicidality (0.93; 95% CI, 0.75–1.15).

A second meta-analysis examined the effect of antidepressants on suicidality in 27 published and unpublished RCTs of pediatric depression and anxiety disorders [20]. When using similar statistical methods as the previous study, this meta-analysis found comparable results, a small but significant increase in overall RR for suicidality for all disorders (1.9; 95% Cl, 1.3–3.0) and for depression (1.9; 95% Cl 1.2–2.9). Since RR analysis is limited to trials with at least one event and several trials had no events, Bridge et al. [20] also assessed risk difference (RD), which permits inclusion of trials with no events. When using random-effects analysis of RD instead of RR, there was a small but significant overall RD for drug compared with placebo (0.7%; 95% CI, 0.1–1.3). No significant difference was found when analyses were limited to studies with depression (0.9%; 95% CI, –0.1–1.9%), OCD (0.5%; 95% CI, –0.4–1.8%), or other anxiety disorders (0.7%; 95% CI, –0.4–1.8%).

The interpretation of these findings and their implications for clinical practice are not clear since there has been a dramatic decline in rate of youth suicide in the U.S. during time of increased usage of SSRIs [81]. Prior to the FDA black box warning on SSRIs, epidemiological studies suggested a positive relationship between the reduction in adolescent suicide rate and use of SSRIs [81–83]. Since U.S. and European regulators issued warnings on SSRIs, there has been a reduction in the rate of SSRI prescriptions to children and adolescents and an increase in completed suicides rates in the U.S. and Netherlands [84]. Thus, epidemiological studies show not only a correlation between increased usage of SSRIs and reduction in suicide rates, but also an association between reduced SSRI usage and increased youth suicide rates.

In summary, spontaneous reports of suicidal ideation or behavior are more common in adolescents treated with SSRIs than placebo. Although this event is rare, some youth experience a new onset or worsening in suicidal ideation or behavior after starting treatment with an SSRI. Thus, it is important to evaluate for the presence of suicidal risk before and carefully after starting treatment with an SSRI (see section below on Monitoring for Adverse Effects).

Long-term impact

The long-term impact of SSRIs is unknown. The effect on brain development and function are often a concern of the child and family for whom SSRI treatment is being considered. It should be noted that the illnesses for which SSRIs are prescribed can be quite serious and can result in substantial morbidity and mortality, so a risk/benefit analysis is indicated. Long-term study of SSRIs is clearly warranted to address concerns about the medication's effect on brain development and other potentially unknown side-effects.

Monitoring for adverse effects

During the first two months of SSRI treatment, the prescribing clinician usually sees patients weekly or twice monthly to monitor for symptoms and adverse effects, to make dose adjustments, as well as to provide education and support. During these visits, we recommend that clinicians inquire about adverse effects including new onset or worsening of suicidal ideation as well as medication adherence.

Withdrawal

Withdrawal and flu-like syndromes can occur when the SSRIs are abruptly discontinued, when SSRIs are taken inconsistently, or when a patient rapidly metabolizes a medication. Somatic symptoms can include: gastrointestinal (for example, nausea or emesis), disequilibrium (for example, dizziness, vertigo, or ataxia), sleep disturbance (for example, insomnia or vivid dreams), flu-like symptoms (for example, fatigue, sedation, myalgia, or chills), and sensory disturbances (for example, paresthesia) [85]. Given the similarity between adverse effects and withdrawal symptoms, it is important to inquire about medication adherence when problems with medication are reported. In studies with adults [86, 87] discontinuation symptoms have been shown to differ among the SSRIs. For example, Baldwin et al. [86] observed significantly fewer discontinuation symptoms with escitalopram compared to paroxetine. Tint et al. [87] reported fewer discontinuation symptoms with fluoxetine compared to short half-life antidepressants (citalopram, fluvoxamine, paroxetine and venlafaxine) and found a similar frequency of discontinuation symptoms with a short taper (three days) compared to a longer taper (14 days). Thus, tapering an SSRI is preferable and some youth may require especially gradual tapering over four-to-six weeks to minimize withdrawal and/or symptom recurrence.

References

1 Findling RL, McNamara NK, Stansbrey RJ et al.: The relevance of pharmacokinetic studies in designing efficacy trials in juvenile major depression. *J Child Adolesc Psychopharmacol* 2006; **16**: 131–45.

2 Wilens TE, Cohen L, Biederman J et al.: Fluoxetine pharmacokinetics in pediatric patients. *J Clin Psychopharmacol* 2002; **22**: 568–75.

3 Hyttel J, Bogeso KP, Perregaard J et al.: The pharmacological effect of citalopram residues in the (S)– (+)– enantiomer. *J Neural Transm* 1992; **88:** 157–60.

4 Perel JM, Axelson DA, Rudolph G et al.: Stereoselective pharmacokinetic/ pharmacodynamic (PK/PD) of ± citalopram in adolescents, comparisons with adult findings [Abstract]. *Clin Pharmacol Therapeut* 2001; **69:** 30.

5 Alderman J, Wolkow R, Chung M et al.: Sertraline treatment of children and adolescents with obsessive-compulsive disorder or depression: pharmacokinetics, tolerability, and efficacy. *J Am Acad Child Adolesc Psychiatry* 1998; **37:** 386–94.

6 Axelson DA, Perel JM, Birmaher B et al.: Sertraline pharmacokinetics and dynamics in adolescents. *Journal of the American Academy of Child and Adolescent Psychiatry* 2002; **41:** 1037–44.

7 Labellarte M, Biederman J, Emslie G et al.: Multiple-dose pharmacokinetics of fluvoxamine in children and adolescents. *Journal of the American Academy of Child and Adolescent Psychiatry* 2006; **43:** 1497–505.

8 Findling RL, Reed MD, Myers C et al.: Paroxetine pharmacokinetics in depressed children and adolescents. *J Am Acad Child Adolesc Psychiatry* 1999; **38:** 952–99.

9 Findling RL, Nucci G, Piergies AA et al.: Multiple dose pharmacokinetics of paroxetine in children and adolescents with major depressive disorder or obsessive-compulsive disorder. *Neuropsychopharmacology* 2006; **31:** 1274–85.

10 Birmaher B, Brent D, Issues AWGoQ et al.: Practice parameter for the assessment and treatment of children and adolescents with depressive disorders. *J Am Acad Child Adolesc Psychiatry* 2007; **46:** 1503–26.

11 Heiligenstein JH, Hoog SL, Wagner KD et al.: Fluoxetine 40–60 mg versus fluoxetine 20 mg in the treatment of children and adolescents with a less-than-complete response to nine-week treatment with fluoxetine 10–20 mg: a pilot study. *J Child Adolesc Psychopharmacol* 2006; **16:** 207–17.

12 Sakolsky DJ, Perel JM, Emslie GJ et al.: Antidepressant exposure as a predictor of clinical outcomes in the treatment of resistant depression in adolescents (TORDIA) Study. *J Clin Psychopharmacol* 2011; **31:** 92–7.

13 Lewinsohn PM, Rohde P, Seeley JR: Major depressive disorder in older adolescents: prevalence, risk factors, and clinical implications. *Clinical Psychology Review* 1998; **18:** 765–94.

14 Birmaher B, Arbelaez C, Brent D: Course and outcome of child and adolescent major depressive disorder. *Child and Adolescent Psychiatric Clinics of North America* 2002; **11:** 619–37.

15 Birmaher B, Ryan ND, Williamson DE et al.: Childhood and adolescent depression: a review of the past 10 years. Part I. *J Am Acad Child Adolesc Psychiatry* 1996; **35:** 1427–39.

16 Lewinsohn PM, Rohde P, Seeley JR et al.: Psychosocial functioning of young adults who have experienced and recovered from major depressive disorder during adolescence. *J Abnorm Psychol* 2003; **112:** 353–63.

17 Birmaher B, Brent DA, Work Group on Quality I: Practice parameter for the assessment and treatment of children and adolescents with depressive disorders. *J Am Acad Child Adolesc Psychiatry* 2007; **46:** 1503–26.

18 Curry J, Rohde P, Simons A et al.: Predictors and moderators of acute outcome in the Treatment for Adolescents with Depression Study (TADS). *J Am Acad Child Adolesc Psychiatry* 2006; **45:** 1427–39.

19 Goodyer I, Dubicka B, Wilkinson P et al.: Selective serotonin reuptake inhibitors (SSRIs) and routine specialist care with and without cognitive behaviour therapy in adolescents with major depression: randomised controlled trial. *BMJ* 2007; **335:** 21.

20 Bridge JA, Iyengar S, Salary CB et al.: Clinical response and risk for reported suicidal ideation and suicide attempts in pediatric antidepressant treatment: a meta-analysis of randomized controlled trials. *JAMA* 2007; **297**: 1683–96. (See the "comment" section.)

21 Emslie GJ, Rush AJ, Weinberg WA et al.: A double-blind, randomized, placebo-controlled trial of fluoxetine in children and adolescents with depression. *Arch Gen Psychiatry* 1997; **54**: 1031–7.

22 Emslie GJ, Heiligenstein JH, Wagner KD et al.: Fluoxetine for acute treatment of depression in children and adolescents: a placebo-controlled, randomized clinical trial. *J Am Acad Child Adolesc Psychiatry* 2002; **41**: 1205–15.

23 March J, Silva S, Vitiello B et al.: The Treatment for Adolescents with Depression Study (TADS): methods and message at 12 weeks. *J Am Acad Child Adolesc Psychiatry* 2004; **45**: 1393–403.

24 Bridge JA, Birmaher B, Iyengar S et al.: Placebo response in randomized controlled trials of antidepressants for pediatric major depressive disorder. *Am J Psychiatry* 2009; **166**: 42–9.

25 Cheung AH, Emslie GJ, Mayes TL: The use of antidepressants to treat depression in children and adolescents. *CMAJ* 2006; **174**: 193–200.

26 Wagner KD, Jonas J, Findling RL et al.: A double-blind, randomized, placebo-controlled trial of escitalopram in the treatment of pediatric depression. *J Am Acad Child Adolesc Psychiatry* 2006; **45**: 280–8.

27 Emslie GJ, Ventura D, Korotzer A et al.: Escitalopram in the treatment of adolescent depression: a randomized placebo-controlled multisite trial. *J Am Acad Child Adolesc Psychiatry* 2009; **48**: 721–9.

28 Wagner KD, Ambrosini P, Rynn M et al.: Efficacy of sertraline in the treatment of children and adolescents with major depressive disorder: two randomized controlled trials. *JAMA* 2003; **290**: 1033–41.

29 Wagner KD, Robb AS, Findling RL et al.: A randomized, placebo-controlled trial of citalopram for the treatment of major depression in children and adolescents. *Am J Psychiatry* 2004; **161**: 1079–83.

30 von Knorring AL, Olsson GI, Thomsen PH et al.: A randomized, double-blind, placebo-controlled study of citalopram in adolescents with major depressive disorder. *J Clin Psychopharmacol* 2006; **26**: 311–15.

31 Berard R, Fong R, Carpenter DJ et al.: An international, multicenter, placebo-controlled trial of paroxetine in adolescents with major depressive disorder. *J Child Adolesc Psychopharmacol* 2006; **16**: 59–75.

32 Emslie GJ, Wagner KD, Kutcher S et al.: Paroxetine treatment in children and adolescents with major depressive disorder: a randomized, multicenter, double-blind, placebo-controlled trial. *J Am Acad Child Adolesc Psychiatry* 2006; **45**: 709–19.

33 Keller MB, Ryan ND, Strober M et al.: Efficacy of paroxetine in the treatment of adolescent major depression: a randomized, controlled trial. *J Am Acad Child Adolesc Psychiatry* 2001; **40**: 762–72.

34 Emslie GJ, Kennard BD, Mayes TL et al.: Fluoxetine versus placebo in preventing relapse of major depression in children and adolescents. *Am J Psychiatry* 2008; **165**: 459–67.

35 Kennard BD, Emslie GJ, Mayes TL et al.: Cognitive-behavioral therapy to prevent relapse in pediatric responders to pharmacotherapy for major depressive disorder. *J Am Acad Child Adolesc Psychiatry* 2008; **47**: 1395–404.

36 Brent D, Emslie G, Clarke G et al.: Switching to another SSRI or to venlafaxine with or without cognitive behavioral therapy for adolescents with SSRI-resistant depression: the TORDIA randomized controlled trial. *JAMA* 2008; **299**: 901–13.

37 Rasmussen SA, Eisen JL: The epidemiology and differential diagnosis of obsessive compulsive disorder. *J Clin Psychiatry* 1994; **55**: 5–10.

38 Nestadt G, Samuels J, Riddle M et al.: A family study of obsessive-compulsive disorder. *Arch Gen Psychiatry* 2000; **57**: 358–363.

39 Pauls DL, Alsobrook JP, 2nd, Goodman W et al.: A family study of obsessive-compulsive disorder. *Am J Psychiatry* 1995; **152**: 76–84.

40 Mancuso E, Faro A, Joshi G, Geller DA: Treatment of pediatric obsessive-compulsive disorder: a review. *J Child Adolesc Psychopharmacol* 2010; **20**: 299–308.

41 Riddle MA, Reeve EA, Yaryura et al.: Fluvoxamine for children and adolescents with obsessive-compulsive disorder: a randomized, controlled, multicenter trial. *J Am Acad Child Adolesc Psychiatry* 2001; **40**: 222–9.

42 Walkup J, Reeve E, Yaryura-Tobias J et al.: Fluvoxamine for childhood obsessive compulsive disorder: long-term treatment. New Clinical Drug Evaluation Unit Program (NCDEU) Abstracts, 38th Annual Meeting, Boca Raton, Florida, 1998.

43 Geller DA, Hoog SL, Heiligenstein JH et al.: Fluoxetine treatment for obsessive-compulsive disorder in children and adolescents: a placebo-controlled clinical trial. *J Am Acad Child Adolesc Psychiatry* 2001; **40**: 773–9.

44 Liebowitz MR, Turner SM, Piacentini J et al.: Fluoxetine in children and adolescents with OCD: a placebo-controlled trial. *J Am Acad Child Adolesc Psychiatry* 2004; **41**: 1431–8.

45 Geller DA, Wagner KD, Emslie G et al.: Paroxetine treatment in children and adolescents with obsessive-compulsive disorder: a randomized, multicenter, double-blind, placebo-controlled trial. *J Am Acad Child Adolesc Psychiatry* 2004; **43**: 1387–96.

46 March JS, Biederman J, Wolkow R et al.: Sertraline in children and adolescents with obsessive-compulsive disorder: a multicenter randomized controlled trial.[Erratum appears in JAMA 2000 Mar 8;283(10):1293]. *JAMA* 2000; **280**: 1752–6.

47 Pediatric OCD Treatment Study Team: cognitive-behavior therapy, sertraline, and their combination for children and adolescents with obsessive-compulsive disorder: the Pediatric OCD Treatment Study (POTS) randomized controlled trial. *JAMA* 2004; **292**: 1969–76.

48 Koran LM, Hanna GL, Hollander E et al.: Practice guideline for the treatment of patients with obsessive-compulsive disorder. *Am J Psychiatry* 2007; **164**(7 Suppl): 5–53.

49 Costello EJ, Egger HL, Angold A: Developmental epidemiology of anxiety disorders. In: Ollendick TH, March JS (eds) *Phobic and Anxiety Disorders in Children and Adolescents: A Clinician's Guide to Effective Psychosocial and Pharmacological Interventions*. New York, NY: Oxford University Press, 2004.

50 Merikangas KR, He J-P, Brody D et al.: Prevalence and treatment of mental disorders among U.S. children in the 2001–2004 NHANES. *Pediatrics* 2001; **125**: 75–81.

51 Brady EU, Kendall PC: Comorbidity of anxiety and depression in children and adolescents. *Psychological Bulletin* 1992; **111**: 244–55.

52 Wood JJ: Effect of anxiety reduction on children's school performance and social adjustment. *Dev Psychol* 2006; **42**: 345–9.

53 Langley AK, Bergman RL, McCracken J et al.: Impairment in childhood anxiety disorders: preliminary examination of the child anxiety impact scale-parent version. *J Child Adolesc Psychopharmacol* 2004; **14**: 105–14.

54 Wood JJ, McLeod BD, Sigman M et al.: Parenting and childhood anxiety: theory, empirical findings, and future directions. *J Child Psychol Psychiatry* 2003; **44**: 134–51.

55 Comment in *Child Psychol Psychiatry* 2007; **48**(12): 1157–9.

56 Beesdo K, Bittner A, Pine DS et al.: Incidence of social anxiety disorder and the consistent risk for secondary depression in the first three decades of life. *Arch Gen Psychiatry* 2007; **64**: 903–12.

57 Bolton JM, Cox BJ, Afifi TO et al.: Anxiety disorders and risk for suicide attempts: findings from the Baltimore Epidemiologic Catchment area follow-up study. *Depress Anxiety* 2008; **25**: 477–81.

58 Buckner JD, Schmidt NB, Lang AR et al.: Specificity of social anxiety disorder as a risk factor for alcohol and cannabis dependence. *J Psychiatr Res* 2008; **42**: 230–9.

59 Connolly SD, Bernstein GA, Work Group on Quality I. Practice parameter for the assessment and treatment of children and adolescents with anxiety disorders. 2007; *J Am Acad Child Adolesc Psychiatry* **46**: 267–83.

60 Walkup JT, Albano AM, Piacentini J et al.: Cognitive behavioral therapy, sertraline, or a combination in childhood anxiety. *N Engl J Med* 2008; **359**: 2753–66.

61 Rynn MA, Siqueland L, Rickels K: Placebo-controlled trial of sertraline in the treatment of children with generalized anxiety disorder. *Am J Psychiatry* 2001; **158**: 2008–14.

62 Birmaher B, Axelson DA, Monk K et al.: Fluoxetine for the treatment of childhood anxiety disorders. *J Am Acad Child Adolesc Psychiatry* 2003; **42**: 415–23.

63 Wagner KD, Berard R, Stein MB et al.: A multicenter, randomized, double-blind, placebo-controlled trial of paroxetine in children and adolescents with social anxiety disorder. *Arch Gen Psychiatry* 2004; **61**: 1153–162.

64 Beidel DC, Turner SM, Sallee FR et al.: SET-C versus fluoxetine in the treatment of childhood social phobia. *J Am Acad Child Adolesc Psychiatry* 2007; **46**: 1622–32.

65 Research Units on Pediatric Psychopharmacology Anxiety Study G, Walkup J, Labellarte M et al. Treatment of pediatric anxiety disorders: an open-label extension of the research units on pediatric psychopharmacology anxiety study. *J Child Adolesc Psychopharmacol* 2002; **12**: 175–88.

66 Clark DB, Birmaher B, Axelson D et al.: Fluoxetine for the treatment of childhood anxiety disorders: open-label, long-term extension to a controlled trial. *J Am Acad Child Adolesc Psychiatry* 2005; **44**: 1263–70.

67 Renaud J, Birmaher B, Wassick SC et al.: Use of selective serotonin reuptake inhibitors for the treatment of childhood panic disorder: a pilot study. *J Child Adolesc Psychopharmacol* 1999; **9**: 73–83.

68 Masi G, Toni C, Mucci M et al.: Paroxetine in child and adolescent outpatients with panic disorder. *J Child Adolesc Psychopharmacol* 2001; **11**: 151–7.

69 Pincus DB, May JE, Whitton SW et al.: Cognitive-behavioral treatment of panic disorder in adolescence. *J Clin Child Adolesc Psychol* 2010; **39**: 638–49.

70 Kessler RC, Sonnega A, Bromet E et al.: Posttraumatic stress disorder in the National Comorbidity Survey. *Arch Gen Psychiatry* 1995; **52**: 1048–60.

71 Cohen JA, Bukstein O, Walter H et al.: Practice parameter for the assessment and treatment of children and adolescents with posttraumatic stress disorder. *J Am Acad Child Adolesc Psychiatry* 2010; **49**: 414–30.

72 Robb A, Cueva J, Sporn J et al.: Efficacy of sertraline in childhood posttraumatic stress disorder. The Scientific Proceedings of the 2008 Annual Meeting of the American Academy of Child and Adolescent Psychiatry. New Research Poster 3.8, 2008.

73 Cohen JA, Mannarino AP, Perel JM et al.: A pilot randomized controlled trial of combined trauma-focused CBT and sertraline for childhood PTSD symptoms. *Journal of the American Academy of Child & Adolescent Psychiatry* 2007; **46**: 811–19.

74 Emslie G, Kratochvil C, Vitiello B, Silva S, Mayes T, McNulty S et al.: Treatment for Adolescents with Depression Study (TADS): safety results. *J Am Acad Child Adolesc Psychiatry* 2006; **45**: 1440–55.

75 Safer DJ, Zito JM: Treatment-emergent adverse events from selective serotonin reuptake inhibitors by age group: children versus adolescents. *J Child Adolesc Psychopharmacol* 2006; **16**: 159–69.

76 Wilens TE, Wyatt D, Spencer TJ: Disentangling disinhibition. *J Am Acad Child Adolesc Psychiatry* 1998; **37**: 1225–7.

77 Boyer EW, Shannon M: The serotonin syndrome. *N Engl J Med* 2005; **352**: 1112–20.

78 Lake MB, Birmaher B, Wassick S et al.: Bleeding and selective serotonin reuptake inhibitors in childhood and adolescence. *J Child Adolesc Psychopharmacol* 2000; **10**: 5–8.

79 Weinrieb RM, Auriacombe M, Lynch KG et al.: Selective serotonin re-uptake inhibitors and the risk of bleeding. *Expert Opin Drug Saf* 2005; **4**: 337–44.

80 Hammad TA, Laughren T, Racoosin J: Suicidality in pediatric patients treated with antidepressant drugs. *Arch Gen Psychiatry* 2006; **63**: 332–9.

81 Olfson M, Shaffer D, Marcus SC et al.: Relationship between antidepressant medication treatment and suicide in adolescents. *Arch Gen Psychiatry* 2003; **60**: 978–82.

82 Gibbons RD, Hur K, Bhaumik DK et al.: The relationship between antidepressant prescription rates and rate of early adolescent suicide. *Am J Psychiatry* 2006; **163**: 1898–904.

83 Valuck RJ, Libby AM, Sills MR et al.: Antidepressant treatment and risk of suicide attempt by adolescents with major depressive disorder: a propensity-adjusted retrospective cohort study. *CNS Drugs* 2004; **18**: 1119–32.

84 Gibbons RD, Brown CH, Hur K et al.: Early evidence on the effects of regulators' suicidality warnings on SSRI prescriptions and suicide in children and adolescents. *Am J Psychiatry* 2007; **164**: 1356–63.

85 Schatzberg AF, Haddad P, Kaplan EM et al.: Serotonin reuptake inhibitor discontinuation syndrome: a hypothetical definition. Discontinuation Consensus panel. *J Clin Psychiatry* 1997; **7**: 5–10.

86 Baldwin DS, Montgomery SA, Nil R et al.: Discontinuation symptoms in depression and anxiety disorders. *Int J Neuropsychopharmacol* 2007; **10**: 73–84.

87 Tint A, Haddad PM, Anderson IM: The effect of rate of antidepressant tapering on the incidence of discontinuation symptoms: a randomised study. *J Psychopharmacol* 2008; **22**: 330–2.

CHAPTER 9

Novel (Atypical) Antidepressants

Heidi R. Bruty, Graham J. Emslie & Paul Croarkin
University of Texas Southwestern Medical Center, Dallas, USA

Novel (atypical) antidepressants

While the selective serotonin-reuptake inhibitors (SSRIs, reviewed in the previous chapter) are the first-line treatment for juvenile depression [1] and anxiety disorders [2], other novel antidepressants not chemically related to the SSRIs, such as bupropion, (Wellbutrin™), duloxetine hydrochloride (Cymbalta™), mirtazapine (Remeron™), trazodone (Desyrel™), venlafaxine (Effexor™), and desvenlafaxine (Pristiq™) have also been prescribed to children and adolescents for unlabeled (non-FDA-approved) indications. Their psychopharmacological profile and relevant pediatric studies are summarized in this chapter. Nefazadone (a mixed serotonin antagonist and reuptake inhibitor) will not be discussed in this chapter as it has been removed from the U.S. drug market due to the risk of hepatotoxicity. Alternative or complimentary treatments, such as St. John's wort, omega-3 fatty acids, thyroid hormones, and S-adenosyl methionine (SAMe) will also be reviewed in this chapter.

General overview

Currently, several of the novel antidepressants have an FDA indication for the treatment of depression and/or generalized anxiety disorder in adults, although none of them are approved for treatment of any disorder in children and adolescents. There appears to be less evidence of efficacy for these medications in the pediatric age group, although they may be good alternatives to SSRIs in some patients, particularly those who fail to respond to first-line treatments.

As with the SSRIs, these antidepressants should be started at low doses and titrated slowly in youth, with the target doses being similar to those used for adults. Generally, the novel antidepressants display a lower side-effect profile than TCAs and monamine oxidase inhibitors (MAOIs),

Pharmacotherapy of Child and Adolescent Psychiatric Disorders, Third Edition.
Edited by David R. Rosenberg and Samuel Gershon.
© 2012 John Wiley & Sons, Ltd. Published 2012 by John Wiley & Sons, Ltd.

Box 9.1   Adverse effects associated with novel antidepressants

Common adverse effects
  Nausea
  Diarrhea
  Dry mouth
  Weight loss
  Headache
  Insomnia
  Drowsiness
  Dizziness or lightheadedness
  Fatigue or asthenia

Less common adverse effects
  Anxiety
  Nervousness
  Behavioral activation
  Increased thoughts of suicide
  Excessive sweating
  Sexual side effects

Rare but serious adverse effects
  Mania or hypomania
  Aggression or significant behavior change
  Suicide attempt

---

and appear to have a higher margin of safety in overdose compared to the TCAs and MAOIs (although some cases of death have been reported with large ingestions). Most side-effects emerge within the first few weeks of treatment, and resolve with time. With the exception of trazodone, they have low or no sexual side-effects. Ideally, these antidepressants are tapered slowly to avoid discontinuation syndrome, which is most pronounced with the use of venlafaxine and desvenlafaxine. Box 9.1 lists the most common side-effects of the novel antidepressants.

All antidepressants, including the ones reviewed in this chapter, have a black-box warning for possible increased risk of suicidal thinking and behavior in children and adolescents. The risk of suicidality for these medications was examined in a pooled analysis of data from acute placebo-controlled studies of nine antidepressants (bupropion, citalopram, fluoxetine, fluvoxamine, mirtazapine, nefazodone, paroxetine, sertraline, venlafaxine) in over 4400 children and adolescents with major depressive disorder, obsessive-compulsive disorder (OCD), or other psychiatric disorders. The analysis revealed an increased risk of suicidal behavior or thinking in pediatric patients receiving antidepressants compared to those receiving placebo (4% versus 2%) [3]. No suicides occurred in the pediatric patients in these studies. In a separate meta-analysis of the risk and benefit of the antidepressants, Bridge and colleagues [4] reported suicidal behavior rates of 3% in active treatment versus 2% in placebo. Furthermore, the authors reported the benefits of the medications out-weighed the risk, with the best risk-benefit ratio found in OCD, followed by non-OCD anxiety disorders and depression [4]. Despite the potential benefits, using antidepressant agents on a child or adolescent patient for any clinical use must balance the potential risk of therapy with the clinical need. Close monitoring of suicidal ideation and behaviors is suggested when starting an antidepressant and at dosage adjustments.

Similar to SSRIs, the novel antidepressants should not be taken con-comitantly with any of the MAOIs (or within two weeks of beginning or discontinuing a MAOI), as the combination of these drugs may lead to confusion, high blood pressure, tremor, hyperactivity and/or death. In addition, concurrent tryptophan with novel antidepressants can cause headaches, nausea, sweating and dizziness associated with serotonin over-load.

All of the antidepressants in this section are category C for pregnancy, which indicates uncertain safety for use in pregnancy, although no human studies or animal studies show adverse effects. Due to the Class C category, any female of child-bearing age should be counseled on the potential risks of the medications on the fetus, and a pregnancy test should be performed before starting these agents.

Information regarding the chemical properties, dosage and administration, pharmacokinetics, treatment indications, potential side-effects, and warnings or precautions about each of the novel antidepressants are re-viewed below.

Bupropion

Chemical properties
Bupropion is an atypical antidepressant unrelated to the TCAs or other currently available antidepressants [5]. It is classified as a monocyclic phenylbutylamine aminoketone, is structurally related to amphetamine, and resembles the sympathomimetic, diethylpropion. Bupropion is a norepinephrine and dopamine reuptake inhibitor with minimal effects on serotonin.

Pharmacokinetics
Bupropion is rapidly absorbed from the GI tract after oral administration. It is primarily metabolized by the liver, and its metabolites, hydroxy-bupropion and threohydrobupropion are excreted in the urine [6, 7]. These metabolites may have particular clinical relevance. Golden and

Table 9.1 Pharmacodynamics and pharmacokinetics of novel antidepressants

Medication	Half-life	Time to steady state	Cytochrome P450 enzyme inhibited	Kinetics
Bupropion	Biphasic: 1.5 hours 14 hours	8 days	2D6 (potent)	Linear
Bupropion SR	21 hours	8 days	2D6 (potent)	Linear
Duloxetine	12.5 hours	3 days	1A2 (potent) 2D6 (potent)	Linear
Mirtazapine	20–40 hours	4 days	No known inhibition substrate for: 1A2, 2D6, 3A4	Linear
Trazodone	Biphasic: 3–6 hours 5–9 hours	Unknown	No known inhibition substrate for: 3A4, 2D6	Nonlinear
Venlafaxine XR	10.3 hours	3 days	2D6 (minimal) 3A4 (minimal)	Linear
Desvenlafaxine	11 hours	4–5 days	2D6 (minimal)	Linear

SR = sustained release; XR = extended release.

associates found that plasma hydroxybupropion concentrations greater than 1250 ng/ml were correlated with a lack of positive clinical response to bupropion therapy [8]. Peak plasma concentrations are achieved within two hours of the conventional or extended release formulation [6, 9]. The half-life of bupropion ranges from eight to 24 hours following single doses [6, 10]. Table 9.1 provides specific pharmacodynamic and pharmacokinetic information for the novel antidepressants.

The only pharmacokinetic study conducted in adolescents with bupropion was in 75 smoking and nonsmoking youth. Females had higher blood levels, larger volume of distribution, and longer half-lives than males. Generally, the pharmacokinetics of bupropion appear to be similar for adolescents and adults, although studies involving bupropion's metabolite, hydroxybupropion, have shown differences between adolescents and adults [11–13].

Dosage and administration

Bupropion has immediate release, sustained release (SR), and extended release (XL) formulations. The immediate release formulation comes in 75 mg and 100 mg tablets; the sustained release formulation is available in 100 mg, 150 mg, and 200 mg tablets; and the extended release formulation is available in 150 mg and 300 mg tablets. Formulations and dosing information for the novel antidepressants are included in Table 9.2.

Table 9.2 Novel antidepressant formulations and dosing

Medication	Formulations	Initial dose	Target dose (children)	Target dose (adolescents)	Max dose
Bupropion, Bupropion SR	*Tab:* 75 mg, 100 mg *Tab ER:* 100 mg, 150 mg, 200 mg	100 mg	150–300 mg	300 mg	300 mg
Bupropion XL	*Tab ER:* 150 mg, 300 mg	150 mg	150–300 mg	450 mg	450 mg
Duloxetine	*Cap:* 20 mg, 30 mg, 60 mg	20 mg bid	40–60 mg	40–60 mg	60 mg
Mirtazapine	*Tab:* 15 mg, 30 mg, 45 mg *Tab Dissolve:* 15 mg, 30 mg, 45 mg	7.5–15 mg	15–5 mg	15–45 mg	45 mg
Trazodone	*Tab:* 50 mg, 100 mg, 150 mg, 300 mg	25–50 mg	100–150 mg	100–150 mg	150 mg
Venlafaxine XR	*Cap:* 37.5 mg, 75 mg, 150 mg	37.5 mg	150–225 mg	150–225 mg	300 mg
Desvenlafaxine*	*Tab:* 50 mg, 100 mg	50 mg	50 mg	50 mg	50 mg

ER = extended release; SR = sustained release; XL = extended release; XR = extended release.
*Currently, there are no data available on dosing of desvenlafaxine in youth. Adult data suggests no additional benefit in doses above 50 mg, so at this time, the authors recommend low dosing for youth until additional dosing data are obtained

Bupropion immediate release is administered three times daily, with six or more hours separating doses [14, 15]. As sustained-release tablets, bupropion is administered twice daily in the morning and mid-day or evening [14, 15]. The extended-release formulation is dosed once daily, typically in the morning. Avoiding bedtime administration of the evening dose may lessen the occurrence of insomnia. Initial dosing of bupropion and bupropion SR is 100 mg, with a target dose for children and adolescents between 150–300 mg. Bupropion XL is initiated at 150 mg, with a target dose of 150–300 mg in children and 300–450 mg in adolescents.

Prior to initiating a bupropion trial, children and adolescents should have a physical and neurologic examination. A baseline screen for abnormal involuntary movements, including tics should be performed. It is important to elicit any family history of motor tic disorders. A thorough drug and alcohol evaluation should be conducted because bupropion should not be started after recent withdrawal from alcohol or benzodiazepines. Use of drugs and alcohol while on bupropion should be discouraged. It is also important to determine the eating habits of patients being considered for bupropion therapy because bupropion is contraindicated in patients with a current or past history of bulimia or anorexia nervosa [16].

Indications

Bupropion is FDA-approved for the treatment of depression in adults (AHFS, 2010). Limited data is available in children and adolescents [17]. An open trial of bupropion in 24 adolescents (ages 11–16) with ADHD and depression was promising [18], and a small open trial suggested that higher plasma levels of bupropion were associated with treatment response in depressed youth (n = 16) [19].

The use of bupropion as a potential second-line treatment for ADHD has been substantiated by several controlled studies [17, 20–23]. Table 9.3 provides information on the randomized controlled trials (RCTs) reported to date for the novel antidepressants. Clay and colleagues [22] used bupropion to treat 30 prepubertal children with diagnosis of ADHD in a double-blind placebo controlled study. The authors found that children with prominent conduct disorder symptoms, or prior stimulant-resistant patients, responded well to bupropion. Optimal doses ranged from 3 to 7 mg/kg/day (100–250 mg/day). Some patients who did not respond well to bupropion responded well to methylphenidate prescribed openly at a later time [22]. Casat and colleagues [21] also found significant improvements with bupropion compared to placebo in 30 children with ADHD. Finally, Conners and collaborators conducted a multisite, double-blind, placebo-controlled trial of bupropion for the treatment of children with ADHD. One-hundred-and-nine children with ADHD (six to 12 years old) were randomized to receive bupropion (3 to 6 mg/kg per day; n = 72) or placebo (n = 37), administered at 7 a.m. and 7 p.m. A significant treatment effect was apparent at day 3 for hyperactivity and conduct dysregulation on the Conners teacher's checklist, and at day 28 for conduct problems and impulsive behavior on the Conners Parent and Teacher Questionnaire. Four children had rash and urticaria requiring discontinuation of the drug [17].

Bupropion has also been used for smoking cessation in adolescents. In an open study of 16 adolescent smokers, there was a significant reduction in cigarette smoking, and 31% of participants were completely abstinent from smoking by the end of six weeks of treatment [24]. Double-blind, placebo-controlled studies have been less consistent. In a study comparing bupropion and placebo, both with and without a contingency management program, bupropion plus contingency management lead to decreased smoking compared to placebo plus contingency management [25]. However, in a study comparing bupropion and placebo in which all participants also received a nicotine patch, the addition of bupropion did not lead to a greater reduction in smoking than the patch plus placebo [26]. It does appear that bupropion may be a potentially effective treatment for smoking cessation in teens.

Table 9.3 Pediatric RCTs for novel antidepressants

Study	Medication	Disorder	N	Age	Study results
Clay et al., 1988 [22]	Buproprion	ADHD	30	6–12	Positive
Simeon et al., 1986 [23]	Bupropion	ADHD	17	7–13	Positive
Casat et al., 1989 [21]	Bupropion	ADHD	30	6–12	Positive
Conners et al., 1996 [17]	Bupropion	ADHD	109	6–12	Positive
Gray et al., 2011 [25]	Bupropion	Smoking Cessation	134	12–21	Positive (both groups also randomized to with and without contingency management)
Killen et al., 2004 [26]	Bupropion	Smoking Cessation	211	15–18	Negative (both groups also had a nicotine patch and skills training sessions)
Reported in Bridge et al., 2007 and Cheung et al., 2005 [4, 46]	Mirtazapine	MDD	126	7–17	Negative
Reported in Bridge et al., 2007 and Cheung et al., 2005 [4, 46]	Mirtazapine	MDD	124	7–17	Negative
Battistella et al., 1993 [59]	Trazodone	Migraines	40	7–18	Negative; however, only those on trazodone in phase 2 continued to report improvement in migraines
Mandoki et al., 1997 [70]	Venlafaxine	MDD	33	8–17	Negative
Emslie et al., 2007 [69]	Venlafaxine	MDD	334	7–17	Negative overall; positive for adolescent age group (data combined from two studies)
Rynn et al., 2007 [72]	Venlafaxine	GAD	320	6–17	Positive
March et al., 2007 [73]	Venlafaxine	Soc phob	293	8–17	Positive

ADHD = attention deficit hyperactivity disorder; GAD = generalized anxiety disorder; MDD = major depressive disorder; RCTs = randomized controlled trials; Soc phob = social phobia.

No reports of RCTs for bupropion or desvenlafaxine. A RCT for duloxetine in adolescents has recently been completed but results are not yet known.

Side-effects

Bupropion has few anticholinergic effects and does not alter cardiac conduction or cause orthostasis. Agitation, restlessness, irritability, headache, insomnia, tremor, constipation and nausea may be common side-effects seen with bupropion therapy [8,27,28]. Weight loss may occur in approximately 25% of patients [28]. Bupropion should be given cautiously to patients with liver or kidney disease.

Bupropion appears to have positive effects on cognitive tasks. Clay and colleagues [22] noted in their study in children with ADHD that bupropion had positive effects on memory performance, which may be unique among the antidepressants. Other antidepressants either have no effect or a negative effect on memory performance. It should be noted, however, that Ferguson and Simeon [23] observed no adverse or positive effects on cognition on a cognitive battery in 17 children with ADHD or conduct disorders receiving bupropion.

Warnings/precautions

Seizure is the side-effect of most concern with bupropion [29]. Seizures have been found to occur in 0.4% of all patients treated with bupropion doses of 450 mg/day or less, which is a four-times increased incidence compared to other available antidepressants [16]. Because of this increased risk it is recommended that daily doses of bupropion should not exceed 450 mg. In addition, no individual dose should be greater than 150 mg, or given more frequently than every 6 hours.

Because of its significantly increased association with seizures [16, 30], bupropion is not recommended in children and adolescents with a history of seizures, head trauma, CNS tumor or other organic brain disease. Although children and adolescents appear to be far less susceptible to severe withdrawal phenomena, including seizures, when alcohol and benzodiazepines are abruptly withdrawn (see substance-abuse chapter), we do not recommend bupropion in such patients because of its increased association with seizures. Caution should be observed with concurrent administration of bupropion and drugs (for example, antidepressants, antipsychotics, lithium, theophylline, corticosteroids) that lower the seizure threshold [16].

In addition, because bupropion crosses the placenta and is secreted in breast milk, it should not be used in pregnant or lactating women.

Duloxetine

Chemical properties

Duloxetine is a dual serotonin and norepinephrine reuptake inhibitor (SSNRI) with a threefold greater potency at the serotonin reuptake transporter than at the norepinephrine reuptake transporter [31]. It has less potent dopaminergic reuptake inhibition, and it has minimal affinity for serotonergic, adrenergic, cholinergic, histaminergic, opioid, dopamine, glutamate, and GABA receptors. It has multiple metabolites, although these do not appear to have any relevant pharmacological activity [32].

Pharmacokinetics

Duloxetine is absorbed from the GI tract following oral administration. Food does not affect the maximum plasma concentration but does delay absorption, and decreases the amount absorbed by about 10% [33]. It can be taken with or without food. The capsules contain enteric-coated pellets that prevent the drug from degrading in the stomach. There is a median delay of about two hours until absorption begins, and peak plasma levels are achieved about six hours after ingestion of the drug [33]. A study on the pharmacokinetics of duloxetine in children and adolescents has been completed (Clinicaltrials.gov # NCT00529789), although the results are not yet published. Additional pharmacodynamic and pharmacokinetic information for duloxetine is available in Table 9.1.

Dosage and administration

Duloxetine is available in 20 mg, 30 mg, and 60 mg capsules. Dosing is initiated at 20 mg twice daily, with a target dose of 40–60 mg in both children and adolescents (Table 9.2). Duloxetine can be taken with or without food.

Indications

Duloxetine is indicated for the treatment of major depressive disorder and diabetic peripheral neuropathic pain in adults. There is significant research data demonstrating that serotonergic-noradrenergic antidepressants possess more effective analgesic properties than noradrenergic antidepressants [34] and, therefore, duloxetine is commonly used for the treatment of depression and co-morbid pain disorders. Two case reports have suggested that duloxetine may improve experience of pain and depressive symptoms in 3 cases of adolescent females with chronic or severe pain and depressive symptoms [35, 36]. Two randomized, controlled trials comparing duloxetine, fluoxetine, and placebo in children and adolescents with depression are under way (Clinialtrials.gov # NCT00849693 and # NCT00849901).

Side-effects

The most common untoward effects of duloxetine reported in adult placebo-controlled clinical trials were nausea, dry mouth, constipation, fatigue, decreased appetite, somnolence and increased sweating. Dulox-etine was associated with a mean blood pressure increase of 2 mm Hg systolic and 0.5 mm Hg diastolic compared to levels with placebo. There are currently no reports on the safety and tolerability of duloxetine in ado-lescents.

Warnings/precautions

Duloxetine is not recommended for patients with severe or end stage renal disease or patients with hepatic failure, as metabolism and elimination are decreased [32]. Potential pharmacokinetic interactions occur with thiori-dazine (increased plasma thioridazine concentrations) which may result in increased risk of serious ventricular arrhythmias and sudden death; con-comitant use it not recommended by manufacturer of duloxetine [37].

Mirtazapine

Chemical properties

Mirtazapine is a piperazino-azepine-derivative antidepressant agent [38, 39]. It differs structurally from selective serotonin reuptake inhibitors, as well as tricyclic antidepressants. Mirtazapine appears to act as an an-tagonist of the central presynaptic alpha2-adrenergic autoreceptors and heteroreceptors, resulting in an antidepressant effect related to enhanced central noradrenergic and serotonergic activity [40]. It is also an antago-nist of 5-HT2 and 5-HT3 receptors, and an enhancer of 5-HT1A-mediated neurotransmission [40]. Mirtazapine antagonizes histamine H1 receptors, which may account for its prominent sedative effect [39], especially in the low dosage range. In addition, mirtazapine exhibits moderate peripheral alpha1-adrenergic blockade reportedly causing occasional orthostatic hy-potension [39].

Pharmacokinetics

Peak plasma concentrations of mirtazapine occur about two hours after ingestion [33]. Its elimination half-life in adults is 20-40 hours [39] and is significantly longer in females (mean, 37 hours) than in males (mean, 26 hours) [33]. Steady-state plasma levels occur within 5 days (Table 9.1), and the drug is eliminated primarily through urinary excretion (75%), with the remainder in feces [33]. Liver and/or renal failure may decrease clearance of mirtazapine by 30–50% [41].

Only one pharmacokinetic study of mirtazapine has been conducted in pediatric patients. Sixteen youth (ages 7–17 years) with depression were given a single dose of 15 mg; maximum plasma concentration decreased with higher ages, and half-life increased with increased weight [42].

Dosage and administration

Mirtazapine is available in 15 mg, 30 mg, and 45 mg tablets (Remeron®; Organon) [16]. It is administered orally as conventional or orally disintegrating tablets. It is often administered at bedtime due to its sedative effects. Food does not appear to affect absorption rates of mirtazapine; thus, it can be administered without regard to meals [39] (Table 9.2). The recommended initial dosage in adults for major depressive disorder is 15 mg daily. Dosage may be increased up to a maximum of 45 mg daily [43] at intervals of 1–2 weeks [39].

Indications

Mirtazapine is FDA approved for the treatment of major depressive disorder in adults [44]. Although a multi-site open label study of mirtazapine demonstrated some efficacy in the treatment of adolescent depression [45], there is not strong data with double-blind, placebo controlled trials available to demonstrate safety and efficacy. In a review of pediatric depression studies, Cheung and colleagues [46] reported on the findings from two double-blind, placebo-controlled trials of mirtazapine in 259 children and adolescents (ages 7–17 years) with major depressive disorder. Mirtazapine and placebo were not significantly different on any of the outcome ratings, although this could in part be due to the high placebo response rate.

No double-blind, placebo-controlled studies have been conducted with mirtazapine in anxiety disorders; however, two open-label studies suggest potential benefit in this population. An eight-week open-label pilot study of mirtazapine in children with social phobia age 8–17 years found that 56% (10/18) responded to treatment, although only 17% (3/18) achieved full remission. However, most patients (61%) did not complete all eight weeks of treatment, with four patients (22%) discontinuing due to adverse effects such as fatigue and irritability [47]. Another open-label study of mirtazapine involved youth with PTSD. Using up to 45 mg/day for eight weeks, the authors reported improvement (>50%) in 50% of the sample when comparing baseline with global ratings at weeks 2, 4, 6 and 8. Improvements in self-rated scales of depression were also noted. The drug was well tolerated with few significant side-effects [48].

Larger controlled trials are needed to further evaluate efficacy and safety of mirtazapine for anxiety disorders.

Due to mirtazapine's sedating effects, it has been suggested that it may be beneficial for insomnia. A study looking at the effect of mirtazapine on sleep architecture reported significantly decreased sleep latency and significantly increased total sleep time and sleep efficiency after one week in six adults (and adolescents) with MDD [49]. Polysomnographic evaluations performed at baseline and after 1 week (on 15 mg at bedtime) and two weeks (30 mg at bedtime) of mirtazapine, showed no significant alteration of rapid-eye-movement sleep parameters [49]. Results of this study could theoretically support the judicious use of this compound in children and adolescents suffering from rebound hyperactivity at bedtime or insomnia secondary to a mood disorder.

Side-effects

Mirtazapine appears to have fewer side-effects than other antidepressants, and is generally well tolerated. One of the most common adverse effects of mirtazapine is sedation [50]. Another common untoward side-effect is increased appetite, often leading to weight gain [33]. Dizziness, dry mouth and constipation are also relatively common [33].

Warnings/precautions

Mirtazapine was associated with the development of severe neutropenia in about 0.1% of patients in premarketing clinical trials [33]. When a patient on mirtazapine develops signs of infection and has a low white blood cell count, mirtazapine should be discontinued and the patient closely monitored.

Trazodone

Chemical properties

Trazodone is a triazolopyridine-derivative antidepressant that is chemically and structurally unrelated to tricyclic or tetracyclic antidepressants or to SSRIs [16]. The precise mechanism of antidepressant action of trazodone is unclear, but the drug has been shown to block the reuptake of serotonin (5-HT) selectively at the presynaptic neuronal membrane [16]. Although trazodone is commonly referred to as a serotonin (5-hydroxytryptamine; 5-HT) uptake inhibitor, its most important pharmacological effect is the antagonism of 5-HT2/1C receptors [51] (Table 9.1).

Pharmacokinetics

Trazodone is rapidly absorbed from the GI tract following oral administration, and achieves peak plasma concentrations in approximately 1–2 hours [16]. These peak plasma levels are achieved more rapidly on an empty stomach, as the total drug absorption may be up to 20% when the drug is taken with food. Plasma concentrations of trazodone decline in a biphasic manner. The half-life of trazodone in the initial phase ($t_{1/2\,a}$) is about 3–6 hours and the half-life in the terminal phase ($t_{1/2\,b}$) is about 5–9 hours

(Table 9.1). Trazodone is metabolized by the liver, and its active metabolite, m-chlorophenyl-piperazine, is excreted by the kidneys [16].

Dosage and administration

Trazodone is available in 50 mg, 100 mg, 150 mg and 300 mg tablets (Desyrel® Dividose®; Apothecon) [16]. The initial adult dosage is typically 150 mg daily given in divided doses, taken shortly after a meal [16]. Dosages may be increased by 50 mg/day every three or four days, depending on therapeutic response and tolerance. The maximum dosage for outpatients usually does not exceed 400 mg daily [16] (Table 9.2).

Indications

Trazodone is approved for the treatment of major depressive disorder in adults [16]. No placebo-controlled trials have been conducted with trazodone in youth with depressive disorders. Trazodone is best known for its sedative effect, and it is therefore often used to treat insomnia, as it increases total sleep time, decreases the number of night-time awakenings, decreases REM sleep, and does not decrease stage IV sleep [52]. In fact, in a survey of child and adolescent psychiatrists, trazodone was the most commonly prescribed insomnia medication in youth with mood and anxiety disorders [53].

However, the safety and efficacy of trazodone in children younger than 18 years of age have not been established. Given the dearth of controlled data, we do not recommend the routine use of trazodone in children and adolescents with major depressive disorder or other psychiatric illnesses. The following are pediatric reports of interest: Levi and Sogos [54] treated a mixed group of 80 pediatric outpatients (ages 9–13) with major depressive disorder, co-morbid with oppositional defiant disorder, generalized anxiety disorder, and learning disorders. These youngsters received weekly blind ratings, while taking 75 mg of trazodone for four months. Trazodone was reportedly safe and effective for over 50% of the sample [54]. The co-morbidity with oppositional defiant disorder was associated with poorer response [54].

A retrospective review of adolescents with major depressive disorder and insomnia, receiving fluoxetine (average 20 mg/day), trazodone (71 mg/day), or a fluoxetine-trazodone combination (fluoxetine 29 mg/day, trazodone 68 mg/day) examined the relative effectiveness of each drug in relieving insomnia [55]. Although the mean time to resolution of insomnia was significantly faster in adolescents treated with trazodone, the median time to insomnia resolution was two days in the trazodone group and four days in the fluoxetine group, questioning the clinical significance of the statistical finding [55].

Zubieta and Alessi conducted an open trial of trazodone in the treatment of severe behavioral disturbances in 22 hospitalized children diagnosed with disruptive behavioral and mood disorders, previously unresponsive to other treatments [56]. Assessed by overall clinical criteria, thirteen children (67%) were considered responders to a mean dose of 185 ± 117 mg/day (given three times/day) for a mean of 27 ± 20 days. Aggressive, impulsive behaviors were symptoms most frequently improved by trazodone. One patient reported painful erections. The most frequent side-effect was orthostatic hypotension. Three nonresponders worsened in symptomatology [56].

The combination of haloperidol and trazodone was evaluated in an open-label trial of ten patients with chronic tics and Tourette's disorder. A mean reduction of symptoms of 59% was found, with a statistically significant difference between the baseline and endpoint treatment conditions, suggesting a potential for using lower doses of haloperidol for the treatment of tics in children [57].

Ten adolescents with bulimia were treated in an open-label, flexible-dose study of trazodone for a mean duration of seven weeks, at a mean maximum dose of 410 mg [58]. The authors reported that the number of binge eating and vomiting episodes was significantly decreased. Pretreatment versus post-treatment mean weight was essentially unchanged. Mild side-effects noted were morning drowsiness and headache [58].

The only placebo-controlled study of trazodone in pediatric patients has been for treatment of migraines. A double-blind, placebo-controlled, crossover trial showed that both trazodone and placebo reduced migraines during the first phase of the trial; however, only those on trazodone during the second phase continued to report improvement in migraines [59].

All of the above reports await replication by controlled studies. In the meantime, the use of trazodone in children and adolescents with major depressive disorder is at best recommended for female youngsters who have failed other first-line agents (such as SSRIs) or who present with insomnia as one of their salient clinical features. Other disorders for which trazodone does not have FDA approval, including bulimia nervosa, tics and impulsive-aggressive behavior, await further replication in pediatric populations before off-label treatment can be suggested.

Side-effects

The incidence and severity of adverse reactions to trazodone in relation to dosage and duration of therapy have not been fully characterized; however, adverse effects appear to occur more frequently at dosages greater than 300 mg/day [16]. Adverse effects appear to be mild to moderate in severity and may decrease after the first few weeks of trazodone therapy. Below is a list of the most common side-effects. However, with the limited available placebo-controlled data in youth, the side-effects included here are based primarily on adults.

Priapism

Priapism is a potential side-effect of trazodone therapy, resulting in a prolonged penile erection [60]. The occurrence of priapism constitutes a medical emergency because it may result in permanent erectile dysfunction even when prompt treatment is received. Priapism may be secondary to trazodone's alpha-adrenergic blocking properties. Adolescent male patients should be questioned concerning prior occurrence of prolonged erections because a past history of delayed detumescence has been reported in approximately 50% of subsequent cases of priapism [60]. This potential side-effect precludes the enthusiastic endorsement of trazodone therapy in male adolescents.

Orthostatic hypotension

In adults, hypotension, including orthostatic hypotension, is the most frequent adverse cardiovascular effect of trazodone, occurring in about 5% of adult patients receiving the drug. In most patients, hypotension is mild and not dose related. This side-effect may be less common in children and adolescents, although there is limited data on trazodone's efficacy and toxicity in this population [16].

Other side-effects

Sedation and dizziness are common, often transient side-effects of trazodone. Conversely, an acute dystonic reaction has also been described in an adolescent taking trazodone [61]. Gastro-intestinal disturbances such as nausea and vomiting can be minimized by taking the medication in divided doses and with meals [16]. Taking the medication with meals slows its absorption and appears to decrease the incidence of dizziness or lightheadedness as well [16]. Although trazodone had little antiarrhythmic effect in preclinical and clinical trials [62] there has been a report that trazodone aggravated arrhythmias in patients with preexisting ventricular conduction disease [63].

Anticholinergic side-effects are generally not seen with trazodone.

Warnings/precautions

Fluoxetine may inhibit the hepatic metabolism of trazodone during concomitant trazodone and fluoxetine therapy, hence increasing plasma trazodone concentrations and causing adverse effects associated with trazodone toxicity [64, 65]. Because trazodone can cause orthostatic hypotension, concomitant administration with clonidine may require a reduction in dosage of the latter agent [16]. In addition, due to the potential for priapism, trazodone should be used with caution in adolescent male patients.

Venlafaxine

Chemical properties

Venlafaxine, a selective serotonin- and norephinephrine-reuptake inhibitor (SNRI), is a phenylethylamine-derivative antidepressant agent and anxiolytic agent [66, 67]. Venlafaxine inhibits 5-HT uptake at low doses, and inhibits the neuronal reuptake of 5HT and NE at high doses [68]. It is a weak inhibitor of dopamine. Its major active metabolite, O-desmethylvenlfaxine (ODV), has similar actions. Venlafaxine and ODV have no clinically meaningful affinity for cholinergic, histaminergic or alpha-adrenergic receptors.

Pharmacokinetics

Venlafaxine is extensively metabolized by the liver to O-desmethylvenlafaxine (ODV), the major metabolite, which is clinically active [33]. Venlafaxine and its metabolites are excreted through the kidneys. The elimination half-life is approximately 11 hours [33] (Table 9.1). A small pharmacokinetic study of six children and six adolescents suggested that children and adolescents have lower exposure to venlafaxine and its major active metabolite than adults [42].

Dosage and administration

Venlafaxine is available in 25 mg, 37.5 mg, 50 mg, and 100 mg tablets (Effexor®; Wyeth-Ayerst), and as 37.5 mg, 75 mg and 150 mg extended-release capsules (Effexor® XR; Wyeth-Ayerst). The recommended initial dosage of venlafaxine in adults is 75 mg daily administered in two or three divided doses or as a single daily dose when using the extended-release capsules [66], an initial dose of 37.5 mg daily as extended release capsules for the first seven days, followed by an increase to 75 mg daily may be considered [67]. The dosage is increased by increments of 75 mg daily at intervals of not less than four days up to 225 mg daily in divided doses or as a single dose when using the extended-release capsules [66, 67]. Outpatient studies have not demonstrated additional benefit from dosages exceeding 225 mg [62]. Dosing in pediatric studies using venlafaxine has followed the same dosing schedule as the recommended adult dosing schedule (Table 9.2). When discontinuing venlafaxine, the dosage should be decreased gradually to reduce the risk of withdrawal symptoms including agitation, fatigue, dizziness, headache or gastro-intestinal discomfort [66, 67].

Venlafaxine is administered orally, and to minimize gastrointestinal intolerance (for example, nausea), should be taken with food. Food does not appear to affect the absolute absorption of the drug, although it may slow the rate of absorption [66,67]. Venlafaxine extended-release capsules should be administered as a single daily dose with food.

Indications

Venlafaxine in its immediate release form is indicated for the treatment of major depressive disorder in adults. Extended release venlafaxine has FDA approval for the treatment of adults with major depressive disorder, generalized anxiety disorder, social phobia and panic disorder [16]. Although not indicated in the pediatric population, there are several note-worthy studies in the literature on the use of venlafaxine in this population (Table 9.3).

The safety, efficacy, and tolerability of venlafaxine extended release (ER) in subjects ages 7 to 17 years with major depressive disorder was evaluated in two recent multicenter, randomized, double-blind, placebo-controlled trials. Analysis of each trial separately showed no statistically signifi-cant difference between venlafaxine ER and placebo on the Children's Depression Rating Scale—Revised. However, a post hoc age subgroup anal-ysis of the pooled data showed greater improvement on the Children's Depression Rating Scale-Revised with venlafaxine ER than with placebo among adolescents (ages 12–17) but not among children (ages 7–11). A high placebo response rate in this study may have minimized the ability to detect a significant difference between treatment groups in the subpopula-tion of children [69]. There were more dropouts due to adverse events in the venlafaxine group than the placebo group, although the only adverse events more commonly reported with venlafaxine were abdominal pain (21% versus 10%) and dizziness (12% versus 6%). There were also sta-tistically significant mean increases from baseline in standing and supine pulse rate in the venlafaxine ER group in this study. Furthermore, signif-icantly greater weight loss was associated with venlafaxine compared to placebo [69].

Another double-blind, placebo-controlled, six-week study compared venlafaxine and placebo in 33 children and adolescents (ages 8–17 years) with depression. In this study, all youth also received therapy. No sig-nificant differences were found between active medication and placebo, although both groups showed improvement over time. Venlafaxine was generally well tolerated [70]. The low dosage used (37.5 mg/day for children; 75 mg/day for adolescents), the lack of baseline observation, inclusion of psychotherapy for all patients, and short duration of the trial may account for the negative findings.

In a study of treatment resistant adolescents with depression, 334 teens (aged 12 to 18 years) who had not responded to a two-month initial treat-ment with an SSRI were randomized to an alternate SSRI, venlafaxine, alternate SSRI plus cognitive behavioral therapy (CBT), or venlafaxine plus CBT. Combination CBT and a switch to another antidepressant resulted in a higher rate of clinical response than medication alone [71]. However, there was no difference in response rates to the alternate SSRI or venlafaxine, regardless of whether CBT was included. The study did show increased skin problems and greater increases in blood pressure and pulse in the venlafaxine group, although these adverse effects were rarely of clinical impact [71]. Thus, it appears that venlafaxine may be a strong second-line treatment in patients who have treatment resistant depression.

Venlafaxine has also been used for treatment of anxiety disorders. A recent report of two randomized, placebo-controlled studies of 320 youth (ages 6–17 years) with generalized anxiety disorder (GAD) demonstrated greater reduction of anxiety symptoms with venlafaxine compared to placebo. Individually, one of the studies was positive on primary and secondary outcomes, although the second study was positive only on some secondary outcomes [72]. Similarly, a study of venlafaxine for social phobia also showed greater reduction in anxiety symptoms for venlafaxine compared to placebo [73]. Thus, venlafaxine appears to be an effective treatment for anxiety disorders in youth.

Venlafaxine has not been studied using randomized controlled trials for any other psychiatric disorders in youth. A five-week open trial of venlafaxine (mean daily dose of 60 mg) conducted in 14 children and adolescents (mean age 11.6 years) with ADHD, showed improvements in ADHD symptoms [74]. However, there were no statistically significant effects of venlafaxine on reaction times or on the number of commission and omission errors on a computerized test of attention. Three subjects displayed a worsening of hyperactivity and required discontinuation of the drug. No effects on blood pressure or heart rate were noticed. Despite an overall improvement in ADHD symptoms, this study suggests that venlafaxine may aggravate hyperactivity [74], requiring cautious use of this drug in children with ADHD.

Side-effects

Except for the potential increase in blood pressure, venlafaxine appears to have a side-effect profile similar to the SSRIs. Dizziness, nervousness, tremor, sedation and sweating have been described as dose-dependent side-effects [75]. The described increase in blood pressure (rare below doses of 225 mg/day) is probably related to venlafaxine's potentiation of NE reuptake inhibition [75]. Blood pressure elevation has occurred both in adult and pediatric populations. In patients that experience a sustained increase in blood pressure during venlafaxine therapy, dosage reduction or discontinuation should be considered. Mydriasis has been reported in association with venlafaxine therapy [16]. Patients with elevated intraocular pressure or those at risk of angle-closure glaucoma should be monitored during treatment with this drug [16].

It does appear that venlafaxine leads to decreased appetite and increased weight loss in youth, as well as potential changes in blood pressure and pulse [16, 69]. Thus, regular monitoring of vitals, including height and weight, during therapy is suggested.

Warnings/precautions

Due to the potential cardiac and blood-pressure changes, obtaining baseline blood pressure and EKG is recommended, with periodic monitoring during treatment. In addition, while all antidepressants carry the black-box warning about potential increased suicidal thoughts and behaviors, venlafaxine was the only individual antidepressant to result in this increased risk [3]. Similarly, in the Treatment Resistant Depression In Adolescents (TORDIA) study, venlafaxine was associated with higher rates of self-harm adverse events in patients who reported higher levels of suicidal ideation [76]. Thus, ongoing monitoring of emergence or worsening of suicidal thoughts and behaviors is necessary during treatment with venlafaxine.

Desvenlafaxine

Desvenlafaxine is the principal active metabolite of venlafaxine, and therefore has similar characteristics to those reviewed with venlafaxine. Additional information specific to desvenlafaxine are included below.

Chemical properties

Desvenlafaxine, or O-desmethylvenlafaxine, the succinate salt of the principal active metabolite of venlafaxine, is a selective serotonin- and norepinephrine inhibitor (SNRI) and an antidepressant agent [77, 78]. Like venlafaxine, desvenlafaxine inhibits the neuronal uptake of serotonin and norepinephrine and has little affinity for muscarinic, cholinergic, histamine H1 and alpha 1-adrenergic receptors [78].

Pharmacokinetics

Desvenlafaxine exhibits a low degree of protein binding (30%), and has a mean elimination half-life of approximately 11 hours (Table 9.2). Elimination is primarily by phase II metabolism to form a glucuronide conjugate metabolite and by renal excretion of unchanged desvenlafaxine [78].

Dosage and administration

Desvenlafaxine is available in 50 mg and 100 mg tablets (Pristiq®; Wyeth), and is administered orally once daily with or without food [77]. The recommended starting dosage in adults is 50 mg daily (Table 9.2). Although efficacy has been established at dosages of 50–400 mg once daily in clinical studies, no additional benefit was observed with dosages greater than 50 mg, and adverse effects were more common at higher dosages. Desvenlafaxine is well absorbed following oral administration. The manufacturer recommends that if desvenlafaxine therapy is to be discontinued, the dosage should be decreased gradually to reduce the risk of withdrawal symptoms including agitation, fatigue, dizziness, headache or gastro-intestinal discomfort [77].

Indications
Desvenlafaxine is FDA approved for the treatment of major depressive disorder in the adult population. To date, there are no clinical studies in the literature on the use of desvenlafaxine in the pediatric population.

Side-effects
In controlled studies of adults, sustained hypertension occurred in 0.7–2.3% of patients receiving desvenlafaxine dosages from 50–400 mg daily, with a higher incidence in those receiving 400 mg [16]. Small increases in heart rate were also reported. Thus, monitoring of blood pressure and pulse is warranted with the use of desvenlafaxine. Mydriasis has been reported in association as well [16]. Therefore, patients with increased intraocular pressure or those at risk of angle-closure glaucoma should be monitored during treatment with this drug. In one double-blind, placebo-controlled study among adult patients with major depressive disorder, the most common treatment emergent adverse events were nausea, insomnia, somnolence, dry mouth, dizziness, sweating, nervousness, anorexia, constipation, asthenia and abnormal ejaculation/orgasm [78]. No studies of the safety and tolerability of desvenlafaxine have been reported in youth.

Warnings/precautions
Desvenlafaxine is not metabolized by the cytochrome P450 pathway. *In vitro* data suggest that it is associated with minimal inhibition of cytochrome P450 enzymes [78]. Due to this and its low protein binding effect, desvenlafaxine has a low risk of drug-drug interactions. However, as with venlafaxine, regular monitoring of blood pressure and EKG is warranted.

Alternative treatments

Despite limited empirical support, alternative or complementary medicines are commonly used as the primary treatment or as augmentation to antidepressant treatment for youth with depression and anxiety disorders.

The most common alternative treatments are St. John's wort, omega-3 fatty acids, thyroid hormones, and S-adenosyl methionine (SAMe).

Some randomized, controlled trials have shown St. John's wort to be effective for adult depression [79, 80] and anxiety disorders [81]. In open studies of SJW, a daily dose between 300 mg and 1800 mg were well tolerated by children. No RTCs of SJW in pediatric depression or anxiety disorders have been published.

One small controlled study with pediatric depression has been done with omega-3 fish oil. Nemets and colleagues [82] reported the data on 20 Israeli children with depression randomized to omega-3 fish oil or placebo for 16-weeks. Seventy percent of children who received 1000 mg daily dose of omega-3 fish oil responded versus 0% responded in the placebo group. The omega-3 fish oil was well tolerated and no significant side-effects were reported [82]. No studies of omega-3 fish oil have been reported in pediatric anxiety disorder.

L-triiodothyronine (T3 or L-triiodothyronine; Cytomel™), the most commonly used thyroid hormone, is used as an adjuvant to an antidepressant medication in an attempt to convert non-responders or partial responders into an antidepressant-responsive patient [83]. More rarely, thyroxin (T4 or levothyroxine; Levoxine™, Levothroid™, and Synthroid™) is sometimes used for the same purpose; however, T3 is believed to be more effective than T4. Several controlled studies have indicated that T3 converts 33% to 75% of antidepressant non-responders to responders, while several other studies have failed to find such a relationship. Most evidence for thyroid hormone augmentation is with TCAs, and there are no studies in children and adolescents [83]. Further studies are necessary before we can recommend this treatment modality in children and adolescents. No pediatric studies in pediatric depressive or anxiety disorders have been done for SAMe.

Summary

In summary, novel antidepressants, such as bupropion, duloxetine, mirtazapine, trazodone, venlafaxine, and desvenlafaxine, may have some use in the treatment of pediatric depression and anxiety disorders, although they are not generally considered first-line treatments. Additional research is needed on the utility of these medications in youth, as there are clear developmental differences in the pharmacokinetics and efficacy compared to adults. As with all psychopharmacological agents, it is essential for clinicians to assess the risk/benefit ratio before initiating medication as a treatment modality and monitor symptom changes and adverse events both prior to and throughout treatment.

References

1 Birmaher B, Brent D, Bernet W et al.: Practice parameter for the assessment and treatment of children and adolescents with depressive disorders. *J Am Acad Child Adolesc Psychiatry* 2007; **46**: 1503–26.

2 Connolly SD, Bernstein GA: Practice parameter for the assessment and treatment of children and adolescents with anxiety disorders. *J Am Acad Child Adolesc Psychiatry* 2007; **46**: 267–83.

3 Hammad TA, Laughren T, Racoosin J: Suicidality in pediatric patients treated with antidepressant drugs. *Archives of General Psychiatry* 2006; **63**: 332–9.

4 Bridge JA, Iyengar S, Salary CB et al.: Clinical response and risk for reported suicidal ideation and suicide attempts in pediatric antidepressant treatment: a meta-analysis of randomized controlled trials. *JAMA* 2007; **297**: 1683–96.

5 Mehta NB: The chemistry of bupropion. *J Clin Psychiatry* 1983; **44**: 56–9.

6 Lai AA, Schroeder DH: Clinical pharmacokinetics of bupropion: a review. *J Clin Psychiatry* 1983; **44**: 82–4.

7 Schroeder DH: Metabolism and kinetics of bupropion. *J Clin Psychiatry* 1983; **44**: 79–81.

8 Golden RN, Rudorfer MV, Sherer MA et al.: Bupropion in depression. I. Biochemical effects and clinical response. *Arch Gen Psychiatry* 1988; **45**: 139–43.

9 Laizure SC, DeVane CL, Stewart JT et al. Pharmacokinetics of bupropion and its major basic metabolites in normal subjects after a single dose. *Clin Pharmacol Ther* 1985; **38**: 586–9.

10 Findlay JW, Van Wyck Fleet J et al. Pharmacokinetics of bupropion, a novel antidepressant agent, following oral administration to healthy subjects. *Eur J Clin Pharmacol* 1985; **21**: 127–35.

11 Daviss WB, Perel JM, Birmaher B et al.: Steady-state clinical pharmacokinetics of bupropion extended-release in youths. *J Am Acad Child Adolesc Psychiatry* 2006; **45**: 1503–9.

12 Hsyu PH, Singh A, Giargiari TD et al. Pharmacokinetics of bupropion and its metabolites in cigarette smokers versus nonsmokers. *J Clin Pharmacol* 1997; **37**: 737–43.

13 Stewart JJ, Berkel HJ, Parish RC et al.: Single-dose pharmacokinetics of bupropion in adolescents: effects of smoking status and gender. *J Clin Pharmacol* 2001; **41**: 770–8.

14 GlaxoSmithKline: Wellbutrin tablets prescribing information. Research Triangle Park, NC: GlaxoSmithKline, 2006.

15 Davidson J: Seizures and bupropion: a review. *J Clin Psychiatry* 1989; **50**: 256–61.

16 AHFS: *American Hospital Formulary Service Drug Information*. Bethesda, MD: American Society of Heatlhy System Pharmacists Inc, 2010.

17 Conners CK, Casat CD, Gualtieri CT et al.: Bupropion hydrochloride in attention deficit disorder with hyperactivity. *J Am Acad Child Adolesc Psychiatry* 1996: **35**: 1314–21.

18 Daviss WB, Bentivoglio P, Racusin R et al.: Bupropion sustained release in adolescents with comorbid attention-deficit/hyperactivity disorder and depression. *J Am Acad Child Adolesc Psychiatry* 2001; **40**: 307–14.

19 Daviss WB, Perel JM, Brent DA et al.: Acute antidepressant response and plasma levels of bupropion and metabolites in a pediatric-aged sample: an exploratory study. *Ther Drug Monit* 2006; **28**: 190–8.

20 Barrickman LL, Perry PJ, Allen AJ et al.: Bupropion versus methylphenidate in the treatment of attention-deficit hyperactivity disorder. *J Am Acad Child Adolesc Psychiatry* 1995; **34**: 649–57.

21 Casat CD, Pleasants DZ, Schroeder DH, Parler DW: Bupropion in children with attention deficit disorder. *Psychopharmacology Bulletin* 1989; **25**: 198–201.
22 Clay TH, Gualtieri CT, Evans RW, Gullion CM: Clinical and neuropsychological effects of the novel antidepressant bupropion. *Psychopharmacol Bull* 1988; **24**: 143–8.
23 Simeon JG, Ferguson HB, Van Wyck Fleet J: Bupropion effects in attention deficit and conduct disorders. *Can J Psychiatry* 1986; **31**: 581–5.
24 Upadhyaya HP, Brady KT, Wang W: Bupropion SR in adolescents with comorbid ADHD and nicotine dependence: a pilot study. *J Am Acad Child Adolesc Psychiatry* 2004; **43**: 199–205.
25 Gray KM, Carpenter MJ, Baker NL et al.: Bupropion SR and contingency management for adolescent smoking cessation. *J Subst Abuse Treat* 2011; **40**: 77–86.
26 Killen JD, Robinson TN, Ammerman S et al.: Randomized clinical trial of the efficacy of bupropion combined with nicotine patch in the treatment of adolescent smokers. *J Consult Clin Psychol* 2004; **72**: 729–35.
27 *Physician's Desk Reference.* 45th edn. Oradell, NJ: Medical Economics Co, 1991.
28 Lineberry CG, Johnston JA, Raymond RN et al.: A fixed-dose (300 mg) efficacy study of bupropion and placebo in depressed outpatients. *J Clin Psychiatry* 1990; **51**: 194–9.
29 Storrow AB: Bupropion overdose and seizure. *Am J Emerg Med* 1994; **12**: 183–4.
30 Tilton P: Bupropion and guanfacine. *J Am Acad Child Adolesc Psychiatry* 1998; **37**: 682–3.
31 Bymaster FP, Lee TC, Knadler MP et al.: The dual transporter inhibitor duloxetine: a review of its preclinical pharmacology, pharmacokinetic profile, and clinical results in depression. *Curr Pharm Des* 2005; **11**: 1475–93.
32 Hunziker ME, Suehs BT, Bettinger TL, Crismon ML: Duloxetine hydrochloride: a new dual-acting medication for the treatment of major depressive disorder. *Clin Ther* 2005; **27**: 1126–43.
33 Green WH: *Child and Adolescent Clinical Psychopharmacology.* 4th edn. Philadelphia, PA.: Lippincott, Williams & Wilkins, 2007.
34 Fishbain DA, Detke MJ, Wernicke J et al.: The relationship between antidepressant and analgesic responses: findings from six placebo-controlled trials assessing the efficacy of duloxetine in patients with major depressive disorder. *Curr Med Res Opin.* 2008; **24**: 3105–15.
35 Desarkar P, Das A, Sinha VK: Duloxetine for childhood depression with pain and dissociative symptoms. *Eur Child Adolesc Psychiatry* 2006; **15**: 496–9.
36 Meighen KG: Duloxetine treatment of pediatric chronic pain and co-morbid major depressive disorder. *J Child Adolesc Psychopharmacol* 2007; **17**: 121–7.
37 Eli Lilly: *Cymbalta Prescribing Information.* Indianapolis, IN: Eli Lilly, 2010.
38 Smith WT, Glaudin V, Panagides J, Gilvary E: Mirtazapine vs. amitriptyline vs. placebo in the treatment of major depressive disorder. *Psychopharmacol Bull* 1990; **26**: 191–6.
39 Organon: Remeron (mirtazapine) tablets prescribing information. West Orange, NJ: Organon, 1999.
40 Gorman JM: Mirtazapine: clinical overview. *J Clin Psychiatry* 1999; **60**: 9–13; discussion 46-8.
41 Timmer CJ, Sitsen JM, Delbressine LP: Clinical pharmacokinetics of mirtazapine. *Clin Pharmacokinet* 2000; **38**: 461–74.
42 Findling RL, McNamara NK, Stansbrey RJ et al.: The relevance of pharmacokinetic studies in designing efficacy trials in juvenile major depression. *J Child Adolesc Psychopharmacol* 2006; **16**: 131–45.

43 Wheatley DP, van Moffaert M, Timmerman L et al.: Mirtazapine: efficacy and tolerability in comparison with fluoxetine in patients with moderate to severe major depressive disorder. *J Clin Psychiatry* 1998; **59**; 306–12.

44 Montgomery SA, Reimitz PE, Zivkov M: Mirtazapine versus amitriptyline in the long-term treatment of depression: a double-blind placebo-controlled study. *Int Clin Psychopharmacol* 1998; **13**: 63–73.

45 Haapasalo-Pesu KM, Vuola T, Lahelma L et al.: Mirtazapine in the treatment of adolescents with major depression: an open-label, multicenter pilot study. *J Child Adolesc Psychopharmacol* 2004; **14**: 175–84.

46 Cheung A, Emslie GJ, Mayes TL: Review of the efficacy and safety of antidepressants in youth depression. *J Child Psychol Psychiatry* 2005; **46**: 735–54.

47 Mrakotsky C, Masek B, Biederman J et al.: Prospective open-label pilot trial of mirtazapine in children and adolescents with social phobia. *J Anxiety Disord* 2008; **22**: 88–97.

48 Connor KM, Davidson JR, Weisler RH, Ahearn E: A pilot study of mirtazapine in post-traumatic stress disorder. *Int Clin Psychopharmacol* 1999; **14**: 29–31.

49 Winokur A, Sateia MJ, Hayes JB et al.: Acute effects of mirtazapine on sleep continuity and sleep architecture in depressed patients: a pilot study. *Biol Psychiatry* 2000; **48**: 75–8.

50 Puzantian T: Mirtazapine, an antidepressant. *Am J Health Syst Pharm* 1998; **55**: 44–9.

51 Marek GJ, McDougle CJ, Price LH et al.: A comparison of trazodone and fluoxetine: implications for a serotonergic mechanism of antidepressant action. *Psychopharmacology (Berl)* 1992; **109**: 2–11.

52 Mouret J, Lemoine P, Minuit MP et al.: Effects of trazodone on the sleep of depressed subjects–a polygraphic study. *Psychopharmacology (Berl)* 1988; **95**(Suppl): S37–43.

53 Owens JA, Rosen CL, Mindell JA et al. Use of pharmacotherapy for insomnia in child psychiatry practice: A national survey. *Sleep Med* 2010; **11**: 692–700.

54 Levi G, Sogos C. Depressive disorder in pre-adolescence: comorbidity or different clinical subtypes? (A pharmacological contribution). *Isr J Psychiatry Relat Sci* 1997; **34**: 187–94.

55 Kallepalli BR, Bhatara VS, Fogas BS et al.: Trazodone is only slightly faster than fluoxetine in relieving insomnia in adolescents with depressive disorders. *J Child Adolesc Psychopharmacol* 1997; **7**: 97–107.

56 Zubieta JK, Alessi NE: Acute and chronic administration of trazodone in the treatment of disruptive behavior disorders in children. *J Clin Psychopharmacol* 1992; **12**: 346–51.

57 Saccomani L, Rizzo P, Nobili L: Combined treatment with haloperidol and trazodone in patients with tic disorders. *J Child Adolesc Psychopharmacol* 2000; **10**: 307–10.

58 Solyom L, Solyom C, Ledwidge B: Trazodone treatment of bulimia nervosa. *J Clin Psychopharmacol* 1989; **9**: 287–90.

59 Battistella PA, Ruffilli R, Cernetti R et al. A placebo-controlled crossover trial using trazodone in pediatric migraine. *Headache* 1993; **33**: 36–9.

60 Thompson JW, Jr., Ware MR, Blashfield RK: Psychotropic medication and priapism: a comprehensive review. *J Clin Psychiatry* 1990; **51**(10): 430–3.

61 Tesler-Mabe CS: Acute dystonic reaction with trazodone. *Can J Psychiatry* 1998; **43**: 1053.

62 Preskorn SH, Janicak PG, Davis JM, Ayd FJJ: Advances in the pharmacotherapy of depressive disorders. In: Janicak PG, editor. *Principles and Practice of Psychopharmacotherapy*. Baltimore, MD: Williams & Wilkins, 1994.

63 Vitullo RN, Wharton JM, Allen NB, Pritchett EL: Trazodone-related exercise-induced nonsustained ventricular tachycardia. *Chest* 1990; **98**: 247–8.

64 Aranow AB, Hudson JI, Pope HG et al.: Elevated antidepressant plasma levels after addition of fluoxetine. *Am J Psychiatry* 1989; **146**: 911–13.

65 Metz A, Shader RI: Adverse interactions encountered when using trazodone to treat insomnia associated with fluoxetine. *Int Clin Psychopharmacol* 1990; **5**: 191–4.

66 Wyeth: Effexor tablets prescribing information. Philadelphia, PA: Wyeth, 2006.

67 Wyeth: Effexor XR extended-release capsules prescribing information. Philadelphia, PA: Wyeth, 2006.

68 Harvey AT, Rudolph RL, Preskorn SH: Evidence of the dual mechanisms of action of venlafaxine. *Arch Gen Psychiatry* 2000; **57**: 503–9.

69 Emslie GJ, Findling RL, Yeung PP et al.: Venlafaxine ER for the treatment of pediatric subjects with depression: results of two placebo-controlled trials. *J Am Acad Child Adolesc Psychiatry* 2007; **46**: 479–88.

70 Mandoki MW, Tapia MR, Tapia MA et al.: Venlafaxine in the Treatment of Children and Adolescents with Major Depression. *Psychopharmacology Bulletin* 1997; **33**, 149–54.

71 Brent D, Emslie G, Clarke G et al.: Switching to another SSRI or to venlafaxine with or without cognitive behavioral therapy for adolescents with SSRI-resistant depression: the TORDIA randomized controlled trial. *JAMA* 2008; **299**: 901–13.

72 Rynn MA, Riddle MA, Yeung PP, Kunz NR: Efficacy and safety of extended-release venlafaxine in the treatment of generalized anxiety disorder in children and adolescents: two placebo-controlled trials. *Am J Psychiatry* 2007; **164**: 290–300.

73 March JS, Entusah AR, Rynn M et al.: A randomized controlled trial of venlafaxine ER versus placebo in pediatric social anxiety disorder. *Biol Psychiatry* 2007; **62**: 1149–54.

74 Olvera RL, Pliszka SR, Luh J, Tatum R: An open trial of venlafaxine in the treatment of attention-deficit/hyperactivity disorder in children and adolescents. *J Child Adolesc Psychopharmacol* 1996; **6**: 241–50.

75 Preskorn SH, Burke M: Somatic therapy for major depressive disorder: selection of an antidepressant. *J Clin Psychiatry* 1992; **53**(Suppl): 5–18.

76 Brent DA, Emslie GJ, Clarke GN et al.: Predictors of Spontaneous and Systematically Assessed Suicidal Adverse Events in the Treatment of SSRI-Resistant Depression in Adolescents (TORDIA) Study. *Am J Psychiatry* 2009; **166**: 418–26.

77 Wyeth: *Pristiq Prescribing Information.* Philadelphia, PA: Wyeth, 2010.

78 DeMartinis NA, Yeung PP, Entsuah R, Manley AL: A double-blind, placebo-controlled study of the efficacy and safety of desvenlafaxine succinate in the treatment of major depressive disorder. *J Clin Psychiatry* 2007; **68**: 677–88.

79 Freeman MP, Mischoulon D, Tedeschini E et al.: Complementary and alternative medicine for major depressive disorder: a meta-analysis of patient characteristics, placebo-response rates, and treatment outcomes relative to standard antidepressants. *J Clin Psychiatry* 2010; **71**(6): 682–8.

80 Linde K: St. John's wort—an overview. *Forsch Komplementmed* 2009; **16**: 146–55.

81 Lakhan SE, Vieira KF: Nutritional and herbal supplements for anxiety and anxiety-related disorders: systematic review. *Nutr J* 2010; **9**: 42.

82 Nemets H, Nemets B, Apter A: Omega-3 treatment of childhood depression: a controlled, double-blind pilot study. *Am J Psychiatry* 2006; **163**: 1098–100.

83 Connolly KR, Thase ME: If at first you don't succeed: a review of the evidence for antidepressant augmentation, combination and switching strategies. *Drugs* 2011; **71**: 43–64.

CHAPTER 10

Antipsychotic Agents

Brieana M. Rowles, John L. Hertzer & Robert L. Findling
Case Western Reserve University, Cleveland, USA

Introduction

Antipsychotic medications—drugs that are generally marketed for the treatment of psychotic disorders in adults—are prescribed for a number of conditions in children and adolescents. There are approximately 20 medications marketed as antipsychotics in the United States. Of the atypicals, only four are approved by the U.S. Food and Drug Administration (FDA) for use in pediatric patients: aripiprazole, olanzapine, quetiapine, risperidone. Table 10.1 lists the typical and atypical antipsychotics and the chemical classes to which they belong.

What makes atypical antipsychotics "atypical" is their reduced propensity to cause neurological side-effects known as extrapyramidal side-effects (EPS) when compared to the older "first generation" antipsychotics (otherwise known as "neuroleptics"). Notably, children appear to be at greater risk of developing EPS than adults. While the atypical antipsychotics have a reduced propensity to cause EPS, use of these medications is frequently associated with fairly significant weight gain. Children tend to experience antipsychotic-related weight gain to a greater degree than adults. In youths, atypical antipsychotics are frequently the first-line treatment for schizophrenia, and their use in the treatment of pervasive developmental disorders, Tourette's disorder, and bipolar disorder is becoming more common.

Antipsychotics have been and continue to be developed for the treatment of adults with schizophrenia and other neuropsychiatric conditions. As such, the amount of data pertaining to antipsychotics in adult patients is substantially greater when compared to what is known about these drugs in youths. However, it is important to recall that what is true about the efficacy and safety of psychotropic agents in adults may not be true in youngsters. Children are not "little adults" and the effects of psychotropic agents on developing systems—particularly the neuronal systems—differ

Pharmacotherapy of Child and Adolescent Psychiatric Disorders, Third Edition.
Edited by David R. Rosenberg and Samuel Gershon.
© 2012 John Wiley & Sons, Ltd. Published 2012 by John Wiley & Sons, Ltd.

Table 10.1 Chemical classes of antipsychotic agents

Typical antipsychotics	Atypical antipsychotics
Butryophenone	*Benzisothiazolyl*
Haloperidol	Ziprasidone
Dibenzoxazepine	*Benzisoxazole*
Loxapine	Aripiprazole
	Iloperidone
	Paliperidone
	Risperidone
Dihydroindolone	*Benzoisothiazol*
Molindone	Lurasidone
Diphenylbutylpiperidine	*Dibenzodiazepine*
Pimozide	Clozapine
Phenothiazine	*Dibenzo-oxepino pyrrole*
Chlorpromazine	Asenapine
Fluphenazine	
Mesoridazine	*Dibenzothiazepine*
Perphenazine	Quetiapine
Thioridazine	
Trifluoperazine	
Thioxanthene	*Thienobenzodiazepine*
Thiothixene	Olanzapine

from the effects in adults [1]. Agents that are effective in adults may not be effective in pediatric patients. Similarly, drug tolerability may differ across the life cycle. Thus, in the absence of pediatric efficacy and tolerability data, particular caution should be exercised when prescribing these medications to this vulnerable population based on adult data.

Chemical properties

Clinical potency of antipsychotic agents correlates best with affinity for dopaminergic receptors [2]. Five types of dopamine receptors have been identified in the central nervous system (D_1–D_5). However, it is the type-2 dopamine receptor (D_2) that is blocked by all antipsychotic agents. Agents with the greatest D_2 receptor binding affinity have a greater propensity for causing some forms of EPS [3]. It is thought that typical agents induce EPS because these agents bind to D_2 in the nigrostriatal region. A compound's affinity for D_2 receptors is proportional to the agent's potency in reducing the positive symptoms of schizophrenia. It is likely that this reduction occurs owing to the modulation of the mesolimbic dopaminergic system.

Atypicals, unlike typical agents, have more significant binding affinity to serotonin (5-HT) receptors. More than a dozen 5-HT receptors have been identified. Atypical antipsychotics predominantly block serotonin $5-HT_{2A}$ receptors in the ventral tegmental area, substantia nigra, limbic regions, basal ganglia, and prefrontal cortex [4]. $5-HT_{2A}$ receptor blockade appears to be responsible for the reduced propensity of atypical antipsychotics to cause EPS. The greater degree of weight gain associated with atypical antipsychotics, when compared to the typicals, may be attributable, in part, to $5-HT_{2C}$ receptor blockade [5].

The typical antipsychotics chlorpromazine and thioridazine, as well as the atypical agents clozapine and olanzapine, have the greatest affinity for muscarinic receptors. Use of agents that block muscarinic cholinergic receptors is associated with a reduced risk of EPS but anticholinergic drugs are associated with other significant adverse events. These adverse events include blurred vision, cognitive dysfunction, constipation, acute onset or exacerbation of narrow-angle glaucoma, sinus tachycardia, urinary retention, and xerostomia. Further, muscarinic cholinergic receptor agonism may lead to sialorrhea, which has been noted during treatment with clozapine [6].

There are two types of α-adrenergic receptors: α_1 and α_2. Chlorpromazine, thioridazine, and risperidone are the agents with the greatest affinity for α_1 blockade. While there are no known beneficial effects associated with α_1-adrenergic receptor antagonism, α_1-adrenergic receptor blockade can lead to hypotension, dizziness, and reflex tachycardia. With the exception of risperidone and clozapine, α_2 blockade is modest for most agents. Similar to α_1-adrenergic receptor antagonism, there are no benefits that have yet to be associated with α_2 receptor antagonism. However, there do not appear to be any side-effects associated with α_2 blockade [7].

Antipsychotics also are associated with histaminergic blockade. Three types of histamine (H) receptors have been isolated. H_1 receptor blockade by antipsychotic agents may be responsible for some of the sedation and weight gain caused by these drugs [3].

Typical antipsychotics

When considering the treatment of schizophrenia, these medications are virtually interchangeable with regard to efficacy. Put in other words, response to one agent is associated with symptom reduction with another. Similarly, treatment nonresponse to one drug is associated with treatment resistance to another typical. Where typical antipsychotics most differ from one another is potency and associated side-effects. As noted above, agents that are given in smaller total daily doses are considered high-potency drugs, and are associated with increased frequency of extrapyramidal side-effects. Lower potency drugs (those given in larger total daily doses) are associated with a greater risk of sedation, orthostasis, and anticholinergic side-effects.

Pharmacokinetics and drug metabolism

Although absorption and metabolism of typical antipsychotics have been extensively studied in adults, scant data are available in children. It is important to note that the pharmacokinetics of any medication may change over the first two decades of life. Based on the few pharmacokinetic studies available in pediatric patients, interindividual variability in metabolism is far greater than the developmental variability seen across age groups.

General indications

Schizophrenia

Since the development of atypical antipsychotics, and based on assumptions of superior efficacy and tolerability, typical antipsychotics are used less frequently in the treatment of early onset schizophrenia. A few randomized, controlled trials in adults comparing treatments for early onset schizophrenia have demonstrated efficacy for typical antipsychotics, but when compared to atypical agents, typical antipsychotics have not shown to be superior.

In the most recent and largest publicly funded trial conducted to date, the Treatment of Early-Onset Schizophrenia Spectrum Disorders (TEOSS) study compared the acute effectiveness and safety of two atypical antipsychotics (olanzapine and risperidone) and one typical antipsychotic (molindone) in youth with early onset schizophrenia spectrum disorders (schizophrenia, schizophreniform disorder, or schizoaffective disorder) [8, 9]. The TEOSS study found that no agent demonstrated superior efficacy, and all three medications were associated with substantial, significant side-effects. Patients treated with either risperidone or olanzapine experienced significantly greater weight gain than patients treated with molindone. Risperidone treatment was associated with elevated prolactin concentrations. Olanzapine showed the greatest risk of weight gain and significant increases in fasting cholesterol, low density lipoprotein, insulin, and liver transamine levels. In fact, randomization to olanzapine treatment was discontinued following an interim analysis which showed a greater increase in weight with olanzapine than molindone or risperidone (without evidence of greater efficacy) by the National Institute of Mental Health's Data and Safety Monitoring Board [8]. Treatment with molindone was associated with more akathisia than treatment with the atypical agents.

Tourette's disorder/tic disorders

Traditional treatments for Tourette's disorder and other tic disorders have included the D_2 antagonists haloperidol, pimozide, or fluphenazine.

Aggression/conduct disorder

Typical antipsychotics have been shown to be helpful in severe aggression appearing specifically in children with conduct disorder and attention-deficit/hyperactivity disorder (ADHD). However, antipsychotics are generally not prescribed to such patients unless both behavioral interventions and standard agents for ADHD (for example, psychostimulants) have failed, and the dysfunction associated with aggressive behaviors is substantial.

Autistic disorder and pervasive developmental disorders

Treatment of children and adolescents with autistic disorder and pervasive developmental disorders (PDD) generally focuses on increasing spontaneous social interaction and communication skills. These core symptoms do not appear to respond to currently available pharmacological agents. However, there are associated symptoms that may respond to medication. These include behavioral impulsivity, hyperactivity, self-injurious behaviors, and compulsive/stereotypic behaviors. Haloperidol has demonstrated effectiveness in reducing symptoms of overactivity, aggression, and stereotypic behavior in children and adolescents with autistic disorder. Pimozide and fluphenazine may also be useful in treating these symptoms in this pediatric population. Despite available clinical trials to suggest that these agents may be useful in the treatment of behavior symptoms associated with autistic disorder and PDD, typical antipsychotics are not recommended as a primary treatment for these disorders.

Adverse effects

Treatment with typical antipsychotics is associated with a wide range of adverse effects, some quite serious. Thus, when prescribing antipsychotic medications to pediatric patients, it is important to minimize the risks associated with these agents.

Anticholinergic effects

Several antipsychotic agents, particularly the phenothiazines (see Table 10.1) and other low-potency neuroleptics, have prominent anticholinergic effects.

Extrapyramidal side-effects

Extrapyramidal side-effects (EPS) are common with antipsychotic medication, both typical and atypical. The most common forms of EPS include those that may occur most commonly early in the course of treatment—acute dystonia, akathisia, and Parkinsonism—as well as those that appear later, such as tardive dyskinesia. The acute effects occur most frequently with high-potency agents such as fluphenazine and haloperidol possessing little or no anticholinergic properties, but can be produced with higher doses of low-potency agents or treatment with pro-phylactic anticholinergic agents (such as benztropine) [10].

Neuroleptic malignant syndrome

Neuroleptic malignant syndrome (NMS) is a rare, medication-induced syndrome that may be a result of dopamine receptor blockade in the basal ganglia. Although specific risk factors are not known, high-potency agents, multiple antipsychotics, and polypharmacy have been implicated. Neuroleptic malignant syndrome is potentially life threatening, and is characterized by hyperthermia, an altered level of consciousness, severe muscular rigidity, autonomic instability, hyper- or hypotension, tachy-cardia, diaphoresis, and pallor. Laboratory findings include leukocytosis and increased levels of creatinine phosphokinase. Clinically, NMS may be mistaken for psychosis, catatonia, EPS, infection, or fever of unknown origin.

Hyperprolactinemia

Prolonged blockade of D_2 receptors in the neurohypophysis associated with treatment with antipsychotic agents can cause increases in plasma prolactin. Amenorrhea, galactorrhea, menstrual changes, breast enlargement, sexual dysfunction, and gynecomastia are associated with hyperprolactinemia.

Cardiovascular side-effects

Several cardiovascular effects are associated with antipsychotic agents. Low-potency agents commonly produce postural hypotension and/or syn-cope, apparently mediated through α_1-adrenergic blockade. Additionally, increases in heart rate that may be the result of hypotension and ventric-ular tachycardia have been reported.

These agents may produce quinidine-like effects on cardiac conduc-tion, and the risk for QTc prolongation during treatment with several typical antipsychotics may be increased. The greatest risk of dose-related QTc changes and arrhythmias appears to be associated with pimozide and thioridazine treatment.

Atypical antipsychotics

Tables 10.2 to 10.7 summarize key clinical trials of atypical antipsychotics conducted from 2000 through 2010. Common adverse events associated with each atypical antipsychotic are listed in Table 10.8. Table 10.9 sum-marizes the recommended clinical use of atypical agents.

Table 10.2 Summary of selected acute trials of clozapine in children and adolescents with psychiatric disorders

Study	N	Age, mean (SD) or range	Inclusion criteria/psychiatric diagnosis	Design	Medication and mean (SD) dose, mg/day	Outcome	Adverse events
Shaw et al. [13]	25	7–16	Schizophrenia (onset prior to age 13)	8 weeks DB-RCT	CLZ: 327 (113) mg OLZ: 18.1 (4.3) mg	SANS: CLZ > OLZ ($p = 0.04$)	CLZ: hypertension supine tachycardia
Kumra et al. [14]	39	15.6 (2.1)	Schizophrenia or schizoaffective disorder	12 weeks DB-RCT	CLZ: 403.1 (201.8) mg OLZ: 26.2 (6.5) mg	†Responder status: CLZ > OLZ ($p = 0.038$)	CLZ: increased salivation sweating
Masi et al. [16]	10	14.8 (1.9)	BP manic or mixed	15–28 days OL	CLZ: 142.5 (73.6) mg	CGI-I of 1 (very much improved) or 2 (much improved): N = 10	increased appetite sedation enuresis sialorrhea

BP = bipolar disorder; CGI-I = Clinical Global Impressions-Improvement scale; CLZ = clozapine; DB = double-blind; OL = open-label; OLZ = olanzapine; RCT = randomized controlled trial; SANS = Scale for the Assessment of Negative Symptoms.

†Response criteria = CGI-I of 1 (very much improved) or 2 (much improved) and ≥ 30% decrease from baseline total BPRS score.

Table 10.3 Summary of selected acute trials of risperidone and paliperidone in children and adolescents with psychiatric disorders

Study	N	Age, mean (SD) or range	Inclusion criteria/ psychiatric diagnosis	Design	Medication and mean (SD) dose, mg/day	Outcome	Adverse events
Risperidone							
Findling et al. [34]	20	9.2 (2.9)	CD	10 weeks DB-RPCT	RIS: 0.028 (0.004) mg/kg	RAAP scale: RIS > PBO ($p < 0.05$)	increased appetite, sedation
Snyder et al. [35]	110	5–12	CD, ODD, or DBD-NOS; NCBRF Conduct Problem ≥24; IQ 36–84; VABS ≤84	6 weeks DB-RPCT	RIS: 0.98 (0.06) mg	NCBRF Conduct Problem subscale: RIS > PBO ($p < 0.01$)	somnolence, headache, increased appetite, dyspepsia
Aman et al. [36]	118	5–12	CD, ODD, or DBD-NOS; NCBRF Conduct Problem ≥24; IQ 36–84; VABS ≤84	6 weeks DB-RPCT	RIS: 1.16 (0.57) mg	NCBRF Conduct Problem subscale: RIS > PBO ($p < 0.001$)	headache, somnolence
McCracken et al. [25]	101	8.8 (2.7)	AD with tantrums, aggression, and/or self-injurious behavior	8 weeks DB-RPCT	RIS: 1.8 (0.7) mg	ABC Irritability subscale: RIS > PBO ($p < 0.001$)	increased appetite, fatigue, drowsiness, dizziness, drooling
Shea et al. [28]	79	5–12	PDD; CARS ≥30	8 weeks DB-RPCT	RIS: 1.17 mg*	ABC Irritability subscale: RIS > PBO ($p \leq 0.001$)	somnolence
Luby et al. [29]	23	2.5–6	AD or PDD-NOS	6 months DB-RPCT	RIS: 1.14 (0.32) mg	CARS: RIS > PBO ($p < 0.05$)	weight gain, hypersalivation

Table 10.3 (*Continued*)

Study	N	Age, mean (SD) or range	Inclusion criteria/ psychiatric diagnosis	Design	Medication and mean (SD) dose, mg/day	Outcome	Adverse events
Miral et al. [30]	30	7–17	AD	12 weeks DB-RCT	HAL: 2.6 (1.3) mg RIS: 2.6 (0.8) mg	ABC: RIS > HAL ($p < 0.05$) Turgay DSM-IV PDD Rating Scale: RIS > HAL ($p < 0.01$)	RIS: constipation nocturnal enuresis upper respiratory tract infection
Sikich et al. [20]	50	14.8 (2.8)	≥ 1 positive psychotic symptom of moderate or greater severity on the BPRS-C	8 weeks DB-RCT	RIS: 4.0 (1.2) mg OLZ: 12.3 (3.5) mg HAL: 5.0 (2.0) mg	BPRS-C: RIS = OLZ = HAL	sedation EPS weight gain
Sikich et al. [8]	116	8–19	Schizophrenia spectrum disorder	8 weeks DB-RCT	MOL: 59.9 (33.5) mg OLZ: 11.4 (5.0) mg RIS: 2.8 (1.4) mg	†Responder status: MOL (50%) = OLZ (34%) = RIS (46%)	sedation irritability anxiety weight gain
Haas et al. [21]	257	13–17	Schizophrenia	8 weeks DB-RCT	RIS 1.5–6.0 mg;§ 4.00 mg	RIS 0.15–0.6 mg;§ 0.4 mg	hypertonia hyperkinesia somnolence tremor weight increase
Haas et al. [22]	160	15.6 (1.3)	Schizophrenia	6 weeks DB-RPCT	RIS 1–3 mg;‡ 3 mg: 82% 2 mg: 12% 1 mg: 6% — RIS 4–6 mg;‡ 6 mg: 66% 5 mg: 23% 4 mg: 11%	PANSS total score: (RIS 1–3 mg/day = RIS 4–6 mg/day) > PBO	somnolence agitation headache EPD dizziness hypertonia
Scahill et al. [33]	34	19.8 (17.01)	TD; YGTSS Total Tic ≥22	8 weeks DB-RPCT	RIS: 2.5 (0.85) mg	YGTSS Total Tic: RIS > PBO ($p = 0.002$)	increased appetite fatigue

(continued)

Table 10.3 (*Continued*)

Study	N	Age, mean (SD) or range	Inclusion criteria/ psychiatric diagnosis	Design	Medication and mean (SD) dose, mg/day			Outcome	Adverse events
Haas et al. [24]	169	10–17	BP-I manic or mixed	3 weeks DB-RPCT	RIS 0.5–2.5 mg:‡ 2.5 mg: 57% 1.5 mg: ~15% 1 mg: ~15% 0.5 mg: ~15%		RIS 3–6 mg:‡ 6 mg: 41% 5 mg: 15% 4 mg: 19% 3 mg: 26%	YMRS: (RIS 0.5–2.5 mg/day = RIS 3–6 mg/day) > PBO	somnolence headache fatigue
Paliperidone									
Singh et al. [45]	201	12–17	Schizophrenia	6 weeks DB-RPCT	PAL low 1.5 mg	PAL med.§ 3 mg or 6 mg	PAL high¥ 6 mg or 12 mg	PANSS total score: PAL 3, 6, and 12 mg/day > PBO	somnolence akathisia tremor

ABC = Aberrant Behavior Checklist; AD = autistic disorder; BP-I = bipolar I disorder; BPRS-C = Brief Psychiatric Rating Scale for Children; CARS = Childhood Autism Rating Scale; CD = conduct disorder; DB = double-blind; DBD-NOS = disruptive behavior disorder not otherwise specified; EPD = extrapyramidal disorder; HAL = haloperidol; IQ = intelligence quotient; MOL = molindone; NCBRF = Nisonger Child Behavior Rating Form; NOS = not otherwise specified; ODD = oppositional defiant disorder; OLZ = olanzapine; PAL = paliperidone; PANSS = Positive and Negative Syndrome Scale; PBO = placebo; PDD = pervasive developmental disorder; RAAP = Rating of Aggression against People and/or Property Scale; RIS = risperidone; RCT = randomized controlled trial; RPCT = randomized, placebo-controlled trial; TD = Tourette's disorder; YGTSS = Yale Global Tic Severity Scale; YMRS = Young Mania Rating Scale.

*Standard deviation not given.

†Response criteria = Clinical Global Impressions-Improvement score of 1 (very much improved) or 2 (much improved) and ≥20% reduction in baseline PANSS score.

‡Mean doses not given. Mode doses are presented for each active treatment group.

§Mean doses not given. Median mode doses are presented for each treatment group.

¥Paliperidone ER daily dose was weight-based. For patients weighing 29 to < 51 kg at baseline, PAL medium = 3 mg and PAL high = 6 mg. For patients ≥ 51 kg, PAL medium = 6 mg and PAL high = 12 mg.

Table 10.4 Summary of selected acute trials of olanzapine in children and adolescents with psychiatric disorders

Study	N	Age, mean (SD) or range	Inclusion criteria/ psychiatric diagnosis	Design	Medication and mean (SD) daily dose	Outcome	Adverse events
Kryzhanovskaya et al. [46]	107	13–17	Schizophrenia	6 weeks DB-RPCT	OLZ: 11.1 mg*	BPRS-C: OLZ > PBO ($p = 0.003$)	increased weight somnolence headache
Tohen et al. [50]	161	13–17	BP manic or mixed	3 weeks DB-RPCT	OLZ: 8.9 mg*	YMRS: OLZ > PBO ($p < 0.001$)	increased appetite sedation increased appetite increased weight somnolence sedation
Hollander et al. [56]	11	6–14	PDD	8 weeks DB-RPCT	OLZ: 10 (2.04) mg	CGI-I of 1 (very much improved) or 2 (much improved): OLZ > PBO ($p = 0.006$)	increased weight increased appetite sedation
Masi et al. [57]	23	13.6 (1.9)	CD	6–12 months CR	OLZ: 8 (3.2) mg	†Responder status: 14/23 (60.9%)	sedation increased appetite
McCracken et al. [58]	12	11.3 (2.4)	TD	6 weeks OL	OLZ: 11.6 (5.6) mg	YGTSS motor: $p = 0.006$ YGTSS vocal: $p = 0.085$ YGTSS total: $p = 0.010$	drowsiness sedation increased weight

BP = bipolar disorder; BPRS-C = Brief Psychiatric Rating Scale for Children; CD = conduct disorder; CGI-I = Clinical Global Impressions-Improvement scale; CR = chart review; DB = double-blind; OL = open-label; OLZ = olanzapine; PBO = placebo; PDD = pervasive developmental disorder; RPCT = randomized, placebo-controlled trial; TD = Tourette's disorder; YGTSS = Yale Global Tic Severity Scale; YMRS = Young Mania Rating Scale.

*Standard deviation not given.

†Response criteria = CGI-I of 1 (very much improved) or 2 (much improved) and ≥ 50% improvement in Modified Overt Aggression Scale total score

Table 10.5 Summary of selected acute trials of quetiapine in children and adolescents with psychiatric disorders

Study	N	Age, mean (SD) or range	Inclusion criteria/ psychiatric diagnosis	Design	Medication and mean dose, mg/day	Outcome	Adverse events
Findling et al. [62]	222	15.41 (1.32)	Schizophrenia	6 weeks DB-RPCT	QUE (titrated to fixed doses): 400 mg 800 mg	PANSS total score: QUE 400 mg > PBO ($p = 0.043$); QUE 800 mg > PBO ($p = 0.009$)	somnolence insomnia headache dizziness
DelBello et al. [65]	30	12–18	BP-I manic or mixed	6 weeks DB-RPCT	DVPX + QUE: DVPX serum level: 104 mg/mL* QUE: 432 mg* DVPX + PBO: DVPX serum level: 102 mg/mL*	YMRS: DVPX + QUE > DVPX + PBO ($p = 0.03$)	sedation (DVPX+QUE > DVPX+PBO)
DelBello et al. [66]	50	12–18	BP-I manic or mixed	4 weeks DB-RCT	QUE: 412 (83) mg DVPX serum level: 101 μg/mL*	YMRS: QUE = DVPX ($p = 0.3$)	sedation dizziness dyspepsia
DelBello et al. [67]	32	12–18	BP-I depressed	8 weeks DB-RPCT	QUE: 403 (133) mg	CDRS-R: QUE = PBO ($p = 0.89$)	dizziness

Study	N	Age	Diagnosis	Duration/Design	Dose	Outcome	Adverse effects
DelBello et al. [64]	20	14.7 (1.7)	Non-BP-I mood disorder; 1° relative with BP-I	12 weeks SB	QUE: 460 (88) mg	†Responder status: 15/20 (75%)	somnolence headache musculoskeletal pain dyspepsia sedation
Mukaddes and Abali [69]	12	11.4 (2.4)	Tourette's disorder	8 weeks OL	QUE: 72.9 (22.5) mg	YGTSS total: Mean change from baseline = 61.91 (18.69)	sedation
Connor et al. [70]	19	12–17	CD	7 weeks DB-RPCT	QUE: 274 (78) mg	CGI-S: QUE > PBO ($p < 0.01$)	sedation social withdrawal weight gain irritability

BP-I = bipolar I disorder; CD = conduct disorder; CDRS-R = Children's Depression Rating Scale-Revised; CGI-S = Clinical Global Impressions Severity scale; DB = double-blind; DVPX = divalproex sodium; OL = open-label; PANSS = Positive and Negative Syndrome Scale; PBO = placebo; QUE = quetiapine; RCT = randomized controlled trial; RPCT = randomized, placebo-controlled trial; SB = single-blind; YGTSS = Yale Global Tic Severity Scale; YMRS = Young Mania Rating Scale

*Standard deviation not given.

†Response criteria = CGI-I of 1 (very much improved) or 2 (much improved)

Table 10.6 Summary of selected acute trials of ziprasidone in children and adolescents with psychiatric disorders

Study	N	Age, mean (SD) or range	Inclusion criteria/ psychiatric diagnosis	Design	Medication and mean dose, mg/day	Outcome	Adverse events
Findling et al. [74]	283	13–17	Schizophrenia	6 weeks DB-RPCT	ZIP: titrated to 120–160 mg, flexibly dosed at 80–160 mg*	BPRS-A: ZIP = PBO (p = 0.153)	somnolence dizziness EPD vomiting insomnia headache fatigue tremor nausea akathisia
DelBello et al. [73]	63	10–17	BP-I manic or mixed, Schizophrenia, or Schizoaffective disorder	27 weeks ROL	ZIP: titrated to 80 mg (low) or 160 mg (high), flexibly dosed at 20–160 mg*	YMRS & BPRS-A: clinically meaningful symptomatic improvements in both patient groups at both low and high ZIP doses	sedation somnolence nausea headache
Biederman et al. [75]	21	10.3 (2.6)	BP	8 weeks OL	ZIP: 56.2 (34.4) mg	†Responder status: 15/21 (71%)	sedation headache
Malone et al. [76]	12	14.5 (1.8)	AD	6 weeks OL	ZIP: 98.3 (40.4) mg	CGI-I of 1 (very much improved) or 2 (much improved); 9/12 (75%)	sedation
Sallee et al. [77]	28	7–17	TD or CTD	8 weeks DB-RPCT	ZIP: 28.2 (9.6) mg	YGTSS total: ZIP > PBO (p = 0.016)	somnolence

AD = autistic disorder; BP = bipolar disorder; BP-I = bipolar I disorder; BPRS-A = Brief Psychiatric Rating Scale–Adolescents; CGI-I = Clinical Global Impression–Improvement scale; CGI-S = Clinical Global Impression–Severity scale; CTD = chronic motor or vocal tic disorder; DB = double-blind; EPD = extrapyramidal disorder; OL = open-label; PBO = placebo; ROL = randomized open-label; RPCT = randomized, placebo-controlled trial; TD = Tourette's disorder; YGTSS = Yale Global Tic Severity Scale; YMRS = Young Mania Rating Scale; ZIP = ziprasidone

*Mean dose not provided.

†Response criteria = CGI-I score of 1 (very much improved) or 2 (much improved) or ≥ 30% reduction from YMRS baseline score.

Table 10.7 Summary of selected acute trials of aripiprazole in children and adolescents with psychiatric disorders

Study	N	Age, mean (SD) or range	Inclusion criteria/ psychiatric diagnosis	Design	Medication and mean dose, mg/day	Outcome	Adverse events
Findling et al. [81]	296	13.4	BP-I manic or mixed	4 weeks DB-RPCT	APZ: titrated to 10 mg/day or 30 mg/day*	YMRS: APZ 10 mg = APZ 30 mg > PBO (p < 0.0001)	EPD somnolence
Tramontina et al. [82]	43	8–17	BP-I or BP-II plus ADHD	6 weeks DB-RPCT	APZ: 13.61 (5.37) mg	†Responder status: APZ > PBO (p = 0.01)	somnolence sialorrhea
Findling et al. [84]	302	13–17	Schizophrenia	6 weeks DB-RPCT	APZ: titrated to 10 mg/day or 30 mg/day*	PANSS total score: APZ 10 mg > PBO (p = 0.05) AZP 30 mg > PBO (p = 0.007)	EPS somnolence tremor
Marcus et al. [86]	218	6–17	AD with tantrums, aggression, and/or self-injurious behavior	8 weeks DB-RPCT	APZ: titrated to 5 mg/day, 10 mg/day or 15 mg/day*	ABC Irritability subscale: APZ > PBO (p 0.05)	sedation
Owen et al. [85]	98	6–17	AD with tantrums, aggression, and/or self-injurious behavior	8 weeks DB-RPCT	APZ at week 8*: 2 mg: N = 2 5 mg: N = 13 10 mg: N = 16 15 mg: N = 8	ABC Irritability subscale: APZ > PBO (p < 0.001)	fatigue somnolence vomiting increased appetite

(continued)

Table 10.7 (*Continued*)

Study	N	Age, mean (SD) or range	Inclusion criteria/ psychiatric diagnosis	Design	Medication and mean dose, mg/day	Outcome	Adverse events
Lyon et al. [89]	11	13.36 (3.33)	TD	10 weeks OL	APZ: 4.5 (3.0) mg	YGTSS total: Mean change from baseline = 16.73 (7.54) ($p = 0.003$)	increased appetite weight gain EPS headache tiredness/fatigue
Murphy et al. [87]	16	12.0 (2.8)	TD or CTD	6 weeks OL	APZ: 3.3 (2.1) mg	YGTSS total: Mean change from baseline = 17.5 (6.2) ($p < 0.0001$)	excitability/restlessness increased irritability weight gain
Findling et al. [79]	23	Children: 8 (2) Adolescents: 14 (1)	CD	15 days OL	APZ final dose: 1 mg/day – 15 mg/day*	CGI-I of 1 (very much improved) or 2 (much improved): - Children = 63.6% Adolescents = 45.5%	somnolence vomiting headache

ABC = Aberrant Behavior Checklist; AD = autistic disorder; ADHD = attention-deficit/hyperactivity disorder; APZ = aripiprazole; BP-I = bipolar I disorder; BP-II = bipolar II disorder; CD = conduct disorder; CGI-I = Clinical Global Impressions-Improvement; CTD = chronic motor or vocal tic disorder; DB = double-blind; EPS = extrapyramidal side-effect; OL = open-label; PANSS = Positive and Negative Syndrome Scale; PBO = placebo; RPCT = randomized, placebo-controlled trial; TD = Tourette's disorder; YGTSS = Yale Global Tic Severity Scale; YMRS = Young Mania Rating Scale

*Mean dose not provided.

†Response criteria = ≥ 50% reduction from YMRS baseline score.

Table 10.8 Adverse events commonly associated with atypical antipsychotic treatment in pediatric patients

Compound	Most commonly reported adverse events	Distinct and potentially serious adverse events
Clozapine	Sedation	Agranulocytosis*
	Excessive salivation	EEG changes & seizures
	Weight gain	Arrhythmia & increased heart rate
Risperidone	Sedation	
	Weight gain	
	Hyperprolactinemia	
Paliperidone	Somnolence	
	Akathisia	
	Tremor	
Olanzapine	Weight gain	
	Metabolic changes	
Quetiapine	Somnolence, nausea	
	Dizziness, vomiting	
	Fatigue, dry mouth	
	Increased appetite,	
	weight gain	
Ziprasidone	Somnolence EPS	QTc interval prolongation
	Insomnia fatigue	
	Nausea dizziness vomiting	
	Headache	
Aripiprazole	EPS, fatigue	
	Somnolence weight gain	
	Headache BMI increase	

*Patients receiving clozapine must have a baseline white blood cell count (WBC) and absolute neutrophil count (ANC) before initiation of treatment, followed by vigilant monitoring of these counts (WBC $\geq$ 3500/mm^3; ANC $\geq$ 2000/mm^3) throughout the course of treatment [105].

Clozapine

Clinical pharmacology

Clozapine interacts with a wide range of different neurotransmitter receptors. Limited data are available on the metabolism of clozapine metabolites, norclozapine, and desmethylclozapine in children. In one small study (N = 6), Frazier et al. [11] found that the average clozapine clearance to be 1.7 L/kg-h over an eight-hour sample period.

Clinical trials: schizophrenia

Since 2000, only a few trials of clozapine treatment in early-onset schizophrenia (EOS) have been published. These trials have replicated the results of a double-blind, parallel-group controlled study of clozapine versus haloperidol performed at the National Institute of Mental Health by

Table 10.9 Recommended clinical use of atypical antipsychotic medications

Compound	Trade name	Pediatric FDA indication (if applicable)	Initial dose	Titration	Target dose	Effective dose range	Recommendations/comments
Clozapine	Clozaril® [105]	SCZ* (adults)	12.5 mg BID	25–50 mg/day	300–450 mg/day (after 2 weeks)	600–900 mg/day	A divided dose schedule reduces risks of hypotension, seizure, and sedation
Risperidone	Risperdal® [106]	SCZ BPD Irritability associated with AD	SCZ, BPD, AD (≥ 20 kg): 0.5 mg/day AD (< 20 kg): 0.25 mg/day	SCZ, BPD: 0.5–1 mg/day AD: 0.25–0.5 mg at ≥ 2 weeks	SCZ: 3 mg/day BPD: 2.5 mg/day AD (< 20 kg): 0.5 mg/day AD (≥ 20 kg): 1 mg/day	SCZ: 1–6 mg/day BPD: 0.5–6 mg/day AD: 0.5–3 mg/day	Patients experiencing persistent somnolence may benefit from once-daily dosing at bedtime or use of a divided dose schedule
Paliperidone	Invega® [107]	SCZ (adults) SAD (adults)	6 mg ER tablet	N/A	N/A	3–12 mg/day	Maximum recommended dose is 12 mg/day
Olanzapine	Zyprexa® [108]	SCZ BPD	2.5–5 mg/day	N/A	10 mg/day	2.5–20 mg/day	When adjustments are necessary, dose increments/decrements of 2.5 or 5 mg are recommended
Quetiapine	Seroquel® [109]	SCZ BPD	25 mg BID	100 mg/day BID	N/A	SCZ: 400–800 mg/day BPD: 400–600 mg/day	Based on response and tolerability, quetiapine may be administered TID

Table 10.9 (Continued)

Compound	Trade name	Pediatric FDA indication (if applicable)	Initial dose	Titration	Target dose	Effective dose range	Recommendations/comments
Ziprasidone	Geodon® [110]	SCZ (adults) BPD (adults)	SCZ: 20 mg/day BID; BPD: 40 mg/day BID	BPD: 60–80 mg/day BID on day 2	SCZ: 80 mg/day BID	SCZ: 80–100 mg/day BID; BPD: 40–80 mg/day BID	The lowest effective dose of ziprasidone should be used
Aripiprazole	Abilify® [111]	SCZ BPD Irritability associated with AD	2 mg/day	N/A	SCZ, BPD: 10 mg/day AD: 5–10 mg/day	N/A	Maximum recommended dose is 30 mg/day for SCZ, BPD; 15 mg/day for AD
Asenapine	Saphris® [91]	SCZ (adults) BPD (adults)	SCZ: 5 mg BID; BPD: 10 mg BID	N/A	SCZ: 5 mg BID; BPD: 5–10 mg BID	N/A	Asenapine is administered sublingually; Maximum recommended dose is 10 mg BID
Iloperidone	Fanapt® [92]	SCZ (adults)	1 mg BID	2 mg BID increases for next 6 days	12–24 mg/day	12–24 mg/day	Titration should occur slowly to avoid orthostatic hypotension
Lurasidone	Latuda® [93]	SCZ (adults)	40 mg once daily	N/A	80 mg once daily	N/A	Lurasidone should be taken with food

AD = autistic disorder; BID = twice daily; BPD = bipolar disorder; ER = extended release; SAD = schizoaffective disorder; SCZ = schizophrenia; TID = thrice daily.

*Clozapine should be reserved for the use of severely ill patients with schizophrenia who fail to show an acceptable response to adequate courses of standard antipsychotic drug treatment [105].

Kumra et al. [12]. Treatment with clozapine was superior to haloperidol on all measures of psychosis in children and adolescents with EOS, but was associated with serious adverse events, including neutropenia and seizures.

Shaw et al. [13] compared clozapine to olanzapine in a double-blind, randomized 8-week controlled trial of 25 children and adolescents (aged 7 to 16 years) with EOS. Although clozapine was associated with a more significant negative symptom reduction than olanzapine, treatment with clozapine was associated with more overall adverse events.

Kumra et al. [14, 15] evaluated the effectiveness and safety of clozapine versus "high-dose" olanzapine in adolescents with treatment-resistant EOS. Significantly more clozapine-treated patients met response criteria than olanzapine-treated patients. Metabolic abnormalities and significant weight-gain were associated with both study medications.

Based on these data, clozapine appears to be a viable treatment option for youths with treatment resistant schizophrenia.

Clinical trials: bipolar disorders
One small, open-label trial of ten adolescent inpatients suffering from a treatment nonresponsive acute manic or mixed episode associated with bipolar disorder was published by Masi et al. [16]. All patients were considered responders to treatment.

Risperidone

Clinical pharmacology
Risperidone has a high affinity for the serotonin $5\text{-}HT_{2A}$ and the dopamine D_2 receptors. It also has a relatively high affinity for H_1 histamine receptors and for α_1-noradrenergic receptors. Risperidone is metabolized by the liver enzyme CYP-2D6 to the active metabolite, 9-hydroxyrisperidone.

Risperidone is FDA approved for the treatment of schizophrenia in adolescents (ages 13 to 17 years), acute management of manic or mixed episodes associated with bipolar I disorder in adolescents (ages 10 to 17 years), and for irritability associated with autism in children and adolescents (ages 5 to 17 years).

Clinical trials: schizophrenia
Since 2000, several open-label and double-blind, randomized trials have compared risperidone with placebo and other medications in the treatment of EOS. When compared with olanzapine and haloperidol [17], olanzapine [18], and olanzapine and quetiapine [19] in an open-label fashion, treatment with risperidone demonstrated little to no advantage. Rather, in each open-label trial, all treatments appeared to be equally effective for

the treatment of EOS. Treatment differences, however, were noted as they related to adverse events. Gothelf et al. [17] found that patients treated with olanzapine or haloperidol experienced fatigue more frequently than those treated with risperidone. Furthermore, treatment with haloperidol was associated with depressive symptoms, as well as more severe EPS than olanzapine or risperidone. Mozes et al. [18] found no differences between treatment with risperidone and treatment with olanzapine on rating scales for EPS. Both groups showed significant weight gain from baseline to endpoint after 12 weeks of treatment. Jensen et al. [19] found that all three treatments were associated with a significant increase in both weight and body mass index.

Randomized, double-blind comparisons of risperidone with other antipsychotics in the treatment of EOS have produced results similar to those described in open-label comparisons. In a pilot study of risperidone, olanzapine, and haloperidol, Sikich et al. [20] randomized 50 patients with psychotic symptoms to eight weeks of double-blind treatment. The authors noted that all treatments reduced symptoms significantly. While the authors concluded that atypical antipsychotics may reduce psychotic symptoms to at least the same degree as the typical antipsychotic haloperidol, they also noted that these young patients suffered from adverse events at a higher rate and to a greater degree than adults with schizophrenia.

The publicly funded TEOSS study compared the acute effectiveness and safety of two atypical antipsychotics (risperidone and olanzapine) and one typical agent (molindone, plus benztropine) in children and adolescents with EOS and current positive psychotic symptoms of at least moderate intensity, as rated on the Positive and Negative Syndrome Scale (PANSS) [8]. Patients who improved during the preliminary eight-week, randomized, double-blind acute trial were then eligible to continue on the same medication for an additional 44 weeks under double-blind conditions [9]. No significant differences were found between treatment groups in response rates (molindone: 50%; olanzapine: 34%; risperidone: 46%) or magnitude of symptom reduction. Both atypical agents were associated with significant weight gain, but patients treated with olanzapine were at the highest risk. Patients treated with molindone reported significantly higher rates of akathisia. Of the 116 pediatric patients randomized in the acute trial, 54 entered maintenance treatment (molindone, N = 20; olanzapine, N = 13; risperidone, N = 21) and 14 completed 44 weeks of treatment [9]. As in the acute trial [8], no agent demonstrated superior efficacy and all were associated with significant adverse events.

Two double-blind, randomized, controlled trials have evaluated the efficacy and safety of varying dose regimens of risperidone in adolescents (ages 13 to 17 years) with schizophrenia [21, 22]. In the first study, 267 patients were randomized to receive risperidone 1.5–6.0 mg/day or risperidone 0.15–0.6 mg/day for eight weeks [21]. The authors found that patients in the higher dose group improved significantly compared with those in the lower dose group. More patients in the higher dose group experienced EPS-related adverse events.

The second study compared two risperidone dose regimens with placebo [22]. Significant improvements occurred in both risperidone groups compared with placebo. Patients treated with risperidone 4–6 mg/day experienced a higher incidence of EPS, hypertonia, and dizziness than those receiving risperidone 1–3 mg/day. The authors concluded that both dose regimens of risperidone were well tolerated and effective but that, owing to a more preferable benefit-risk profile, a risperidone dose of 1–3 mg/day may be optimal for the treatment of acute psychotic symptoms in adolescent schizophrenia.

Clinical trials: bipolar disorders
The potential of risperidone as a treatment for pediatric bipolar disorder was evaluated by Biederman et al. [23] in an open-label trial. Additionally, Haas et al. [24] evaluated the efficacy, safety, and tolerability of risperidone monotherapy at two dose levels for the treatment of an acute manic or mixed episode in pediatric patients with bipolar I disorder. Compared to placebo, both risperidone-treated groups experienced significantly greater reductions in the Young Mania Rating Scale (YMRS) score. Owing to a better benefit-risk profile, the authors suggested that risperidone 0.5–2.5 mg/day may be preferable for the treatment of acute manic or mixed episodes of bipolar I disorder in pediatric patients.

Clinical trials: pervasive developmental disorders
Several randomized, double-blind, placebo-controlled trials of risperidone treatment have described both acute and long-term benefit in children with autistic disorder and other PDDs. In 2002, the Research Units on the Pediatric Psychopharmacology (RUPP) Autism Network randomized 101 children [25]. Treatment with risperidone was associated with a significant reduction in irritability, as well as a significant, positive response to treatment.

Responders to treatment (N = 63) were enrolled in an additional four-month, open-label extension, followed by a placebo-controlled discontinuation trial lasting up to eight weeks [26]. The mean risperidone dose was 1.96 mg/day at baseline of the open-label phase and was maintained with only a 6% increase (maximum mean dose of 2.10 mg/day at week 12) over the 16-week treatment period. During open treatment, the mean reduction in irritability (according to the Aberrant Behavior Checklist (ABC) irritability subscale) remained stable. Of the 63 patients receiving open-label risperidone, 38 enrolled in the discontinuation phase.

A statistically significant difference ($p = 0.01$) was noted in relapse rates between those randomized to gradual placebo substitution (62.5%) and those receiving continued risperidone treatment (12.5%). Throughout the first two phases, treatment with risperidone was associated with weight gain significantly greater than the amount expected based on developmental norms [25, 26]. Adverse events most commonly included increased appetite, fatigue, and/or drowsiness.

A similar set of studies were conducted by Troost et al. [27] in 36 children (ages 5 to 17 years) with pervasive developmental disorder (autistic disorder, Asperger's disorder, or PDD-not otherwise specified (NOS)) and clinically significant, serious behavior problems. Following an eight-week open-label phase in which patients received a maximum daily dose of 2.5 mg to 3.5 mg risperidone, 26 treatment responders continued to receive open-label risperidone for an additional 16 weeks. After 24 weeks of open-label treatment, all of the ABC subscale scores had decreased significantly, and 69% of the children were considered "much improved" or "very much improved" on the Clinical Global Impressions-Scale of Symptom Change (CGI-SC). Notably, two children discontinued treatment owing to weight gain. The remaining 24 patients continued in an eight-week double-blind, placebo-controlled discontinuation phase. Children randomized to gradual placebo substitution were significantly more likely to experience symptom relapse ($p = 0.049$) and an increase in irritability (as measured by the ABC; $p = 0.043$) than those children receiving continued treatment with risperidone. In addition to weight gain, the most common side-effect was increased appetite.

Data from two additional randomized, double-blind, placebo-controlled trials in pediatric patients with autistic disorder and other PDDs have been published [28, 29] but with differing results. Shea et al. [28] found that eight weeks of treatment with risperidone was associated with a significantly greater mean decrease on the irritability subscale of the ABC compared to treatment with placebo in children ages 5 to 12 years. In a younger group of children (ages 2.5 to 6 years), risperidone treatment was associated with only minimally greater improvement in the amelioration of disruptive behavioral symptoms and social deficits compared to placebo [29].

Risperidone has also been reported to be more effective than haloperidol in the treatment of children and adolescents with autistic disorder [30, 31]. Miral et al. [30] randomized 30 pediatric patients (ages 7 to 17 years) with autistic disorder to receive double-blind treatment with either risperidone or haloperidol for 12 weeks, 28 of which completed the study. Overall, both treatments were associated with improvements on outcome measures. However, between-group comparisons, demonstrated that risperidone treatment was superior to haloperidol treatment. After this double-blind study, patients were given open-label treatment with the same medication for an additional 24 weeks [31]. Medication doses remained close to those in the double-blind study, with a mean haloperidol dose of 2.7 (1.3) mg/day and a mean risperidone dose of 2.5 (0.7) mg/day. Owing to a lower incidence of adverse events and comparisons of outcome measure scores, the authors concluded that risperidone may be safer and more effective than haloperidol in the long-term maintenance treatment of children and adolescents with autistic disorder [31].

Clinical trials: Tourette's disorder

A six-week, open-label study of risperidone in the treatment of chronic tic disorder or Tourette's disorder described the effectiveness and safety of this medication in pediatric patients [32]. Scahill et al. [33] evaluated the efficacy and safety of risperidone in 26 children and eight adults (mean age of 19.7 (17.0) years) with Tourette's disorder in an eight-week, randomized, double-blind, placebo-controlled trial. The authors noted a 32% improvement in tic severity in patients treated with risperidone compared to a 7% improvement in patients treated with placebo. A mean increase in body weight of 2.8 kg was observed in the risperidone group, while patients receiving placebo did not experience weight gain. Notably, no EPS were observed during this study.

Clinical trials: disruptive behavior disorders

Since 2000, three double-blind, randomized, placebo-controlled acute trials [34–36]—two of which were followed by long-term open-label extensions—and five additional studies have described the efficacy, safety, and tolerability of treatment with risperidone.

Snyder et al. [35] randomized 110 children with a disruptive behavior disorder and subaverage intelligence to treatment with either risperidone or placebo. Risperidone-treated patients showed significant improvement compared with placebo. Seven (13.2%) of the patients treated with risperidone reported side-effects related to EPS. Study participants who completed at least two weeks of the double-blind treatment were eligible to enroll in a 48-week open-label extension study of risperidone [37]. The most commonly reported adverse events were somnolence (51.9%), headache (37.7%), and weight gain (36.4%). The response to risperidone in the extension study remained stable for those patients who were treated with active medication in the double-blind study. Further, risperidone-naïve patients experienced significant symptomatic improvement.

Similar results to Snyder et al. [35] were reported by Aman et al. [36] in another six-week double-blind, placebo-controlled study of risperidone for the treatment of disruptive behaviors in children with subaverage intelligence. In a 48-week open-label extension study of Aman et al. [36],

Findling et al. [38] reported that long-term risperidone treatment was generally safe and effective. The most commonly reported adverse events in this study were somnolence (33%), headache (33%), rhinitis (28%), and weight gain (21%), similar to those reported by Turgay et al. [37].

Following the trials by Aman et al. [36] and Findling et al. [38], Croonenberghs et al. [39] and the Risperidone Disruptive Behavior Study Group studied the long-term safety and effectiveness of risperidone for severe disruptive behaviors in children with subaverage intelligence. In this one-year, open-label study, 504 patients (ages 5–14 years) were treated with a mean (modal) dose of 1.6 (0.03) mg/day for an average of 307.3 (5.0) days. Adverse events were generally mild or moderate, the most common of which were somnolence (30%), rhinitis (27%), and headache (22%). Weight gain led to study withdrawal in nine patients. Overall, treatment with open-label risperidone was associated with significant improvement in disruptive behaviors. Of the 367 patients who completed this trial, 48 enrolled in an additional year of open-label treatment with risperidone [40]. The authors noted that the efficacy benefits seen in Croonenberghs et al. [39] were maintained over the course of this study, and that the overall safety and tolerability of the study drug were good, with the number of adverse events decreasing in the extension trial. A subset (N = 35) of children (ages 6 to 16 years) who completed the open-label extension trial described by Reyes et al. [40] were followed for an additional two years of treatment with risperidone [41]. As in the previous one-year study [40], the beneficial effects of risperidone were maintained during this two-year follow-up period, and the reported adverse events were of a similar type and severity [41]. It was concluded that continuing low-dose risperidone (0.048 (0.014) mg/kg/day) for up to three years appears to be both tolerable and effective in this pediatric population.

Additionally, one randomized, double-blind, placebo-controlled trial of risperidone maintenance versus withdrawal in children and adolescents with disruptive behavior disorders has reported that continuous treatment with risperidone is more beneficial than placebo [42]. Pediatric patients (N = 335; mean age of 11.1 (2.95) years) with disruptive behavior disorders who had responded to weight-based, flexibly dosed risperidone treatment over 12 weeks were randomized to six months of double-blind treatment with either risperidone or placebo. Symptom recurrence occurred more frequently ($p \doteq 0.002$) and more rapidly ($p < 0.001$) in patients treated with placebo compared to those receiving maintenance risperidone. Of these 335 randomized patients, 232 entered a one-year open-label extension study of risperidone treatment [43]. Regardless of previous treatment and whether symptom occurrence had been experienced [42], clinical improvement in disruptive behaviors was noted. Further, risperidone was generally well tolerated.

Paliperidone

Clinical pharmacology

Paliperidone is the major active metabolite of risperidone, 9-hydroxyrisperidone (9-OHR). Like risperidone, paliperidone is a centrally active dopamine D_2 antagonist with predominant serotonin $5HT_{2A}$ activity [44].

Clinical trials

Paliperidone was approved in 2006 by the FDA for the acute and maintenance treatment of schizophrenia, as well as the acute treatment of schizoaffective disorder as monotherapy and as an adjunct to mood stabilizers and/or antidepressants in adult patients. Only one randomized, double-blind, placebo-controlled trial of paliperidone treatment has reported efficacy in young patients. Singh et al. [45] randomized 201 adolescents (ages 12–17) with schizophrenia to receive either placebo or one of three weight-based, fixed-doses of paliperidone extended-release (ER) (low = 1.5 mg; medium = 3 or 6 mg; high = 6 or 12 mg). The authors found that doses of 3, 6, and 12 mg/day (but not 1.5 mg/day) of paliperidone ER were superior to treatment with placebo in the reduction of both positive and negative symptoms of schizophrenia.

Olanzapine

Clinical pharmacology

Olanzapine, a thienobenzodiazepine derivative antipsychotic agent, chemically and pharmacologically similar to clozapine, is approved for the treatment of schizophrenia and bipolar I disorder (manic or mixed episodes) in adolescents ages 13 to 17 years.

Clinical trials: schizophrenia

In 2009, olanzapine was approved by the FDA for the treatment of schizophrenia in adolescents 13 to 17 years of age. Kryzhanovskaya et al. [46] randomized 107 inpatient and outpatient adolescents to six weeks of double-blind treatment with either olanzapine or placebo. Compared with placebo-treated patients, olanzapine-treated patients had significantly greater improvement than placebo-treated youths.

Several open-label studies have evaluated the effectiveness and tolerability of olanzapine in younger patients with childhood-onset schizophrenia [17, 18]. To reiterate, olanzapine (mean dose of 8.18 (4.41) mg/day) and risperidone (mean dose of 1.62 (1.02) mg/day) were found to be efficacious in improving baseline and endpoint PANSS total and subscale scores [18].

A one-year prospective, open-label trial to assess response in naturalistic treatment settings found that olanzapine appears to be useful in the treatment of childhood-onset schizophrenia in school-age children [47]. Notably, four of the five patients who discontinued study participation cited weight gain as the reason for discontinuation. A few international studies have also described the effectiveness of olanzapine treatment in childhood-onset schizophrenia [48, 49].

Clinical trials: bipolar disorders

Olanzapine is also FDA approved for the acute treatment of manic or mixed episodes associated with bipolar I disorder and maintenance treatment of bipolar I disorder in adolescents ages 13 to 17 years. Tohen et al. [50] described the efficacy of olanzapine in this population in a three-week, randomized, double-blind, placebo-controlled trial. Two additional, open-label studies have assessed olanzapine's efficacy and tolerability in the treatment of bipolar disorder in children and adolescents [51, 52].

To determine whether the co-administration of topiramate with olanzapine resulted in less weight gain and better symptom amelioration than olanzapine monotherapy in children and adolescents with a bipolar disorder, Wozniak et al. [52] treated 17 patients with olanzapine monotherapy and 23 patients with olanzapine augmented with topiramate. While those receiving combination pharmacotherapy gained significantly less weight than those receiving olanzapine monotherapy, there was no difference in response between the two groups based on YMRS or CGI-I scores. Both groups experienced a statistically significant reduction in YMRS scores after eight weeks of open-label treatment.

Clinical trials: pervasive developmental disorders

A few studies have described differing results regarding the use of olanzapine in children and adolescents with autistic disorder and other PDDs [53, 54]. When compared to open-label treatment with haloperidol, open-label treatment with olanzapine was associated with a slight, non-significant advantage in clinical improvement (based on CGI-I scores) [55].

One double-blind, placebo-controlled pilot study of olanzapine in childhood/adolescent PDD has been published. Hollander et al. [56] randomized 11 patients aged six to 14 years with a diagnosis of autism, Asperger's syndrome, or PDD-NOS to eight weeks of double-blind treatment with either olanzapine or placebo. The primary efficacy measure was CGI-I score at eight weeks, and three of the six olanzapine-treated patients, as well as one of the five placebo-treated patients were considered responders to treatment.

Clinical trial: other disorders

One published retrospective study has suggested that olanzapine may improve behavior in adolescents with severe and treatment-refractory conduct disorder (Table 10.4) [57]. A prospective, open-label study to evaluate the effectiveness and tolerability of olanzapine on motor and vocal tics in children and adolescents with Tourette's disorder was conducted by McCracken et al. [58]. Olanzapine treatment was associated with a significant decrease in tic severity.

Quetiapine

Clinical pharmacology

Quetiapine is FDA-approved for the treatment of schizophrenia in adolescents, ages 13 to 17 years, and monotherapy or adjunct to lithium or divalproex for manic or mixed episodes associated with bipolar I disorder in children and adolescents (ages 10 to 17). Overall, the pharmacokinetic profile of quetiapine in pediatric patients is similar to the profile reported in adults [59]. A summary of key studies of quetiapine in youths can be found in Table 10.5.

Clinical trials: schizophrenia

Before larger scale studies were undertaken, several open-label treatment studies described the effectiveness of quetiapine for the treatment of schizophrenia [60, 61]. In a double-blind study with three parallel arms, PANSS total score improved significantly more from baseline to endpoint in two quetiapine treatment groups compared to the placebo group [62]. Following six weeks of acute treatment, the long-term effects of quetiapine were evaluated in a 26-week open-label extension study [63]. Patients previously treated with placebo during the acute trial showed the greatest changes from baseline in efficacy variables. Further, efficacy was maintained and continued to improve after 26 weeks of treatment in those patients treated with quetiapine 400 mg/day or quetiapine 800 mg/day in the acute trial.

Clinical trials: bipolar disorders

Several trials have evaluated both the effectiveness and efficacy of quetiapine as monotherapy or adjunctive pharmacotherapy in several populations with bipolar disorders. Effectiveness for quetiapine has been described in studies of adolescents at high risk for developing bipolar I disorder [64] and as an adjunct to divalproex in teens with bipolarity [65]. In a head-to-head comparison, no statistically significant group differences in YMRS scores were found between quetiapine and divalproex [66]. However, for the treatment of depressive episodes in adolescents with bipolar I disorder, quetiapine has been found to be no more effective than placebo [67].

The efficacy of quetiapine in the treatment of manic episodes associated with bipolar I disorder in children and adolescents (10 to 17 years of age) was demonstrated in a three-week multicenter double-blind, placebo-controlled trial [68]. Subsequent open-label treatment with quetiapine was associated with maintenance of efficacy for those patients who received quetiapine during the acute study. Further, patients previously treated with placebo during the acute study experienced significant improvement from baseline during open-label treatment [63].

Clinical trials: other disorders

One international open-label trial has investigated the short-term effectiveness and safety of quetiapine in the treatment of children and adolescents with Tourette's disorder [69]. Also, in a randomized, double-blind, placebo-controlled pilot study, quetiapine demonstrated superiority to placebo in the treatment of adolescent conduct disorder [70].

Ziprasidone

Clinical pharmacology

Ziprasidone has a high ratio of 5-HT_{2A} to D_2 receptor antagonism, and has high affinity for the 5-HT_{1A} receptor subtype [71]. Comparable to adult data, ziprasidone exhibits linear pharmacokinetics and dose-related exposure [72].

Clinical trials: schizophrenia

Two trials—one randomized, open-label study [73] and one randomized, double-blind, placebo-controlled trial [74]—of ziprasidone treatment in pediatric patients with schizophrenia have been published. DelBello et al. [73] randomized 63 children and adolescents (aged 10 to 17 years) with either bipolar I disorder, schizophrenia, or schizoaffective disorder to receive open-label treatment with either 80 mg/day (low) or 160 mg/day (high) ziprasidone for three weeks, followed by a 24-week, flexible-dose (20–160 mg/day) period. The authors noted clinically meaningful symptomatic improvement in both diagnostic groups at both low and high doses of ziprasidone. Further, no significant effects on QTc interval were noted. Findling et al. [74] examined the efficacy, safety, and tolerability of ziprasidone in 283 adolescents (ages 13 to 17 years) with schizophrenia and found that flexibly dosed (80–160 mg/day) ziprasidone was not superior to placebo in the reduction of psychotic symptomatology.

Clinical trials: bipolar disorders

In addition to the open-label trial published by DelBello et al. [73] one prospective open-label treatment trial of ziprasidone monotherapy in children and adolescents with a bipolar disorder has been published [75]. Ziprasidone was associated with clinically and statistically significant improvement in mean YMRS score, was well-tolerated, and was not associated with an increase in QTc interval.

Clinical trials: other disorders

Ziprasidone has been reported to reduce symptoms associated with autism in an open-label pilot study in 12 adolescents [76]. Sallee et al. [77] evaluated the efficacy and tolerability of ziprasidone in children and adolescents with Tourette's disorder and chronic tic disorders. Ziprasidone treatment was associated with significant reductions in tic severity and frequency.

Aripiprazole

Clinical pharmacology

Aripiprazole is a partial agonist at D_2 and $5\text{-}HT_{1A}$ receptors, and antagonist activity at $5\text{-}HT_{2A}$ receptors. It is FDA-approved for the treatment of schizophrenia in adolescents (ages 13 to 17 years), acute management manic or mixed episodes associated with bipolar I disorder in adolescents (ages 10 to 17 years), and, most recently, for irritability associated with autism in children and adolescents (ages 6 to 17 years). Pharmacokinetics of aripiprazole in pediatric populations are linear and comparable to previous pharmacokinetic observations in adults [78, 79].

Clinical trials: bipolar disorders

An eight-week, open-label, prospective study of aripiprazole monotherapy conducted by Biederman et al. [80] described the benefit of aripiprazole in the treatment of mania in 19 pediatric patients with bipolar disorder. Aripiprazole was associated with clinically and statistically significant improvement in mean YMRS scores.

The efficacy of aripiprazole in the treatment of bipolar I disorder in pediatric patients (ages 10 to 17 years) was evaluated in a four-week placebo-controlled trial of 296 children and adolescents currently experiencing a manic or mixed episode associated with bipolar I disorder (Table 10.7) [81]. Both aripiprazole doses were superior to placebo on the primary efficacy variable. The most commonly reported adverse events occurred at higher rates at the 30 mg/day aripiprazole dose than the 10 mg/day dose.

In 43 children and adolescents diagnosed with bipolar disorder and comorbid ADHD, aripiprazole (13.61 (5.37) mg/day) was superior to placebo in reducing manic symptoms and improving global functioning after six weeks of treatment [82]. A subset of this study population (N = 16) participated in a randomized crossover trial of methylphenidate and placebo (two weeks each) combined with aripiprazole [83]. Significant improvement in depressive symptoms was observed during adjunctive treatment with methylphenidate but no significant differences between the effects of methylphenidate and placebo were noted in ADHD or manic symptoms.

Clinical trials: schizophrenia

A multiple-center, randomized, double-blind, placebo-controlled study conducted by Findling et al. [84] evaluated the efficacy of aripiprazole in 302 adolescents (ages 13 to 17 years) with schizophrenia. Both aripiprazole doses showed statistically significant differences from placebo in reduction in PANSS total score. Both active treatment groups had significantly greater reductions in prolactin than the placebo group.

Clinical trials: pervasive developmental disorders

The efficacy of aripiprazole in the treatment of irritability associated with autistic disorder was established in two eight-week, placebo-controlled trials in pediatric patients ages 6 to 17 years [85, 86].

Clinical trials: Tourette's disorder and tic disorders

A few prospective, open-label studies of aripiprazole for the treatment of tics associated with Tourette's disorder and tic disorders have been published [87–90]. The most commonly reported adverse events in these four studies were nausea, sedation/hypersomnia/tiredness/fatigue, headache, EPS/akathisia, increased appetite, and weight gain.

Clinical trials: conduct disorder

An open-label study of aripiprazole to evaluate the pharmacokinetics, tolerability, and effectiveness of aripiprazole in the treatment of children and adolescents with conduct disorder was conducted by Findling et al. [79]. Overall, improvements in aggressive behavior were noted during the course of the study.

Asenapine

The dibenzo-oxepino pyrrole asenapine recently received FDA approval as monotherapy in adults for the acute treatment of schizophrenia and for manic or mixed episodes associated with bipolar I disorder with or without psychotic features [91]. The safety and effectiveness of asenapine have not been established in pediatric populations.

Iloperidone

Iloperidone, a newly approved atypical antipsychotic for the treatment of schizophrenia in adults, is a piperidinyl-benzisoxazole derivative with higher affinity for the serotonin 5-HT$_{2A}$ than dopamine D$_2$ receptors [92]. The effectiveness and safety of iloperidone has not yet been studied in pediatric patients.

Lurasidone

Lurasidone is a benzoisothiazol derivative recently approved by the FDA for the treatment of adult patients with schizophrenia [93]. The efficacy and safety of lurasidone has not been evaluated in pediatric populations.

Ethical issues: treatment of at-risk populations

Early identification and treatment of schizophrenia and bipolar disorder can alleviate symptoms, delay the onset of illness, and improve outcome [94]. Prior to the onset of frank psychosis or mania, a period of subsyndromal illness representing change from premorbid functioning—prodrome—is frequently experienced by patients.

With both schizophrenia and bipolar disorder, there is recognition that treatment delays impact prognosis. Longer duration of untreated psychosis is associated with poorer response to antipsychotic treatment, incomplete remission of symptoms, increased risk of relapse, depression, suicide, substance use, family burden, and treatment costs [94]. Earlier intervention is associated with a greater response to treatment, prevents biological and psychosocial deterioration, and reduces hospitalizations as well as costs [95]. Similarly, treatment delays with bipolar disorder lead to a more difficult course as an adult, more recurrences, treatment resistance (particularly with depression), chronicity, and suicide [96].

To date worldwide, seven randomized controlled trials were identified evaluating the efficacy of treatment approaches in reducing the transition rate from "ultra-high risk" (UHR) symptoms to psychosis in patients ages 12 to 45 years [97–103]. The atypical antipsychotics evaluated in these trials were risperidone, olanzapine, and amisulpride (not available in the United States), and active treatment phases lasted three, six, or 12 months, and after active treatment, follow-up durations lasted six, nine, or 12 months. From these trials, a final conclusion about efficacy and safety of interventions cannot be drawn.

While optimal methods to classify high-risk patients for bipolar disorder have yet to be determined, the importance of such identification is unequivocal. Retrospective data have shown that treating children with mood stabilizers early in bipolar development can delay the onset of the first full manic episode [104]. Earlier age of onset in bipolarity is a poor prognostic factor owing in part to the delays to the first treatment in those children and adolescents with manic, mixed, or depressive episodes.

In short, early identification and treatment of schizophrenia and bipolar disorder can alleviate symptoms, delay the onset of illness, and improve outcome. Future research that focuses on more accurate early detection/prevention as well as therapeutic interventions holds the promise for substantially reducing the human suffering that these conditions bring.

Conclusions

When compared with adult data, much less is known about the safety and effectiveness of atypical antipsychotics in pediatric patients. Based on the data that are available, longer term studies of the efficacy and safety of atypical antipsychotic treatment are warranted for this vulnerable patient group. Pivotal studies for newer agents, as well as trials comparing atypical agents and medications from different drug classes are also recommended. Safe and effective treatments are needed to improve the outcomes of children and adolescents suffering from psychiatric disorders. Although it is fortunate that more research in pediatric populations has been performed in the recent past than in previous years, there is much more research that needs to be done.

References

1 Wiznitzer M, Findling RL: Why do psychiatric drug research in children? *Lancet* 2003; **361**: 1147–8.
2 Peroutka SJ, Snyder SH: Relationship of neuroleptics drug effects at brain dopamine, serotonin, α-adrenergic, and histamine receptors to clinical potency. *Am J Psychiatry* 1980; **137**: 1518–22.
3 Sekine Y, Rikihisa T, Ogata H et al.: Correlations between in vitro affinity of antipsychotics to various central neurotransmitter receptors and clinical incidence of their adverse drug reactions. *Eur J Clin Pharmacol* 1999; **55**: 583–7.
4 Davanzo PA: Antipsychotic agents. In: Rosenberg DR, Davanzo PA, Gershon S (eds) *Pharmacotherapy for Child and Adolescent Psychiatric Disorders*, 2nd edn. Wiley-Blackwell, New York, 2002, pp. 355–414.
5 Lader M: Some adverse effects of antipsychotics: prevention and treatment. *J Clin Psychiatry* 1999; **60**: 18–21.
6 Findling RL, McNamara NK, Gracious BL: Antipsychotic agents: traditional and atypical. In: Martin A, Scahill L, Charney DS, Leckman JF (eds): *Pediatric Psychopharmacology: Principles and Practice*, Oxford UP, New York, 2003, pp. 328–40.
7 Richelson E: Receptor pharmacology of neuroleptics: relation to clinical effects. *J Clin Psychiatry* 1999; **60**: 5–14.

8 Sikich L, Frazier JA, McClellan J et al.: Double-blind comparison of first- and second-generation antipsychotics in early-onset schizophrenia and schizo-affective disorder: findings from the Treatment of Early-Onset Schizophrenia Spectrum Disorders (TEOSS) study. *Am J Psychiatry* 2008; **165:** 1420–31.

9 Findling RL, Johnson JL, McClellan J et al.: Double-blind maintenance safety and effectiveness findings from the Treatment of Early-Onset Schizophrenia Spectrum (TEOSS) study. *J Am Acad Child Adolesc Psychiatry* 2010; **49:** 583–94.

10 Keepers GA, Clappison VJ, Casey DE: Initial anticholinergic prophylaxis for neuroleptic-induced extrapyramidal syndromes. *Arch Gen Psychiatry* 1983; **40:** 1113–17.

11 Frazier JA, Cohen LG, Jacobsen L et al.: Clozapine pharmacokinetics in children and adolescents with childhood-onset schizophrenia. *J Clin Psychopharmacol* 2003; **23:** 87–91.

12 Kumra S, Frazier JA, Jacobsen LK et al.: Childhood-onset schizophrenia: a double-blind clozapine-haloperidol comparison. *Arch Gen Psychiatry* 1996; **53:** 1090–7.

13 Shaw P, Sporn A, Gogtay N et al.: Childhood-onset schizophrenia: a double-blind, randomized clozapine-olanzapine comparison. *Arch Gen Psychiatry* 2006; **63:** 721–30.

14 Kumra S, Kranzler H, Gerbino-Rosen G et al.: Clozapine and "high-dose" olanzapine in refractory early-onset schizophrenia: a 12-week randomized and double-blind comparison. *Biol Psychiatry* 2008; **63:** 524–9.

15 Kumra S, Kranzler H, Gerbino-Rosen G et al.: Clozapine versus "high-dose" olanzapine in refractory early-onset schizophrenia: an open-label extension study. *J Child Adolesc Psychopharmacol* 2008; **18:** 307–16.

16 Masi G, Mucci M, Millepiedi S: Clozapine in adolescent inpatients with acute mania. *J Child Adolesc Psychopharmacol* 2002; **12:** 93–9.

17 Gothelf D, Apter A, Reidman J et al.: Olanzapine, risperidone and haloperidol in the treatment of adolescent patients with schizophrenia. *J Neural Transm* 2003; **110:** 545–60.

18 Mozes T, Ebert T, Michal SE et al.: An open-label randomized comparison of olanzapine versus risperidone in the treatment of childhood-onset schizophrenia. *J Child Adolesc Psychopharmacol* 2006; **16:** 393–403.

19 Jensen JB, Kumra S, Leitten W et al.: A comparative pilot study of second-generation antipsychotics in children and adolescents with schizophrenia-spectrum disorders. *J Child Adolesc Psychopharmacol* 2008; **18:** 317–26.

20 Sikich L, Hamer RM, Bashford RA et al.: A pilot study of risperidone, olanzapine, and haloperidol in psychotic youth: a double-blind, randomized, 8-week trial. *Neuropsychopharmacology* 2004; **29:** 133–45.

21 Haas M, Eerdekens M, Kushner S et al.: Efficacy, safety and tolerability of two risperidone dosing regimens in adolescent schizophrenia: double-blind study. *Br J Psychiatry* 2009; **194:** 158–64.

22 Haas M, Unis AS, Armenteros J et al.: A 6-week, randomized, double-blind, placebo-controlled study of the efficacy and safety of risperidone in adolescents with schizophrenia. *J Child Adolesc Psychopharmacol* 2009; **19:** 611–21.

23 Biederman J, Mick E, Wozniak J et al.: An open-label trial of risperidone in children and adolescents with bipolar disorder. *J Child Adolesc Psychopharmacol* 2005; **15:** 311–17.

24 Haas M, DelBello MP, Pandina G et al.: Risperidone for the treatment of acute mania in children and adolescents with bipolar disorder: a randomized, double-blind, placebo-controlled study. *Bipolar Disord* 2009; **11:** 687–700.

25 McCracken JT, McGough J, Shah B et al.: Risperidone in children with autism and serious behavioral problems. *N Engl J Med* 2002; **347**: 314–21.

26 Research Units on Pediatric Psychopharmacology (RUPP) Autism Network: Risperidone treatment of autistic disorder: longer-term benefits and blinded discontinuation after 6 months. *Am J Psychiatry* 2005; **162**: 1361–9.

27 Troost PW, Lahuis BE, Steenhuis MP et al.: Long-term effects of risperidone in children with autism spectrum disorders: a placebo discontinuation study. *J Am Acad Child Adolesc Psychiatry* 2005; **44**: 1137–44.

28 Shea S, Turgay A, Carroll A et al.: Risperidone in the treatment of disruptive behavioral symptoms in children with autistic and other pervasive developmental disorders. *Pediatrics* 2004; **114**: e634–e641.

29 Luby J, Mrakotsky C, Stalets MM et al.: Risperidone in preschool children with autistic spectrum disorders: an investigation of safety and efficacy. *J Child Adolesc Psychopharmacol* 2006; **16**: 575–87.

30 Miral S, Gencer O, Inal-Emiroglu FN et al.: Risperidone versus haloperidol in children and adolescents with AD: a randomized, controlled, double-blind trial. *Eur Child Adolesc Psychiatry* 2008; **17**: 1–8.

31 Gencer O, Emiroglu FN, Miral S et al.: Comparison of long-term efficacy and safety of risperidone and haloperidol in children and adolescents with autistic disorder: an open label maintenance study. *Eur Child Adolesc Psychiatry* 2008; **17**: 217–25.

32 Kim BN, Lee CB, Hwang JW et al.: Effectiveness and safety of risperidone for children and adolescents with chronic tic or Tourette disorders in Korea. *J Child Adolesc Psychopharmacol* 2005; **15**: 318–24.

33 Scahill L, Leckman JF, Schultz RT et al.: A placebo-controlled trial of risperidone in Tourette syndrome. *Neurology* 2003; **60**: 1130–5.

34 Findling RL, McNamara NK, Branicky LA et al.: A double-blind study of risperidone in the treatment of conduct disorder. *J Am Acad Child Adolesc Psychiatry* 2000; **39**: 509–16.

35 Snyder R, Turgay A, Aman M et al.: Effects of risperidone on conduct and disruptive behavior disorders in children with subaverage IQs. *J Am Acad Child Adolesc Psychiatry* 2002; **41**: 1026–36.

36 Aman MG, DeSmedt G, Derivan A et al.: Double-blind, placebo-controlled study of risperidone for the treatment of disruptive behaviors in children with subaverage intelligence. *Am J Psychiatry* 2002; **159**: 1337–46.

37 Turgay A, Binder C, Snyder R et al.: Long-term safety and efficacy of risperidone for the treatment of disruptive behavior disorders in children with subaverage IQs. *Pediatrics* 2002; **110**: e34.

38 Findling RL, Aman MG, Eerdekens M et al.: Long-term, open-label study of risperidone in children with severe disruptive behaviors and below-average IQ. *Am J Psychiatry* 2004; **161**: 677–84.

39 Croonenberghs J, Fegert JM, Findling RL et al.: Risperidone in children with disruptive behavior disorders and subaverage intelligence: a 1-year, open-label study of 504 patients. *J Am Acad Child Adolesc Psychiatry* 2005; **44**: 64–72.

40 Reyes M, Croonenberghs J, Augustyns I et al.: Long-term use of risperidone in children with disruptive behavior disorders and subaverage intelligence: efficacy, safety, and tolerability. *J Child Adolesc Psychopharmacol* 2005; **16**: 260–72.

41 Reyes M, Olah R, Csaba K et al.: Long-term safety and efficacy of risperidone in children with disruptive behaviour disorders: results of a 2-year extension study. *Eur Child Adolesc Psychiatry* 2006; **15**: 97–104.

42 Reyes M, Buitelaar J, Toren P et al.: A randomized, double-blind, placebo-controlled study of risperidone maintenance treatment in children and adolescents with disruptive behavior disorders. *Am J Psychiatry* 2006; **163:** 402–10.

43 Haas M, Karcher K, Pandina GJ: Treating disruptive behavior disorders with risperidone: a 1-year, open-label safety study in children and adolescents. *J Child Adolesc Psychopharmacol* 2008; **18:** 337–45.

44 Chwieduk CM, Keating GM: Paliperidone extended release: a review of its use in the management of schizophrenia. *Drugs* 2010; **70:** 1295–317.

45 Singh J, Vijapurkar U, Robb A et al.: Efficacy, safety, and tolerability of paliperidone ER in adolescent patients with schizophrenia. Poster presented at the 57th Annual Meeting of the American Academy of Child and Adolescent Psychiatry, Oct 26–31, 2010, New York, NY.

46 Kryzhanovskaya L, Schulz SC, McDougle C et al.: Olanzapine versus placebo in adolescents with schizophrenia: a 6-week, randomized, double-blind, placebo-controlled trial. *J Am Acad Child Adolesc Psychiatry* 2009; **48:** 60–70.

47 Ross RG, Novins D, Farley GK et al.: A 1-year open-label trial of olanzapine in school-age children with schizophrenia. *J Child Adolesc Psychopharmacol* 2003; **13:** 301–9.

48 Dittmann RW, Meyer E, Freisleder FJ et al.: Effectiveness and tolerability of olanzapine in the treatment of adolescents with schizophrenia and related psychotic disorders: results from a large, prospective, open-label study. *J Child Adolesc Psychopharmacol* 2008; **18:** 54–69.

49 Mozes T, Greenberg Y, Spivak B et al.: Olanzapine treatment in chronic drug-resistant childhood-onset schizophrenia: an open-label study. *J Child Adolesc Psychopharmacol* 2003; **13:** 311–17.

50 Tohen M, Kryzhanovskaya L, Carlson G et al.: Olanzapine versus placebo in the treatment of adolescents with bipolar mania. *Am J Psychiatry* 2007; **164:** 1547–56.

51 Frazier JA, Biederman J, Tohen M et al.: A prospective open-label treatment trial of olanzapine monotherapy in children and adolescents with bipolar disorder. *J Child Adolesc Psychopharmacol* 2001; **11:** 239–50.

52 Wozniak J, Mick E, Waxmonsky J et al.: Comparison of open-label, 8-week trials of olanzapine monotherapy and topiramate augmentation of olanzapine for the treatment of pediatric bipolar disorder. *J Child Adolesc Psychopharmacol* 2009; **19:** 539–45.

53 Kemner C, Willemsen-Swinkels SH, De Jonge M et al.: Open-label study of olanzapine in children with pervasive developmental disorder. *J Clin Psychopharmacol* 2002; **22:** 455–60.

54 Fido A, Al-Saad S: Olanzapine in the treatment of behavioral problems associated with autism: an open-label trial in Kuwait. *Med Princ Pract* 2008; **17:** 415–18.

55 Malone RP, Cater J, Sheikh RM et al.: Olanzapine versus haloperidol in children with autistic disorder: an open pilot study. *J Am Acad Child Adolesc Psychiatry* 2001; **40:** 887–94.

56 Hollander E, Wasserman S, Swanson EN et al.: A double-blind placebo-controlled pilot study of olanzapine in childhood/adolescent pervasive developmental disorder. *J Child Adolesc Psychopharmacol* 2006; **16:** 541–8.

57 Masi G, Milone A, Canepa G et al.: Olanzapine treatment in adolescents with severe conduct disorder. *Eur Psychiatry* 2006; **21:** 51–7.

58 McCracken JT, Suddath R, Chang S et al.: Effectiveness and tolerability of open label olanzapine in children and adolescents with Tourette syndrome. *J Child Adolesc Psychopharmacol* 2008; **18:** 501–8.

59 McConville BJ, Arvanitis LA, Thyrum PT et al.: Pharmacokinetics, tolerability, and clinical effectiveness of quetiapine fumarate: an open-label trial in adolescents with psychotic disorders. *J Clin Psychiatry* 2000; **61**: 252–60.

60 Shaw JA, Lewis JE, Pascal S et al.: A study of quetiapine: efficacy and tolerability in psychotic adolescents. *J Child Adolesc Psychopharmacol* 2001; **11**: 415–24.

61 Schimmelmann BG, Mehler-Wex C, Lambert M et al.: A prospective 12-week study of quetiapine in adolescents with schizophrenia spectrum disorders. *J Child Adolesc Psychopharmacol* 2007; **17**: 768–78.

62 Findling RL, Kline K, McKenna K et al.: Efficacy and safety of quetiapine in adolescents with schizophrenia: a 6-week, double-blind, randomized, placebo-controlled trial. Poster presented at the 55th Annual Meeting of the American Academy of Child and Adolescent Psychiatry, October 28–November 2, 2008, Chicago, IL.

63 DelBello MP, Findling RL, Earley W et al.: Safety and tolerability of quetiapine in children and adolescents with bipolar I disorder and adolescents with schizophrenia: a 26-week, open-label study. Poster presented at the 55th Annual Meeting of the American Academy of Child and Adolescent Psychiatry; October 28–November 2, 2008, Chicago, IL.

64 DelBello MP, Adler CM, Whitsel RM et al.: A 12-week single-blind trial of quetiapine for the treatment of mood symptoms in adolescents at high risk for developing bipolar I disorder. *J Clin Psychiatry* 2007; **68**: 789–95.

65 DelBello MP, Schwiers ML, Rosenberg HL et al.: A double-blind, randomized, placebo-controlled study of quetiapine as adjunctive treatment for adolescent mania. *J Am Acad Child Adolesc Psychiatry* 2002; **41**: 1216–23.

66 DelBello MP, Kowatch RA, Adler CM et al.: A double-blind randomized pilot study comparing quetiapine and divalproex for adolescent mania. *J Am Acad Child Adolesc Psychiatry* 2006; **45**: 305–13.

67 DelBello MP, Chang K, Welge JA et al.: A double-blind, placebo-controlled pilot study of quetiapine for depressed adolescents with bipolar disorder. *Bipolar Disord* 2009; **11**: 483–93.

68 DelBello MP, Findling RL, Earley WR et al.: Efficacy of quetiapine in children and adolescents with bipolar mania: a 3-week double-blind, randomized, placebo-controlled trial. Poster presented at the 54th Annual Meeting of the American Academy of Child and Adolescent Psychiatry, October 24–29, 2007, Boston, MA.

69 Mukaddes NM, Abali O: Quetiapine treatment of children and adolescents with Tourette's disorder. *J Child Adolesc Psychopharmacol* 2003; **13**: 295–9.

70 Connor DF, McLaughlin TJ, Jeffers-Terry M: Randomized controlled pilot study of quetiapine in the treatment of adolescent conduct disorder. *J Child Adolesc Psychopharmacol* 2008; **18**: 140–56.

71 Sallee FR, Gilbert DL, Vinks AA et al.: Pharmacodynamics of ziprasidone in children and adolescents: impact on dopamine transmission. *J Am Acad Child Adolesc Psychiatry* 2003; **42**: 902–7.

72 Sallee FR, Miceli JJ, Tensfeldt T et al.: Single-dose pharmacokinetics and safety of ziprasidone in children and adolescents. *J Am Acad Child Adolesc Psychiatry* 2006; **45**: 720–8.

73 DelBello MP, Versavel M, Ice K et al.: Tolerability of oral ziprasidone in children and adolescents with bipolar mania, schizophrenia, or schizoaffective disorder. *J Child Adolesc Psychopharmacol* 2008; **18**: 491–9.

74 Findling RL, Cavus I, Pappadopulos E et al.: A placebo-controlled trial to evaluate the efficacy and safety of flexibly dosed oral ziprasidone in adolescent subjects with schizophrenia. [abstract] *Schizophr Res* 2010; **117**: 437.

75 Biederman J, Mick E, Spencer T et al.: A prospective open-label treatment trial of ziprasidone monotherapy in children and adolescents with bipolar disorder. *Bipolar Disord* 2007; **9**: 888–94.

76 Malone RP, Delaney MA, Hyman SB et al.: Ziprasidone in adolescents with autism: an open-label pilot study. *J Child Adolesc Psychopharmacol* 2007; **17**: 779–90.

77 Sallee FR, Kurlan R, Goetz CG et al.: Ziprasidone treatment of children and adolescents with Tourette's syndrome: a pilot study. *J Am Acad Child Adolesc Psychiatry* 2000; **39**: 292–9.

78 Findling RL, Kauffman RE, Sallee FR et al.: Tolerability and pharmacokinetics of aripiprazole in children and adolescents with psychiatric disorders: an open-label, dose-escalation study. *J Clin Psychopharmacol* 2008; **28**: 441–6.

79 Findling RL, Kauffman R, Sallee FR et al.: An open-label study of aripiprazole: pharmacokinetics, tolerability, and effectiveness in children and adolescents with conduct disorder. *J Child Adolesc Psychopharmacol* 2009; **19**: 431–9.

80 Biederman J, Mick E, Spencer T et al.: An open-label trial of aripiprazole monotherapy in children and adolescents with bipolar disorder. *CNS Spectr* 2007; **12**: 683–9.

81 Findling RL, Nyilas M, Forbes RA et al.: Acute treatment of pediatric bipolar I disorder, manic or mixed episode, with aripiprazole: a randomized, double-blind, placebo-controlled study. *J Clin Psychiatry* 2009; **70**: 1441–51.

82 Tramontina S, Zeni CP, Ketzer CR et al.: Aripiprazole in children and adolescents with bipolar disorder comorbid with attention-deficit/hyperactivity disorder: a pilot randomized clinical trial. *J Clin Psychiatry* 2009; **70**: 756–64.

83 Zeni CP, Tramontina S, Ketzer CR et al.: Methylphenidate combined with aripiprazole in children and adolescents with bipolar disorder and attention-deficit/hyperactivity disorder: a randomized controlled trial. *J Child Adolesc Psychopharmacol* 2009; **19**: 553–61.

84 Findling RL, Robb A, Nyilas M et al.: A multiple-center, randomized, double-blind, placebo-controlled study of oral aripiprazole for treatment of adolescents with schizophrenia. *Am J Psychiatry* 2008; **165**: 1432–41.

85 Owen R, Sikich L, Marcus RN et al.: Aripiprazole in the treatment of irritability in children and adolescents with autistic disorder. *Pediatrics* 2009; **124**: 1533–40.

86 Marcus RN, Owen R, Kamen L et al.: A placebo-controlled, fixed-dose study of aripiprazole in children and adolescents with irritability associated with autistic disorder. *J Am Acad Child Adolesc Psychiatry* 2009; **48**: 1110–19.

87 Murphy TK, Mutch PJ, Reid JM et al.: Open label aripiprazole in the treatment of youth with tic disorders. *J Child Adolesc Psychopharmacol* 2009; **19**: 441–7.

88 Yoo HK, Choi SH, Park S et al.: An open-label study of the efficacy and tolerability of aripiprazole for children and adolescents with tic disorders. *J Clin Psychiatry* 2007; **68**: 1088–93.

89 Lyon GJ, Samar S, Jummani R et al.: Aripiprazole in children and adolescents with Tourette's disorder: an open-label safety and tolerability study. *J Child Adolesc Psychopharmacol* 2009; **19**: 623–33.

90 Seo WS, Sung HM, Sea HS et al.: Aripiprazole treatment of children and adolescents with Tourette disorder or chronic tic disorder. *J Child Adolesc Psychopharmacol* 2008; **18**: 197–205.

91 SAPHRIS® prescribing information: September 2010. Available from http://www.spfiles.com/pisaphrisv1.pdf, accessed July 27, 2011.

92 FANAPT® prescribing information: August 2010. Available from http://www.pharma.us.novartis.com/product/pi/pdf/fanapt.pdf, accessed July 27, 2011.

93 LATUDA® prescribing information: October 2010. Available from http://www. latuda.com/LatudaPrescribingInformation.pdf, accessed July 27, 2011.

94 Ruhrmann S, Schultze-Lutter F, Maier W et al.: Pharmacological intervention in the initial prodromal phase of psychosis. *Eur Psychiatry* 2005; **20:** 1–6.

95 Francey SM, Nelson B, Thompson A et al.: Who needs antipsychotic medication in the earliest stages of psychosis? A reconsideration of benefits, risks, neurobiology and ethics in the era of early intervention. *Schizophr Res* 2010; **119:** 1–10.

96 Post RM, Leverich GS, Kupka RW et al.: Early-onset bipolar disorder and treatment delay are risk factors for poor outcome in adulthood. *J Clin Psychiatry* 2010; **71:** 864–72.

97 McGorry PD, Yung AR, Phillips LJ et al.: Randomized controlled trial of interventions designed to reduce the risk of progression to first-episode psychosis in a clinical sample with subthreshold symptoms. *Arch Gen Psychiatry* 2002; **59:** 921–8.

98 Morrison AP, French P, Parker S et al.: Three-year follow-up of a randomized controlled trial of cognitive therapy for the prevention of psychosis in people at ultra-high risk. *Schizophr Bull* 2007; **33:** 682–7.

99 McGlashan TH, Zipursky RB, Perkins D et al.: Randomized, double-blind trial of olanzapine versus placebo in patients prodromally symptomatic for psychosis. *Am J Psychiatry* 2006; **163:** 790–9.

100 Bechdolf A, Phillips LJ, Francey SM et al.: Recent approaches to psychological interventions for people at risk of psychosis. *Eur Arch Psychiatry Clin Neurosci* 2006; **256:** 159–73.

101 Amminger GP, Schäfer MR, Papageorgiou K et al.: Long-chain omega-3 fatty acids for indicated prevention of psychotic disorders: a randomized, placebo-controlled trial. *Arch Gen Psychiatry* 2010; **67:** 146–54.

102 Yung AR, Nelson B, Stanford C et al.: Validation of "prodromal" criteria to detect individuals at ultra high risk of psychosis: 2 year follow-up. *Schizophr Res* 2008; **105:** 10–17.

103 Ruhrmann S, Schultze-Lutter F, Salokangas RK et al.: Prediction of psychosis in adolescents and young adults at high risk: results from the Prospective European Prediction of Psychosis Study. *Arch Gen Psychiatry* 2010; **67:** 241–51.

104 Chang KD, Saxena K, Howe M et al.: Psychotropic medication exposure and age at onset of bipolar disorder in offspring of parents with bipolar disorder. *J Child Adolesc Psychopharmacol* 2010; **20:** 25–32.

105 CLOZARIL® prescribing information: January 2010. http://www.pharma.us. novartis.com/product/pi/pdf/Clozaril.pdf, accessed July 27, 2011.

106 RISPERDAL® prescribing information: April 2010. Available from http://www. risperdal.com/sites/default/files/shared/pi/risperdal.pdf, accessed July 27, 2011.

107 INVEGA® prescribing information: January 2010. Available from http://www. invega.com/assets/prescribing-information.pdf, accessed July 27, 2011.

108 ZYPREXA® prescribing information: May 2010. Available from http://pi.lilly. com/us/zyprexa-pi.pdf, accessed July 27, 2011.

109 SEROQUEL® prescribing information: May 2010. Available from http://www1. astrazeneca-us.com/pi/Seroquel.pdf, accessed July 27, 2011.

110 GEODON® prescribing information: November 2009. Available from http:// labeling.pfizer.com/ShowLabeling.aspx?id=584, accessed July 27, 2011.

111 ABILIFY® prescribing information: December 2010. Available from http:// packageinserts.bms.com/pi/pi_abilify.pdf, accessed July 27, 2011.

CHAPTER 11

Lithium

Garrett M. Sparks & David A. Axelson
University of Pittsburgh Medical Center, Pittsburgh, USA

Introduction

In his seminal 1949 publication in the *Medical Journal of Australia*, John Cade described the case histories of patients with acute mania who had a robust response to treatment with lithium [1]. Cade's initial work was extended by Mogens Schou and other investigators, leading to the clear demonstration that lithium has efficacy for the treatment of acute mania episodes and for prevention of new mood episodes in adults with bipolar disorder.

Controlled data regarding lithium treatment in children and adolescents is limited. Lithium has FDA-approved indications for the treatment of acute mania and for maintenance treatment in bipolar youth aged 12 years or older. However, the scientific support for these indications is based primarily on extrapolation from studies of bipolar adults, as most of the studies in children and adolescents are small, lack rigorous control, and use heterogeneous populations. Larger randomized controlled trials of lithium for the treatment of acute mania in youth are under way or have been recently completed so that more definitive results will be available in the near future. In addition to studies in bipolar youth, several small randomized controlled trials have examined the efficacy of acute lithium therapy for the treatment of severe aggression in youth with conduct disorder, with the majority of studies indicating that lithium may have short-term efficacy for the reduction of aggression in this population. Lithium has a narrow therapeutic index and can cause permanent damage or death in overdose, so cautious dosing and monitoring of blood levels are required. Lithium also has several potential long-term side-effects which require ongoing monitoring when it is used as a maintenance treatment.

Pharmacotherapy of Child and Adolescent Psychiatric Disorders, Third Edition.
Edited by David R. Rosenberg and Samuel Gershon.
© 2012 John Wiley & Sons, Ltd. Published 2012 by John Wiley & Sons, Ltd.

Pharmacology

Lithium carbonate (Li_2CO_3) is a very soluble cation salt which is rapidly absorbed by the gastrointestinal tract. Peak serum levels are typically achieved about 2 hours after administration of the immediate release formulations and about four to five hours after administration of the extended release formulations [2]. Lithium circulates unbound to protein and crosses the lipophilic blood-brain barrier after about one day.

In adults, the half-life of lithium is typically reported as approximately 24 hours. One study with a small subject size found that the half-life in children aged 10–12 (17.9 ± 7.9 hours) was shorter than in adults (21.4 ± 6.3 hours) (this difference was not statistically significant). Children have a greater volume of distribution and glomerular filtration rate than adults and may require an increased lithium dose per body mass. As a result, children may also reach steady state faster than adults [3]. A more recent study examining children aged 7–17 found marked variability in lithium elimination, mostly related to fat-free mass rather than age [4]. Lithium elimination is almost exclusively through the kidney, and it competes with the reabsorption of sodium in the proximal renal tubules.

Potential mechanisms of action

No single mechanism of action has been proposed for lithium that accounts for its efficacy as a treatment for bipolar disorder, though a substantial body of work has suggested numerous likely mechanisms, many of which may in part explain its mood stabilizing effects. A recent review [5] suggests that many of lithium's most clinically significant mechanisms of actions may be best understood as neurotrophic effects (effects related to survival, growth, and development of neurons) in treating manic and depressive symptoms, though the effects of lithium on the circadian system must also be considered.

Lithium is known to exert biochemical and molecular effects on receptor-mediated signaling, signal transduction cascades, ion transport, and gene expression [6]. It has demonstrated diverse molecular effects reversing increased oxidative stress, programmed cell death, inflammation, environmental stress, glial dysfunction, neurotrophic factor dysfunction, excitotoxicity, mitochondrial and endoplasmic reticulum dysfunction, and disruption in epigenetic mechanisms.

Lithium acts as an inhibitor of glycogen synthase kinase 3β (GSK-3β). GSK-3β regulates diverse cellular processes, such as gene transcription, synaptic plasticity, circadian rhythm, and programmed cell death, each of which has been implicated in the pathophysiology of bipolar disorder. In a knock-out mouse model, the deletion of a single copy of GSK-3β resulted in antidepressant effects akin to administration of lithium [7]. A polymorphism of this gene has been associated with earlier onset of bipolar disorder [8]. GSK-3β inhibition influences gene transcription, protecting against programmed cell death and improving cellular structural stability. It also regulates the dopaminergic, serotonergic, and glutamatergic neurotransmitter systems.

The phosphoinositol pathway facilitates signal transduction from G-protein-coupled receptors to a variety of intracellular processes, including activation of phosphokinase C isozymes (PKC) as well as release of calcium from intracellular stores relevant to mitochondrial function. Phosphokinase C isozymes influence a variety of cellular processes throughout the body, though they are highly enriched in the brain, where they play a significant role in the regulation of pre- and postsynaptic neurotransmission. The ratios of membrane-bound to cytosolic PKC activities are elevated during a manic episode [9], and the expression of specific PKC isozymes is significantly decreased in the platelets of adults with bipolar disorder [10]. Lithium has been shown to significantly increase PKC activity in patients with pediatric bipolar disorder [11] and acts through complicated mechanisms to cumulatively downregulate PKC isoenzymes through reduction of myoinositol. Diverse brain areas have shown increased myoinositol levels during manic and depressive episodes of bipolar disorder, which are not observed during euthymia or following treatment with lithium [12]. However, this latter finding may be less of a contributor to lithium's effect in children and adolescents [13].

Other significant targets for lithium's mood stabilizing effects include a variety of enzymes and substrates in second messenger systems with intricate cytosolic, mitochondrial, and nuclear activity. Bcl-2, a neuronal neuroprotective factor, down-regulates calcium release in the endoplasmic reticulum. Lithium increases Bcl-2 levels, and lithium induces a similar primary effect. Both brain derived neurotrophic factor (BDNF) and cAMP response element binding protein (CREB) are heavily involved with the above pathways and cross-talk between them, further mediating lithium's alterations of phospholipid pathways. While increased concentrations of neuronal mitochondrial N-Acetyl-Aspartate (NAA), thought to increase Blc-2 expression and inhibit GSK-3β, have been demonstrated in adults with bipolar disorder treated with lithium, this same finding has not been consistently replicated in youth [14].

Strengthening the notion that lithium acts through neurotrophic mechanisms, structural neuroimaging studies have consistently demonstrated an association between lithium treatment and increased gray matter volume in areas related to cognition and emotional control, including the anterior cingulate gyrus, the amygdala, and the hippocampus [15]. The hippocampus of patients with bipolar disorder treated with lithium has been shown to be larger than that of either healthy controls or unmedicated patients with bipolar disorder [16]. Increases in total gray matter volume in the prefrontal cortex and the subgenual prefrontal cortex correlate well with treatment response [17], and these same gray matter volume changes were not observed in patients treated with valproate with similar treatment response [18].

As the role of circadian rhythm functioning has become increasingly important in the pathophysiology of bipolar disorder, it has become similarly evident that lithium's therapeutic action may somehow mediate this process as well. The CLOCK protein, the central transcriptional activator of molecular rhythms, regulates circadian rhythm in the hypothalamus, and genetic variations in the CLOCK gene have been associated with manic symptoms. Mice with a mutation in the CLOCK gene resulting in decreased expression in the ventral tegmental area exhibit some manic-like behaviors [19]. Administration of therapeutic doses of lithium for ten days reversed these behaviors to normal, suggesting yet another mechanism by which lithium may have mood-stabilizing properties. Administration of lithium has been shown to improve phase signaling in the nucleus accumbens, correlating with improvements in behavior of CLOCK mutant rats [20].

Bipolar disorder in children and adolescents

Clinicians once believed that bipolar disorder was a rare phenomenon in child and adolescent populations, while more recent data, consistent with Kraepelin's early descriptions, suggests that nearly one-third of adults with bipolar disorder recall significant symptoms by the age of 13, while nearly two-thirds recall significant symptoms before the age of 18 [21]. Adults with onset of bipolar disorder during childhood or adolescence have a greater burden of mood symptomatology over prospective follow-up when adults as compared to those with onset after age 18. Children and adolescents diagnosed with pediatric bipolar disorder are at high risk for suicide, psychosis, and substance abuse, and they struggle with behavioral, academic, social, and legal problems.

Children and adolescents with bipolar disorder often present with short but frequent periods of syndromal mania, hypomania, or depression that can switch back and forth between depressive and manic symptoms. Syndromal episodes usually present in the context of chronic subsyndromal mood symptomatology and irritability. In addition, comorbid psychiatric disorders are present in a substantial majority of bipolar youth. Because of these features, bipolar youth tend to present with chronic psychopathology and impairment, and discerning clear, sustained episodes of mania or hypomania can be difficult. Distinguishing manic symptomatology from other common psychiatric presentations in their developmental contexts remains a diagnostic challenge, and DSM-IV criteria do not provide clear adaptations for making the diagnosis in children and adolescents. However with careful assessment, most often in conjunction with longitudinal follow-up, distinct mood episodes meeting DSM-IV criteria for manic, mixed or hypomanic episodes can be identified in a subset of youth presenting with potential manic symptomatology.

Given the significant challenges in making a diagnosis of pediatric bipolar disorder and the implications for both development and psychosocial functioning, a clinician must establish a thoughtful differential diagnosis based upon a thorough assessment including an interview with the patient and family, review of family history, and medical evaluation with laboratory testing when appropriate. Some studies have shown that symptoms of bipolar disorder typically precede correct diagnosis and proper treatment by an average of ten years [22].

Epidemiology

A recent large U.S. study of adolescents aged 13–17 found the estimated prevalence of BP-I and -II to be 2.3% (1.0% BP-I; 1.3% BP-II). Approximately 4% of adolescents were also found to exhibit subthreshold symptoms of bipolar disorder that did not meet criteria for BP-I or -II [23]. Other community studies have found the combined prevalence rates of BP-I and II ranging from 0–2.8% [24–27]. The prevalence of bipolar disorder in prepubertal children has not been systematically studied.

The diagnosis of bipolar disorder in youth has increased significantly in both inpatient and outpatient clinical settings [28–30], with one study estimating a fortyfold increase in the number of outpatient appointments listing a bipolar diagnosis on insurance claims from 1994 to 2003 [31]. As these data are generated largely from billing claims, they must be interpreted with exceptional caution. Despite this apparent increase, it is not clear that children and adolescents are being diagnosed with bipolar disorder at a higher rate than would be expected from rigorous epidemiological studies. These data are unable to demonstrate that youth with bipolar disorder are being diagnosed correctly, or that youth who suffer from other psychiatric illnesses are not misdiagnosed as having bipolar disorder. Further research will be necessary to clarify these important diagnostic questions.

Comorbidity

Making the diagnosis of bipolar disorder in children and adolescents is complicated by high rates of psychiatric comorbidity and symptom overlap with other common disorders in this same population such as ADHD,

ODD, CD, and anxiety disorders [32]. Estimates of rates of comorbid disorders vary substantially among studies based upon the age of the child, sample selection (clinical versus community), and methods used to discern disorders (different instruments used; structured versus clinical interviews; assessment of child, parent, or both, etc.). There are also differences among studies in how to count symptoms that overlap multiple disorders. The range of comorbidity has been reported as 11–75% for ADHD, 46–75% for ODD, 6–37% for CD, 13–56% for anxiety disorders, and 0–40% for substance abuse disorders. Children with earlier onset of bipolar disorder have higher rates of ADHD than do adolescents, while adolescents with bipolar disorder have higher rates of substance abuse disorders. Pediatric bipolar disorder can also be comorbid with autism spectrum disorders.

Clinical characteristics

As the rates of diagnosis of pediatric bipolar disorder has increased, so has the energy expended by researchers to better characterize the clinical characteristics of the presentation of bipolar disorder in children and adolescents. It is clear that some children and adolescents meet full DSM-IV criteria for bipolar disorder. While researchers have made progress in the phenomenological study of pediatric bipolar disorder, substantial debate remains regarding issues such as the diagnostic primacy of elated mood and grandiosity, the role of irritable mood, the distinctness of mood episodes, cycling patterns, and the prognostic significance of manic symptoms that do not meet the DSM-IV symptom or duration thresholds for manic, hypomanic, or mixed episodes.

When examining a pediatric patient, a clinician must consider diagnostic criteria in relation to the developmental context, as many normal behaviors could be wrongly interpreted as symptoms of a mental illness. A seven year old boy in a clearly elevated mood who says he cannot get to sleep on Christmas Eve and who is running through the house speaking quickly and loudly would most likely be the subject of fond memories, and most certainly would not be considered to be suffering from a mental illness. A 14-year-old girl who becomes hyper and stays up all night "bouncing off the walls" during a slumber party, but otherwise does not display such behaviors, similarly is behaving within expected developmental parameters.

Many common screening questions used in adults are not going to be relevant in children, as a nine-year-old girl will likely not be driving recklessly, going on shopping sprees, making bad business decisions, or having sex with multiple partners. That same child might, however, demonstrate inappropriate sexuality for her age (touching others inappropriately, masturbating publicly, touching other children) or participate in uncharacteristically dangerous behaviors in playing, such as trying to fly by jumping from a high place or trying to perform very dangerous tricks on her bicycle [33]. In order to meet DSM-IV criteria for a manic episode, the child must experience marked impairment of functioning, which must be judged within the child's developmental context as a student at school, a member of a family, and a peer with friends. While criteria for a hypomanic episode do not require marked impairment, for a diagnosis of pediatric bipolar disorder to be made, there must be a clear and inarguable change from the patient's baseline level of functioning observable by others.

Symptomatology

Across studies of pediatric bipolar disorder, a meta-analysis has demonstrated that increased energy is present in approximately 90% of cases. Irritability, elated mood, and grandiosity are each present in nearly 80% of cases, and most other conventional symptoms of mania will be present in 70–85% of cases, with the exception of "flight of ideas" and hypersexuality, which are present in 56% and 38% of cases of pediatric bipolar disorder, respectively [34]. However, the greatest controversies in diagnosis remain in discrepant rates of elevated or elated mood across studies, likely due to differences in assessment techniques in research studies.

Some researchers advocate that elated mood (with or without grandiosity) should be a *sine qua non* of pediatric bipolar disorder and elevated, expansive and/or elated mood is generally present in rates about 80% in the majority of phenomenology studies of pediatric bipolar disorder [34, 35]. Such an approach would inevitably lead to the risk of misdiagnosis of the subset of pediatric bipolar disorder patients who do not exhibit this symptom, and it is not required by the DSM-IV criteria. Evaluating whether a child or adolescent has elated mood outside of the normal developmental context in frequency, intensity, and duration can be very difficult and it is important to clarify whether elevated mood is truly beyond what would be expected for the child's developmental level or is simply an expected reaction to a highly stimulating environment or situation. True elation is highly specific to mania, but does not necessarily account for a significant portion of the decreased functioning experienced by children and adolescents with bipolar disorder and may not even be considered a primary cause for concern by family members.

Irritable mood is also a very common symptom of pediatric mania. However, irritability is not at all specific to mania and can commonly occur in other disorders frequently in the differential diagnosis in these clinical scenarios. Irritability that intensifies in the context of other manic symptoms is more suggestive of pediatric bipolar disorder, while chronic irritability independent of changes in energy, activity level, sleep, rate of speech and cognition is less likely to be evidence for a bipolar diagnosis. Assessment of irritability typically requires collateral information from family, as patients will typically under-report this symptom. Irritability is also part of the diagnostic criteria for oppositional defiant disorder, major depressive disorder, generalized anxiety disorder, and post-traumatic stress disorder, and is a common component of attention deficit hyperactivity disorder and autistic spectrum disorders. Substantial controversy remains based on a subset of published reports as to whether chronic presentations of severe, explosive irritability alone may represent the primary mood disturbance in pediatric bipolar disorder in some instances. However, evidence from phenomenological, neurobiological, and longitudinal outcome studies indicate that youth with severe chronic irritability plus ADHD-like symptoms, such as motor hyperactivity, rapid speech, intrusiveness and distractibility, differ substantially from youth that have classic, episodic bipolar I disorder [36, 37].

Further complicating the diagnosis of pediatric bipolar disorder is the fact that several of the most common symptoms present in a manic episode overlap diffusely with symptoms present in other common psychiatric disorders in this population. For example, there are minimal differences in the rates of irritability (98% BP versus 72% ADHD), accelerated speech (97% versus 82%), distractibility (94% versus 96%) or unusual energy (100% versus 95%) [38]. As such, symptoms should only be attributed to pediatric bipolar disorder if there is a clear concurrent temporal association with the elevated, expansive, or irritable mood state. Chronic irritability plus non-specific symptoms, such as distractibility and hyperactivity, which do not significantly intensify with change in mood state, are much more suggestive of a diagnosis other than pediatric bipolar disorder.

Much of the focus remains on questions about the nature of manic symptomatology in pediatric bipolar disorder, but depressive symptoms and episodes are prominently noted in most phenomenological studies. Adults with bipolar disorder frequently recall having significant depressive symptoms in their youth [22, 39, 40]. As is true for adults with bipolar disorder, youth with bipolar disorder may have discrete episodes of depression which meet full criteria for a major depressive episode (MDE). Over 50% of BP youth had a prior history of a MDE in a recent report [35]. A major depressive episode with or without preceding subthreshold manic or hypomanic symptoms may be the chief complaint when a youth with bipolar disorder initially presents for treatment, which may lead to misdiagnosis as well as treatment with pharmacologic agents that may worsen rather than treat depressive symptoms or trigger manic symptoms.

Mood episodes in pediatric bipolar disorder: chronicity and cycling

There has been significant debate regarding the chronicity of episodes and mood cycling in pediatric bipolar disorder, reflecting both disagreements in how to define what constitutes a mood episode as well as differences in assessment techniques and instruments used in research studies. Some groups report manic or mixed episodes lasting 3–4 years [41,42], while others report that while children and adolescents with pediatric bipolar disorder may have some chronic symptoms, pediatric bipolar disorder remains an episodic illness with mood episodes that meet full diagnostic criteria for mania, hypomania or mixed state lasting considerably shorter than 3–4 years in most cases [43,44]. A key feature of DSM-IV criteria for manic, mixed, or hypomanic episodes requires a distinct period of abnormal mood, which calls into question whether symptoms persisting chronically meet this definition and can be used to make a diagnosis of bipolar disorder [45]. Comorbid disorders, frequent shifts between manic and depressive symptoms, as well as subthreshold mood symptomatology complicate the identification of distinct mood episodes. Children and adolescents with bipolar I disorder spend more time over prospective follow-up with mood symptoms that do not meet DSM-IV criteria for a mood episode than with full syndromal mood episodes [46]. Youth with bipolar disorder have high rates of comorbid ADHD, anxiety disorders, and disruptive behavioral disorders, which may remain present regardless of fluctuation in mood. Though symptoms that overlap between other Axis I disorders and pediatric bipolar disorder, such as irritability, rapid speech, psychomotor agitation, and distractibility may fluctuate somewhat over time, they generally do not present in the distinct episodic pattern associated with bipolar disorder. While depressive and manic episodes in bipolar disorder in youth represent a shift from baseline, given the high rate of comorbid disorders, bipolar youth may frequently continue to experience significant symptoms between mood episodes. Others may continue to experience significant subthreshold symptoms in between mood episodes, while some may return to a baseline relatively free of symptoms for extended periods of time. At this time, it is not clear what implications extended periods of remission have for the bipolar diagnosis into adulthood.

Sub-threshold bipolar disorder in youth

A common presentation of pediatric bipolar disorder in clinical settings involves significant manic symptomatology that does not meet criteria for bipolar type I or bipolar type II disorders according to strict DSM-IV criteria. The American Academy of Child and Adolescent Psychiatry (AACAP) Practice Parameters [47] recommend that youth be given a diagnosis of Bipolar Disorder Not Otherwise Specified (BP-NOS) when they have clear manic symptoms that do not meet the DSM-IV duration criteria for a manic, mixed or hypomanic episode, or they have manic symptoms that do not present in distinct episodes. The prognostic and treatment implications of these two different types of BP-NOS are not clear, as evidence noted above indicates that nonepisodic presentations may not be likely to evolve into bipolar I or II. However longitudinal follow-up of a cohort of BP-NOS cases with primarily recurrent, brief episodes (for example, 1–3 days) demonstrated that nearly 40% converted to bipolar I or bipolar II disorder over an average of four years of follow-up [46]. Therefore, paying particular attention to recurrent, brief, distinct episodes of manic symptoms may be indicated.

At-risk populations

The single best predictive factor associated with the risk of developing bipolar disorder is high family loading for the disorder [32, 48, 49]. Twin and adoption studies have demonstrated that bipolar disorder has some of the highest heritability of any psychiatric disorder [32, 48, 50]. The risk of bipolar disorder in first-degree relatives of adults with BP is increased eight- to tenfold [32, 50–52].

The significance of family history seems to be especially robust in children and adolescents. In a study comparing offspring with a parent with bipolar disorder to offspring of healthy community controls and community controls with psychopathology other than bipolar disorder, the risk of a bipolar spectrum disorder in school-aged offspring of a parent with bipolar disorder was increased fourteenfold [53]. However, even with such elevated levels of risk, the majority of children with a bipolar parent will not develop bipolar disorder.

The first mood episode in pediatric bipolar disorder may be a depressive episode [43], and most depressed youth seen at psychiatric clinics are experiencing their first episode of depression [54]. There are no clear risk factors at this juncture that help a clinician delineate who will eventually develop a bipolar spectrum disorder following the major depressive episode. Careful assessment for history of manic or hypomanic symptoms may provide some guidance, and the presence of recurrent brief episodes of manic symptoms, psychosis, family history of BP, and pharmacological induced mania/hypomania may indicate susceptibility to develop BP [46, 55–58].

To date, there is not sufficient evidence to guide treatment decisions for depressed youth at elevated risk to develop bipolar disorder, and there is very little research about treatment considerations for children and adolescents at high risk for bipolar disorder. An early study of prepubertal children (mean age 10.7) with major depressive disorder with family history of bipolar disorder demonstrated that lithium was no better than placebo in treating depressive symptoms [59]. One small single-blind study of 20 high-risk adolescents who had a mood disorder other than bipolar disorder type I or II as well as a first-degree relative with bipolar disorder were treated for 12 weeks with quetiapine. Many of these subjects had been treated in the past with antidepressants or stimulants and had poor treatment response. Subjects did show some improvements in symptoms of mania and depression [60].

Two studies have examined the use of valproate in high risk populations. In the first, 24 children diagnosed with ADHD, MDD, dysthymic disorder, or cyclothymic disorder with current affective symptomatology, and who also had at least one parent with bipolar disorder, were treated with divalproex for 12 weeks. Of the 23 subjects who finished the protocol, 18 were considered responders based on study criteria [61]. In contrast, 56 children diagnosed with bipolar disorder NOS or cyclothymia, who also had at least one parent with bipolar disorder, were randomized to treatment with divalproex or placebo for up to five years. Both treatment and placebo group improved over time, though there were no significant differences between the two in functioning or in discontinuation of treatment, suggesting divalproex was well tolerated but not necessarily effective in treating this population [62]. No other controlled treatment studies of youth with BP-NOS have been published.

Given that significant investigations remain to characterize the early clinical presentation of pediatric bipolar disorder as well as both clinical and biological markers of progression of prodromal symptoms to a diagnosable psychiatric disorder, there remains significant ambiguity as to how to treat children and adolescents at high risk for bipolar disorder. Researchers focusing on psychotic disorders have long struggled with the ethics and practicality of treating the prodromal phases of schizophrenia [63], given that current pharmacologic interventions are not without significant risks.

The treatment of children and adolescents at-risk for development of bipolar disorder depends upon careful assessment and very close monitoring of treatment. Psychosocial treatments should be maximized whenever possible and pharmacological intervention should be reserved for at-risk youth who are clearly significantly impaired by symptoms. Assessment should include thorough inquiry into past symptoms of hypomania or mania in patients presenting with other mood disorders, anxiety disorders, ADHD, disruptive behavior disorders, substance abuse disorders, and autism spectrum disorders, as well as a family history of a bipolar spectrum disorder, including intolerance of antidepressant medications or stimulants. If history does not uncover clear evidence of manic or hypomanic episodes, then pharmacological treatment should focus on target symptoms, such as depression, anxiety, ADHD symptoms or severe aggression. Monitoring of symptoms following the initiation of antidepressant or stimulant medications should include regular inquiry into the onset or worsening of mood or manic symptoms and a low threshold for discontinuing agents that appear to be worsening the child's clinical presentation. If manic symptomatology is present and causes significant impairment, but does not meet diagnostic criteria for mania or hypomania, an antimanic medication can still be considered, especially if other treatments have failed. While the clinical presentation of pediatric bipolar disorder provides a unique diagnostic challenge, close monitoring of treatment response and clinical course will be helpful in clarifying diagnosis and an optimal treatment plan over time.

Evidence for the use of lithium in children and adolescents

Extensive research and clinical practice has demonstrated the effectiveness of lithium in adults for treating the symptoms of acute mania as well as in preventing manic and mixed episode relapse [64, 65]. The FDA has established that lithium is indicated for acute mania as well as maintenance treatment in patients with bipolar disorder older than 12 years of age. Small sample size, varying assessment protocols without adequate controls and other methodologic concerns characterize much of the early literature, but more recent studies with larger samples and more rigorous methodologies suggest that lithium may be an effective treatment for youth with bipolar disorder. Questions regarding predictors of response based on clinical profile are largely unanswered or are addressed only cursorily in the literature. This may reflect ambiguity in the literature regarding how best to define bipolar phenotypes in children and adolescents other than bipolar disorder type I, for which the most evidence seems to be available.

According to recent treatment guidelines for children and adolescents with bipolar disorder, lithium is a recommended treatment for acute manic or mixed states with or without psychosis in youth with bipolar disorder based on studies conducted in youth, as well as for depression in youth with bipolar disorder based upon studies conducted in adults [66]. Recommendation for use of lithium as maintenance treatment for bipolar disorder in youth is based primarily on studies conducted in adults.

Early studies
Early evidence for the use of lithium in children and adolescents with bipolar disorder consisted mainly of case series or double-blinded crossover studies with very small numbers or diagnostically mixed samples. An early survey of these trials suggested that the positive response rate in open trials of lithium in children with bipolar disorder was around 66%, similar to lithium-treated adults with bipolar disorder [67]. Further review of lithium's use in other diagnoses early after publication of DSM-III suggested that lithium was an effective treatment for children with bipolar disorder, emotionally unstable character disorder (a diagnosis not included

in DSM-III, but which shared characteristics with borderline personality disorder, disruptive behavior disorders, and bipolar spectrum disorders), and diagnostically unclear children with parents who had responded to lithium [68].

Four early controlled trials of lithium in children and adolescents with bipolar disorder (combined N = 46) featured cross-over designs [69–72]. These studies used daily dosages ranging from 600–1200 mg/day to achieve blood levels of 0.3–1.3 mEq/L and yielded response rates ranging from 33–80%.

Mania and mixed episodes

Lithium is the oldest and possibly the most extensively studied mood stabilizer in adults for the treatment and prevention of manic and mixed episodes, with placebo controlled-studies dating back to Morgens Schou in 1954 [73], though the methodologies of many of these controlled trials limit their applicability to clinical practice. The most modern of these studies demonstrated significant improvement at day 21 for 49% of patients receiving lithium [74]. Various trials against placebo, other mood stabilizers, and neuroleptics have yielded response rates from 32–88% [75]. Monotherapy with lithium has been shown to be comparable to monotherapy treatment with haloperidol or the second generation antipsychotics [76]. The applicability of this data to children and adolescents is not entirely clear.

A rigorous chart review was conducted of 59 patients exhibiting manic-like symptoms who were initially assessed by structured clinical interview using the Schedule for Affective Disorders and Schizophrenia for School Age Children, Epidemiologic Version (K-SADS-E) [77]. Survival analysis of this data suggested that 65% of children with manic-like symptoms would improve over two years if treated with lithium.

Geller et al. [78] conducted a controlled prospective study of adolescents utilizing more current diagnostic criteria for bipolar disorder in 1998, though with several characteristics that might limit the generalizability of the study. Twenty-five subjects with bipolar disorder (bipolar I, bipolar II, but also MDD youth at-risk for bipolar disorder) and secondary substance abuse disorders were randomized to treatment with lithium or placebo. The average age of mood symptoms predated substance abuse disorders by approximately six years. Those treated with lithium (mean serum level 0.9 mEq/L) demonstrated significant improvements in global functioning and reduction in positive urine drug samples. The response rate at six weeks was somewhat lower than would be expected at 46% using a cut-off on the Children's Global Assessment Scale, calling into question whether lithium might be as effective in this population compared to other mood stabilizers. Mood symptoms measured by KSADS did not appear to improve differentially between the treatment and placebo groups. Notably, these participants were not experiencing an episode of acute mania at the time of entry to the study.

In a subsequent study, Kowatch et al. [79] randomized 42 outpatients (mean age 11.4, range 6–18 years) in acute manic or mixed episodes to treatment with lithium, valproate, or carbamazepine over six weeks (no placebo arm). Measuring response as a 50% decrease in symptoms on the Young Mania Rating Scale (Y-MRS) and improvement in the Clinical Global Impression (CGI), response rates were 46% for valproate, 42% for lithium, and 34% for carbamazepine. Each was well tolerated. These response rates corresponded to effect sizes (measured by Cohen's d) of 1.63 for valproate, 1.06 for lithium, and 1.00 for carbamazepine, suggesting that lithium and the other mood stabilizers had a large effect in open treatment of acute mixed or manic episodes in the pediatric population. The authors also suggested that a treatment period of eight weeks is adequate for assessing treatment response to lithium (compared to six weeks for valproate).

A large open trial of 100 adolescents (age 12–18) yielded a response rate of 63% at four weeks using a 33% decrease in the Y-MRS or improvement in the CGI [80]. Depressive features, age at first manic episode, and comorbidity with ADHD did not predict response. Subsequently, 40 of the lithium-responsive subjects were randomized to either continued treatment with lithium or placebo [81]. At two weeks, there were no differences between rates of symptom exacerbation, though the rate of exacerbation was high in both groups.

In a series of papers using open combination treatment with lithium and valproate, investigators attempted to improve upon the rates of monotherapy using either lithium or valproate [82–84]. Youths between five and 17 with history of at least one hypomanic or manic episode were identified using the Schedule for Affective Disorders and Schizophrenia for School-Age Children—Present and Life-time (K-SADS-PL) or K-SADS-E. At the time of entry to the study, subjects variably met criteria for mixed [39] manic [34], depressed [8], hypomanic [5], or euthymic episodes [4]. At approximately 11 weeks, 47% of the 90 subjects met criteria for remission, including 44% in mixed episodes at the time of entry and 47% in manic episodes. Mean valproate levels were 79.8 and mean lithium levels were 0.9. Fifteen of the patients were withdrawn from the study due to side-effects, 12 of which were attributed to lithium (ataxia, thyroid disease, proteinuria, enuresis, emesis, or dysphoria). There was no comparison to monotherapy with either agent, although this did not appear to be a significant improvement over monotherapy in prior studies.

In addition to the above, several studies have suggested some clinical characteristics that might predict differential response to lithium compared to other treatment options, including family treatment history. In a study of adult bipolar relatives, having a bipolar family member who was a lithium responder strongly predicted a response to lithium [85]. A study of the bipolar offspring (aged 10–25) of bipolar parents who were responsive or nonresponsive to lithium suggested that the offspring of lithium responders had better premorbid functioning and manifested classical mood disorders with episodic course, while offspring of non-responders had a more chronic course with worse premorbid functioning [86]. A small case series of this same study group demonstrated that treatment response in patients who met criteria for bipolar disorder as adolescents highly correlated with membership in either a lithium-responsive or lithium non-responsive family [87].

In the adult literature, earlier research suggested that valproate may be more effective than lithium in bipolar disorder with rapid cycling and mixed episodes, though this finding appears to be less supported by more recent data from the same research group [88].

A more recent retrospective naturalistic case series compared 266 youth with bipolar disorder who were treated initially with valproate, lithium, or an atypical antipsychotic. Ninety of the subjects were treated initially with lithium monotherapy. Response to lithium monotherapy did not seem to be related to bipolar disorder type (I versus II) or the presence of psychotic symptoms or conduct disorder. Younger age at onset of treatment and co-morbid ADHD did predict less response to lithium [89].

In an open-label trial of risperidone augmentation to lithium nonre-sponders, predictors of insufficient response to lithium included severity of ADHD symptoms, a history of physical or sexual abuse, and preschool age at time of study [90]. These findings were consistent with earlier data by also suggesting that comorbid ADHD predicted negative response to lithium [91]. Also, a case-control study of adolescents with bipolar disorder type 1 suggested that prepubertal onset of manic symptoms might predict poorer response to lithium [92].

A recent meta-analysis suggested that monotherapy with second generation antipsychotics may be more effective in treating pediatric mania than monotherapy with traditional mood stabilizers, including lithium [93]. Given the challenges in treating mania in children and adolescents as well as the side-effect profile of second generation antipsychotics in children, lithium remains an important treatment option in appropriate patients.

In adults, evidence supports augmentation of lithium with an SGA, with trials supporting the use of risperidone [94, 95], olanzapine [96], quetiapine [97, 98], aripiprazole [99], and ziprasidone [100]. In the pediatric literature, there is only one study of lithium augmentation with a second generation antipsychotic. The trial compared treatment with lithium to treatment with lithium plus risperidone in lithium non-responders. Out of 38 subjects, 17 responded with lithium monotherapy. Of the 21 remaining, 18 responded to treatment with lithium and risperidone [90].

Bipolar depression

The efficacy of lithium in the treatment of bipolar depression in children and adolescents has not been well established in prospective studies. However, success with lithium in treating depressed adults with bipolar disorder (with a partial response rate of 79%, and a full response rate of 36%) [101, 102] as well as clinical experience, the AACAP treatment guidelines for bipolar disorder [66] recommended lithium as a treatment option for bipolar depression in children and adolescents.

A retrospective chart review, described earlier, suggested that mood stabilizers (lithium, carbamazepine, and valproate) were in general not effective in treatment of bipolar depression in children and adolescents [103]. Though no control arm was present, five out of eight subjects who were experiencing a depressive episode at the time of initiation of the study who received combination treatment with lithium and valproate experienced remission of symptoms [82]. In an open-label trial of 27 adolescents with bipolar depression, the response rate was 48% and the remission rate was 30% using lithium titrated to a serum level of 1.0–1.2 mEq/L [104].

Bipolar maintenance

In adults, the BALANCE trial compared lithium and valproate combination treatment with monotherapy with either agent alone for the prevention of manic and depressive episodes over a two-year period [105]. Lithium monotherapy and combination treatment with lithium and valproate were found to be more effective than valproate monotherapy in preventing any mood episode, though the study was unable to distinguish between combination treatment and lithium monotherapy. Recent trials comparing lamotrigine and lithium in bipolar maintenance against placebo found that lithium was superior to placebo in time to intervention (about six months) for a mood episode and for prevention of a manic, hypomanic, or mixed episode, though, unlike lamotrigine (which was not effective for preventing manic, hypomanic, or mixed episodes), was not more effective than placebo for prevention of depressive episodes [106]. Further studies have suggested that lithium is about as effective as olanzapine in preventing relapse of depressive episodes, though olanzapine was more effective at preventing manic or mixed episodes [107]. Also in adults, lithium may also significantly reduce the risk of completed suicide and suicide attempts [108].

A naturalistic 18-month follow-up study comparing relapse rates of bipolar disorder type 1 in adolescents stabilized on lithium who discontinued treatment suggested a relapse rate nearly three times higher (92% versus 38%) compared to patients who continued lithium maintenance treatment without interruption [109]. Following up on previous work with lithium and valproate, Findling et al. [83] randomized 60 youth previously treated with combination lithium and valproate combination treatment to receive either lithium or valproate monotherapy for maintenance treatment. Time to mood episode relapse did not differ between lithium and valproate over follow-up of up to 76 weeks using survival analysis. Average time to discontinuation due to mood symptoms was 114 days (SE ± 57 days) for subjects randomized to lithium. In a third study of this cohort [84], 38 of the 60 youth who relapsed while treated with lithium or valproate monotherapy were again treated with the combination of lithium and depakote following relapse. Of the 38 subjects, 34 were restabilized on combination treatment.

The AACAP treatment guidelines [66] recommend that medication tapering can be considered if the patient has achieved remission for a minimum of 12 to 24 consecutive months, though the risk for relapse must be calculated against the risk associated with continued pharmacotherapy, and particular care should be taken with patients who have a history of suicidal behavior, severe aggression, and/or psychosis.

Mania with psychosis

A study of ten prepubertal children with bipolar disorder found that lithium alone (mean dose 1270 mg/day, up to 1800 mg/day) was an effective treatment for acute manic episodes with psychotic features, although improvement took an average of 11 days [110]. As combination treatment of lithium and some typical antipsychotics (notably haloperidol) is associated with an increased risk for extrapyramidal symptoms compared to the use of a typical antipsychotic alone, the avoidance of even short-term use of antipsychotic medication was preferable.

The AACAP guidelines on treatment of bipolar disorder recommend combination of a traditional mood stabilizer (lithium, valproate, carbamazepine) and an atypical antipsychotic in the treatment of a manic or mixed episode with psychotic features. Of the traditional mood stabilizers, only lithium is supported by published data, as lithium with an adjunctive atypical antipsychotic was found to be effective for acute mania and psychosis in an open trial [111].

Unipolar depression

In adults, evidence supports that lithium may be a useful adjunctive agent for unipolar depression in patients treated with TCAs, SSRIs, and SNRIs [112, 113]. Lithium augmentation was modestly helpful in treatment-resistant unipolar depression in STAR*D [114]. As mentioned previously, lithium may significantly reduce the risk of completed suicide and suicide attempts [108] independent of its effects on mood. However, these findings have not been replicated in children and adolescents. Lithium was investigated as a potential treatment for MDD in adolescents with a family history of bipolar disorder who did not respond to treatment with tricyclic antidepressants [115], as well as in prepubertal (mean age 10.7) children with MDD with a family history of bipolar disorder [59]. In each trial, lithium was no better than placebo.

In a case review of 14 adolescents with MDD who were partial responders to treatment with a tricyclic antidepressant, six of the subjects experienced significant improvement of symptoms with TCA/lithium combination treatment (mean level 0.65 mEq/L) [116]. In a second study with a control group, 10 out of 24 adolescents showed at least partial improvement with lithium augmentation following partial response to imipramine, compared to only 1 out of 10 control partial responders to imipramine [117], during a three-week trial.

There are no available studies of lithium augmentation of SSRIs or other newer antidepressants for MDD in children and adolescents.

Severe mood dysregulation (SMD)

Some researchers have operationalized a diagnosis of severe nonepisodic irritability and hyperarousal, in contrast to the episodic nature of bipolar disorder in youth, as detailed above. Twenty-five youth who met research criteria for SMD were randomized to a six-week double-blind trial of lithium or placebo with measurements of clinical outcomes as well as magnetic resonance spectroscopy (MRS) outcomes including myoinositol, N-acetyl-aspartate, and combined glutamate/glutamine. No significant between-group differences were found relating to any clinical or MRS outcome measures in subjects receiving lithium or placebo [118].

Aggression and conduct disorder

Lithium has been shown to decrease aggressiveness and violence in animal models [119] as well as in humans [120], seemingly independent of primary psychiatric disorders. In human studies, lithium has been shown to be an effective treatment for aggression associated with mood disorders, disruptive behavior disorders, and autistic spectrum disorders. Much of the early data consists of small case studies and open trials that did not use DSM criteria to distinguish comorbid disorders, which may have accounted for the violent behavior or possible treatment response and did not use similar instruments to measure aggression. Delong and Aldershof [68] used lithium to treat children with behavioral disorders who had a variety of concomitant neurological disorders including mental retardation and noted a significant decrease in aggression, explosive outbursts, and encopresis. Lithium was used to treat severe aggression and destructive behaviors in 17 children aged 3–12 who were refractory to haloperidol and aggressive psychosocial interventions [121]. Thirteen of

the 18 children exhibited decreased aggressiveness, though maximal efficacy was only seen after treatment of up to six months.

Several double-blind placebo-controlled studies suggest that lithium is
effective in treating aggression associated with conduct disorder [122].
Lithium was also found to be just as effective and better tolerated than
haloperidol in a placebo-controlled randomized trial of 61 treatment-
resistant hospitalized patients with conduct disorder aged 5–13 [123]. A
double-blind, placebo-controlled study randomized 50 inpatient children
aged 5–12 with aggressive behavior and conduct disorder to lithium or
placebo, and found that lithium (mean serum level 1.1 mEq/L) was effective in reducing aggressive behavior after six weeks [124]. In contrast,
Rifkin et al. [125] found that lithium was not beneficial for reducing
aggression, as measured using the Overt Aggression Scale (OAS), in 33
hospitalized children with conduct disorder in older children aged 12–17
randomized to lithium or placebo after two weeks of treatment [125].
In another study using the OAS, 40 inpatients (mean age 12.5), 16
of 20 subjects treated with lithium were responders on the Consensus
scales used in the study, compared to 6 of 20 treated with placebo, and
significant improvement on the OAS was observed in subjects taking
lithium in a 4 week trial [126].

Future directions

Given concerns regarding the stringency of methodologies in the above
studies, the FDA issued a Written Request pertaining to the study of
lithium in pediatric mania to the National Institute of Child Health and
Human Development (NIHCD) in 2004. The Collaborative Lithium Trials
(CoLT) aim to establish evidence-based dosing strategies for lithium, characterize the pharmacokinetics and biodisposition of lithium, examine the
acute efficacy of lithium in pediatric bipolarity as well as the long-term effectiveness of lithium treatment, and characterize the short- and long-term
safety of lithium through multi-phase, multisite studies [127].

Future work clarifying the best use of lithium in bipolar depression in
children and adolescents, as well as predictors of clinical response based
on clinical profile, are needed to inform the safe and effective optimal use
of lithium in children and adolescents.

Dosing and drug monitoring

Available preparations

Lithium carbonate is currently available as a generic medication. Immediate release capsules are available at doses of 150 mg, 300 mg, and 600 mg.
Extended release tablets are available at 300 mg and 450 mg doses. Brand

name lithium formulations include Lithobid® (300 mg extended release tablet), Eskalith® (300 mg immediate release capsule), and Eskalith CR® (450 mg extended release tablet).

Lithium citrate is available as a liquid with concentration of 8 meq/5 ml of syrup; 300 mg of lithium carbonate contains 8 meq of lithium and is equivalent to 5 ml of the syrup. The syrup is sugar-free and is available in a raspberry flavor.

Note that the bioavailability of the liquid, immediate release and extended release preparations may vary within individuals, so close monitoring for side-effects and checking serum levels may be necessary when changing a patient from one preparation to another.

Initiating therapy and monitoring

Prior to prescribing lithium, children and adolescents should have a preliminary medical evaluation to determine whether lithium is an appropriate medication for the patient, including a complete history and physical examination performed by a primary care physician. Laboratory investigations including a complete blood count, a comprehensive metabolic profile including electrolytes, blood urea nitrogen and creatinine, urinalysis, and thyroid stimulating hormone should be checked for baseline levels and to assess whether lithium is appropriate for the patient. An electrocardiogram can be considered routinely or in a patient with a history of cardiac disease or a family history of arrhythmia or sudden cardiac death.

A variety of initial dosing regimens are proposed in the literature based on age and/or weight. Others suggest using pharmacokinetic nomograms based on a single test dose and subsequent serum level 24 hours later [128], but the practicality of this approach is limited in outpatient settings. Though dose is somewhat proportional to fat-free body mass, lithium clearance varies widely among the population; therefore, initial dosing should be conservative and titration can be based on steady-state serum levels. One reasonable outpatient dosing strategy outlined in Table 11.1

Table 11.1 Sample dosing strategy

Weight	Starting dose (for two days)	Target dose
20–30 kg	150 mg in the evening	150 mg twice per day
30–39 kg	150 mg twice per day	150 mg in the morning and 300 mg in the evening
40–49 kg	150 mg twice per day	300 mg twice per day
50–59 kg	150 mg in the morning and 300 mg in the evening	300 mg in the morning and 450 mg in the evening
≥60 kg	300 mg in the morning and evening	300 mg in the morning and 600 mg in the evening

uses two days of low doses to assess initial tolerability, followed by a target dose of 15 mg/kg/day.

By convention, lithium levels should be checked 10–12 hours after the evening dose is administered and before the next dose is administered. Serum levels should be checked after 4–5 days of initiation and dose adjusted to clinical effect and tolerability while continuing to monitor serum levels. Serum levels should be drawn after each dose adjustment until initial target levels of 0.6–1.0 meq/L are obtained, though individuals may respond or have side-effects to lower levels, while others may need levels of 1.1–1.3 mEq/L if clinical response is inadequate. Lithium generally has linear pharmacokinetics, so that serum levels change proportionally with dose. It is reasonable to increase the dose proportionally based on the ratio of the target serum level to the last serum level when targeting levels below 1.0 mEq/L; higher levels may require more cautious dose increases. However it is important that medication adherence and the time interval between the last dose and when the serum level was drawn has been determined, as missed doses and/or levels drawn well outside the 10–12 hour interval may affect whether the level can be used to accurately predict proper dose adjustments. Side-effects can occur at presumably therapeutic levels, so close clinical monitoring is necessary throughout the titration process.

A variety of factors may influence the aggressiveness of the dosing regimen and titration, including treatment setting (inpatient versus outpatient), acuteness of symptoms, and physician experience. Once daily dosing is popular in adults for improving compliance as well as possibly decreasing polyuria and the long-term risk of renal toxicity [129–131], but it is unclear whether this regimen is safe or effective in children and adolescents. Twice-daily dosing is generally acceptable in children and adolescents, particularly when the extended release preparations are used. There may be some circumstances where three times per day dosing might be preferable if side-effects are present with twice per day dosing.

After a stable dose has been determined, lithium levels should be rechecked every 3–6 months, though there is not agreement on a definitive standard. Some clinicians check levels monthly for the first several months to assess for any abrupt unexpected changes in pharmacokinetics. Some clinicians have noted that acutely manic patients require and tolerate higher lithium levels so that dosage decreases may be required as the patient reaches euthymia. The serum level for prophylaxis of new mood episodes may or may not be the same as what was required for acute response. Some authors advocate monitoring using salivary samples. Serum and salivary lithium ratios vary substantially between subjects, limiting the utility of monitoring using salivary lithium levels [132]. A device is now commercially available that allows for point-of-care lithium levels to be determined using blood from a fingerstick, though more data regarding its reliability may be necessary before it could be recommended without qualification [133].

Thyroid function and kidney functions should be monitored after the first three months, and then every four to six months. In adults, some authors place emphasis upon estimating glomerular filtration rate using various published estimation equations rather than simply serum creatinine [134, 135]. While such an approach has not been directly validated in children and adolescents, estimation and tracking of glomerular filtration rate by use of the Schwartz equation, which considers age, gender, and height, may be helpful in identifying patients in whom lithium is no longer an appropriate treatment or who should be referred to nephrology for further assessment [136]. Online calculators can be found using major search engines.

Contraindications, precautions, and drug interactions

Black box warning

The FDA black box warning on lithium states that lithium toxicity is closely related to serum lithium levels, and can occur at doses close to therapeutic levels (see side-effects—toxicity). Facilities for prompt and accurate serum lithium determinations should be available before initiating therapy, and referral for emergent clinical evaluation should be made when significant symptoms of lithium toxicity are present.

Contraindications and precautions

The only absolute contraindication to use of lithium is a previous allergic drug reaction. A variety of conditions suggest the need to consider an alternate agent when appropriate or to increase the frequency of monitoring serum lithium levels.

Several conditions significantly raise the risk of lithium toxicity in children and adolescents:

- Severe dehydration or sodium depletion dramatically alters lithium secretion. Lithium itself decreases sodium reabsorption, which may itself cause sodium depletion resulting in an increased risk for lithium toxicity.
- Children experiencing fever from a viral illness or other infection are particularly at risk for dehydration and subsequent lithium toxicity.
- Lithium has been associated with atrioventricular nodal blockade and other alterations in cardiac conduction. Lithium should be used with caution in patients with cardiovascular disease in consultation with the physicians involved in treatment of the cardiac issues.

- As lithium is excreted primarily through the kidneys, significant renal impairment increases the risk of lithium toxicity and may have primary effects on renal disease progression.
- An inability to appropriately monitor blood levels precludes the use of lithium, as unmonitored use significantly raises the risk of not detecting an elevated level.

Particular caution should be used in several clinical scenarios:
- While lithium levels correlate highly with clinical efficacy and toxicity, patients can experience lithium toxicity at putatively normal serum levels.
- Patients may tolerate higher doses of lithium while in an acute manic phase than when symptoms have largely improved, requiring a decrease in a previously well-tolerated dosage.
- Thyroid disease is not clearly a contraindication but careful monitoring of thyroid function and treatment with supplemental thyroid hormone as indicated is particularly important in patients with premorbid thyroid disease or who develop thyroid disease while using lithium.

Significant drug interactions

Lithium has potential pharmacokinetic and pharmacodynamic interactions with many medications. Patients and families should always make sure other treatment providers are aware that the child is taking lithium. Drug interactions should be specifically checked using updated sources whenever lithium is combined with other medications. Any medication that changes renal function could affect lithium clearance. The most common significant interactions are listed below.

Diuretics

Extreme caution should be used when a patient is taking diuretics affecting the distal renal tubule (loop and thiazide diuretics), as these agents decrease the renal excretion of lithium and can increase serum lithium levels. Diuretics that act at the proximal tubule (such as acetazolamide) can potentially decrease serum lithium levels. Although not an absolute contraindication, changes in doses of diuretics should prompt close monitoring of lithium levels and precautions to prevent toxicity.

ACE-inhibitors and ARBs

There is risk of increase in lithium levels with angiotensin converting enzyme inhibitors (ACE inhibitors) and angiotensin receptor blockers (ARBs). Angiotensin II vasoconstricts the efferent arteriole at the glomerulus, increasing glomerular filtration rate (GFR). ACE-inhibitors and ARBs block this process, decreasing GFR and the excretion of lithium.

NSAIDs

NSAIDs inhibit prostaglandin synthesis. In the kidney, this prevents vasodilation of the afferent arterioles, decreasing GFR and the excretion of lithium. There are notable inconsistencies in this effect among NSAID agents as well as within individuals [137]. Aspirin and sulindac do not appear to affect lithium concentrations in the blood [138]. In general, we recommend use of acetaminophen when not otherwise contraindicated. We also consider holding the next one or two doses of lithium after accidental brief use of NSAIDs. Repeated and/or erratic use may require dose reduction and close monitoring of serum levels as well as clinical monitoring for symptoms of lithium toxicity.

Caffeine

Caffeine, which acts as a diuretic by inhibiting the binding of antidiuretic hormone, increases the excretion of lithium. Increased use of caffeine may lower lithium levels, or abrupt discontinuation of caffeine may lead to lithium toxicity.

Calcium-channel blockers

Concomitant use of nondihydropyridine calcium channel blockers (verapamil, diltiazem) may decrease lithium levels or precipitate or worsen mania through unclear mechanisms, though likely through altered calcium ion transport. Neurotoxicity may be more pronounced, and this combination could also worsen delay of atrioventricular transmission, leading to AV block.

Desmopressin

Desmopressin may decrease renal clearance of lithium and increase lithium serum levels.

Metronidazole

Metronidazole can significantly reduce the renal excretion of lithium leading to increased serum concentrations and acute toxicity as well as signs of renal damage up to six months later [139].

Antibiotics

Certain antibiotics such as tetracycline, doxycycline, and trimethoprim can in rare cases cause renal dysfunction that could raise serum lithium levels.

Carbamazepine

Neurotoxic effects of lithium, such as weakness, tremor, nystagmus, or asterixis, may be increased when used concomitantly with carmabazepine independent of serum lithium levels. Cardiac conduction effects may also be potentiated with combined treatment.

Serotonergic agents

Lithium may interact with serotonergic agents to increase the risk of serotonin syndrome. These include selective serotonin reuptake inhibitors (SSRIs), serotonin-norepinephrine reuptake inhibitors (SNRIs), monoamine oxidase inhibitors (MAO-Is), some tricyclic antidepressants (TCAs), buspirone, triptans, and ergot alkaloids. However, these agents have been combined with lithium without difficulty in many patients, so use with cautious dosing and close monitoring may be appropriate in some cases.

Phenothiazines and haloperidol

Through an unclear mechanism, lithium may increase the neurotoxicity of phenothiazine neuroleptics, putting patients at increased risk for extrapyramidal symptoms.

Theophylline

Theophylline may decrease lithium serum concentrations.

Topiramate

Topiramate may increase lithium serum concentrations in some patients.

Pregnancy and women's health

Lithium is an FDA Pregnancy Rating Category D Drug, meaning there is positive evidence of human fetal risk, but the benefits from use in pregnant women may be acceptable despite the risk (for example, if the drug is needed in a life-threatening situation or for a serious disease for which safer drugs cannot be used or are ineffective). In animal models, the teratogenic effects of lithium have been well described, including CNS, craniofacial, skeletal, and cardiac abnormalities [140]. The most well-known fetal abnormality associated with lithium use is a downward displacement of the tricuspid valve known as Ebstein's abnormality, which typically occurs in 1 in 20 000 births. Data from 225 subjects in the Lithium Baby Registry found 18 cardiac abnormalities, six of which were Ebstein abnormalities, suggesting a very high relative risk compared to the risk in the general population. Subsequent retrospective and prospective data have suggested the risk of cardiac abnormalities is much lower, though an accurate estimate of the relative risk remains elusive, and some authors have speculated that lithium may not confer any increased risk of fetal abnormality in humans [141]. Regardless, adolescents should be educated about the possible risks to the fetus should they become pregnant, and be given appropriate education in contraceptive methods if they are sexually active. The possible teratogenic effects of lithium are theoretically most significant during the first trimester, so avoidance of the agent especially during this time would be recommended. However, given the risk of untreated bipolar disorder to the fetus, the risks and benefits of using lithium compared to other mood stabilizer options must be considered carefully by the physician and patient.

Lithium is excreted into breast milk, such that a breastfeeding child is at risk for lithium toxicity. Mothers taking lithium should avoid breastfeeding, or an alternate agent could be considered when appropriate for a breastfeeding mother.

Side-effects

Toxicity

As previously reviewed, lithium toxicity is closely related to serum lithium levels, and can occur at doses close to therapeutic levels. Toxicity can occur in cases of patients taking excessive lithium or in changes in fluid status, including major dietary changes, especially with regards to salt intake, significant sudden decrease in caffeine intake, dehydration from exercise, being out in the hot sun for too long, decreased oral intake of fluids, running a fever from a viral illness or other infection, or the use of medications such as diuretics or NSAIDs, which may increase lithium levels.

Suspicion of lithium toxicity should prompt an immediate clinical evaluation and prompt clinicians to obtain a new serum lithium level to assess for an increase from baseline. Obvious signs of lithium toxicity require referral for emergent evaluation. Data pooled from three early studies suggest that younger children tend to experience higher rates of side-effects with lithium administration than adolescents, even after adjusting for weight and serum lithium levels [142]. Side-effects may be particularly common in children under age six, correlating with higher serum levels, higher dose per kilogram, and early phase of treatment [143].

If a thorough history does not reveal a clear reason for lithium toxicity, laboratory investigations focusing on change in kidney function, including electrolytes, urinalysis, and serum creatinine should be obtained, and nephrology consultation sought if indicated.

Mild lithium toxicity may be associated with gastrointestinal distress and dizziness and resolve with increased hydration and correcting the underlying process that lead to the change in metabolism and by holding doses until levels return to therapeutic ranges. More severe toxicity may manifest as nausea, vomiting, polyuria, ataxia, slurred speech, a gross tremor, muscle weakness, confusion/delirium, hallucinations, seizure, acute renal failure, diarrhea, and neuromuscular flaccidity [144]. Severe toxicity may require admission to the hospital for hydration, sodium repletion, and frequent monitoring of levels. In the most severe cases of renal failure with decreased urine output, hemodialysis may be necessary.

In cases of more chronic lithium toxicity, symptoms may not correlate well with serum levels, as lithium ions do not rapidly cross the lipophilic blood-brain barrier. Neurologic symptoms of tremor, delirium, ataxia, and memory problems may persist for days even after the serum level has apparently returned to the normal therapeutic range while the lithium level in the CNS continues to decrease.

Gastrointestinal side-effects

Gastrointestinal (GI) side-effects are among the most common experienced by patients taking lithium [145]. Symptoms can include nausea, vomiting, diarrhea, or vague abdominal discomfort. These effects are thought to be related to a rapid absorption through the GI tract, as lithium is directly irritating to the gastric mucosa, and rapid increase in plasma lithium levels. Strategies for lessening these effects include giving lithium with meals as well as switching to the time release formulation. Immediate release formulations may have a tendency to cause more nausea and vomiting, while delayed release formulations may cause more diarrhea.

As children and adolescents can have nausea, vomiting, diarrhea and decreased fluid intake due to gastroenteritis from infections and other sources, clinicians must caution families to be aware of the possibility that this could affect lithium levels. Typically, we hold lithium doses if the patient is not able to hold down fluids. It is also important to differentiate whether lithium toxicity is playing a role in the etiology of the GI distress.

Neurological

Patients treated with lithium can complain of a "cognitive dulling" associated with diminished processing speeds and working memory, though studies disagree as to how common, severe, or independent of psychiatric illness these effects may be [146–148]. A fine postural and digital/hand tremor is often seen during early lithium treatment and can be present even at therapeutic levels [145]. Low dose treatment with propanolol may be helpful in managing this symptom if it becomes bothersome to the patient and lithium is otherwise fairly well tolerated. Headache can be a common complaint with lithium treatment. Though rare, lithium can be associated with increased intracranial pressure leading to pseudotumor cerebri [144, 149] and complaints of headaches and blurred vision should be investigated further. An ophthalmologic exam should be obtained for evidence of papilledema.

Renal

Acquired nephrogenic diabetes insipidus is one of the most common major side-effects associated with the use of lithium, occurring in up to 40% of patients [150]. Increased water and sodium diuresis leads to mild dehydration, hyperchloremic metabolic acidosis and renal tubular acidosis, and can occur just a few weeks after initiation of lithium treatment [151]. Such disturbances of water homeostasis may lead to electrolyte abnormalities that must be monitored along with renal function. Many of these effects may be reversible with reduction of lithium dose or discontinuation of lithium treatment. Following chronic administration of lithium (usually 10–20 years) [152, 153], an irreversible tubulointerstitial nephritis can develop, which may be evident on renal biopsy and associated with decreased glomerular filtration rate and chronic kidney disease [154]. The frequency of kidney disease induced by chronic lithium exposure is not clear. Consultation with a nephrologist is necessary if significant change in renal function is detected, as lithium may or may not play a role in the etiology of the change.

Substantial evidence suggests that the nephrotoxic effects of lithium are due to cytotoxic concentrations of lithium that accumulate in the principal cells of the collecting duct, leading to downregulation of aquaporin 2, a water channel in the collecting duct, leading to significant water diuresis [155]. Lithium enters the principal cell through the epithelial sodium channel (ENaC) on the apical membrane and inhibits intracellular signaling pathways involving GSK-3β. Amiloride, an inhibitor of ENaC, may be useful for reversing lithium-induced nephrogenic diabetes insipidus [156] but it is unclear whether it is useful for treating the effects of chronic lithium administration.

Endocrine

Lithium can cause goiter and hypothyroidism in approximately 20–30% of patients [157]. Goiter and hypothyroidism usually occur within the first two years of lithium therapy [158]. Female gender and increasing age seem to increase the risk of lithium-induced hypothyroidism [159]. In a study of youth treated with combination lithium and valproate, 24% of patients showed significant elevations in thyroid stimulating hormone (TSH) [160]. The effect appeared to be dose-related. However, long-term studies of lithium's effect on thyroid function have not been performed, and it is not clear if all TSH elevations will be sustained over time.

Lithium interferes with the production of thyroid hormones through several mechanisms, including the inhibition of TSH-responsive adenylate cyclase and protein kinase C in thyroid cells [161], leading to a decrease in release of T3 and T4 [162–164]. Lithium also inhibits the uptake of iodine directly into thyroid cells as well as the iodination of tyrosine. Patients who develop hypothyroidism after exposure to lithium may have subclinical autoimmune thyroiditis prior to treatment, as pretreatment anti-thyroid antibodies seem to predict the development of hypothyroidism [165]. Hypothyroidism that develops during lithium use may be treated with hormone replacement if the risks of discontinuing lithium are unacceptable. Consultation with an endocrinologist may be indicated, especially if other etiologies for thyroid dysfunction are possible, or physical symptoms of thyroid dysfunction are present.

Lithium may also lead to increased serum calcium not attributable to hyperparathyroidism, although the rate of hyperparathyroidism may be elevated in lithium treated individuals as well [166]. The mechanism of hypercalcemia is not clearly understood.

Cardiac

Use of lithium is associated with EKG changes, such as T-wave inversions or flattenings, which are usually benign and reversible. However, lithium can slow down cardiac conduction at the AV node and may result in arrhythmias. A careful personal and family medical history assessing for history of arrhythmias or sudden unexplained death are requisite prior to initiation of treatment with lithium.

Other side-effects

Tables 11.2 and 11.3 provide a comprehensive list of common and major side-effects. Mild side-effects during initiation of treatment can often be managed by slow titration of dose and may be transient. Ongoing side-effects may be managed by dose reduction. If dose reduction adversely

Table 11.2 Common side-effects

General	Fatigue, drowsiness, dry mouth, edema
Weight gain	Nearly half of 100 adolescents taking lithium for 4 weeks gained weight ranging from 1 to 12 pounds [80]
Cardiovascular	T-wave inversions and flattening on electrocardiogram (EKG), relatively benign conduction abnormalities
Gastrointestinal	Poor appetite, nausea and vomiting (may be worse with immediate-release formulations, may be sign of toxicity), diarrhea (may be worse with delayed-release formulations)
Musculoskeletal	Muscle irritability, weakness
Neurologic	Postural tremor (fine tremor common at therapeutic levels), headaches, diffuse slowing on electroencephalogram (EEG)
Renal	Polyuria, polydyspia, enuresis, albuminuria, glycosuria
Hematologic	Leukocytosis
Dermatologic	Worsening of acne, psoriasis. Males may be more susceptible [167] Hair loss (with regrowth upon discontinuation of lithium) [168]

Table 11.3 Major side-effects

Renal	Nephrogenic diabetes insipidus, electrolyte abnormalities, tubulointerstitial nephritis which may be irreversible; renal biopsy may reveal permanent injury
Cardiovascular	Atrioventricular block, severe bradyarrhythmias, ventricular arrhythmias, hypotension, sinus node dysfunction
Endocrine	Hypothyroidism, hyperparathyroidism, papillary thyroid carcinoma
Neurologic	Ataxia, coma, pseudotumor cerebri, increased intracranial pressure and papilledema, seizure
Ophthalmic	Blurred vision, transient visual field scotoma
Otic	Tinnitus (with severe toxicity)

affects efficacy, then the clinician, patient and family together must weigh the benefits of lithium treatment, whether the side-effects can be ameliorated by other means or safely tolerated, and whether other treatment options are available.

References

1 Cade J: Lithium salts in the treatment of psychotic excitement. *Med J Aust* 1949; **11**: 349–51.

2 Jefferson JW, Greist JH, Ackerman DL: *Lithium Encyclopedia for Clinical Practice.* Washington, DC: American Psychiatric Press, 1987.

3 Vitiello B, Behar D, Malone R et al.: Pharmacokinetics of lithium carbonate in children. *J Clin Psychopharmacol* 1988; **8**: 355–9.

4 Findling RL, Landersdorfer CB, Kafantaris V et al.: First-dose pharmacokinetics of lithium carbonate in children and adolescents. *J Clin Psychopharmacol* 2010; **30**: 404–10.

5 Machado-Vieira R, Manji HK, Zarate Jr CA: The role of lithium in the treatment of bipolar disorder: convergent evidence for neurotrophic effects as a unifying hypothesis. *Bipolar Disord* 2009; **11**: 92–109.

6 Manji HK, Lenox RH: Signalling: cellular insights into the pathophysiology of bipolar disorder. *Biol Psychiatry* 2000; **48**: 518–30.

7 O'Brien WT, Harper AD, Jove F et al.: Glycogen synthase kinase-3beta haploinsufficiency mimics the behavioral and molecular effects of lithium. *J Neurosci* 2004; **24**: 6791–8.

8 Benedetti F, Serretti A, Colombo C et al.: A glycogen synthase kinase 3-beta promoter gene single nucleotide polymorphism is associated with age at onset and response to total sleep deprivation in bipolar depression. *Neurosci Lett* 2004; **368**:123–6.

9 Friedman E, Hoau Yan W, Levinson D et al.: Altered platelet protein kinase C activity in bipolar affective disorder, manic episode. *Biol Psychiatry* 1993; **33**: 520–5.

10 Pandey GN, Dwivedi Y, SridharaRao J et al.: Protein kinase C and phospholipase C activity and expression of their specific isozymes is decreased and expression of MARCKS is increased in platelets of bipolar but not in unipolar patients. *Neuropsychopharmacology* 2002; **26**: 216–28.

11 Pandey GN, Ren X, Dwivedi Y et al.: Decreased protein kinase C (PKC) in platelets of pediatric bipolar patients: effect of treatment with mood stabilizing drugs. *J Psychiatric Res*. 2008; **42**: 106–16.

12 Silverstone PH, McGrath BM, Kim H: Bipolar disorder and myo-inositol: a review of the magnetic resonance spectroscopy findings. *Bipolar Disord* 2005; **7**: 1–10.

13 Patel NC, DelBello MP, Cecil KM et al.: Lithium treatment effects on Myo-inositol in adolescents with bipolar depression. *Biol Psychiatry* 2006; **60**: 998–1004.

14 Patel NC, DelBello MP, Cecil KM et al.: Temporal change in N-acetyl-aspartate concentrations in adolescents with bipolar depression treated with lithium. *J Child Adolesc Psychopharmacol* 2008; **18**: 132–9.

15 Phillips ML, Travis MJ, Fagiolini A et al.: Medication effects in neuroimaging studies of bipolar disorder. *Am J Psychiatry* 2008; **165**: 313–20.

16 Bearden CE, Thompson PM, Dalwani M et al.: Greater cortical gray matter density in lithium-treated patients with bipolar disorder. *Biol Psychiatry* 2007; **62**: 7–16.

17 Moore GJ, Cortese BM, Glitz DA et al.: A longitudinal study of the effects of lithium treatment on prefrontal and subgenual prefrontal gray matter volume in treatment-responsive bipolar disorder patients. *J Clin Psychiatry* 2009; **70**: 699–705.

18 Lyoo IK, Dager SR, Kim JE et al.: Lithium-induced gray matter volume increase as a neural correlate of treatment response in bipolar disorder: a longitudinal brain imaging study. *Neuropsychopharmacology* 2010; **35**: 1743–50.

19 Roybal K, Theobold D, Graham A et al.: Mania-like behavior induced by disruption of CLOCK. *Proc Natl Acad Sci U S A* 2007; **104**: 6406–11.

20 Dzirasa K, Coque L, Sidor MM et al.: Lithium ameliorates nucleus accumbens phase-signaling dysfunction in a genetic mouse model of mania. *J Neurosci* 2010; **30**: 16214–3.

21 Perlis RH, Dennehy EB, Miklowitz DJ et al.: Retrospective age at onset of bipolar disorder and outcome during two-year follow-up: results from the STEP-BD study. *Bipolar Disord* 2009; **11**: 391–400.

22 Egeland JA, Shaw JA, Endicott J et al.: Prospective study of prodromal features for bipolarity in well Amish children. *J Am Acad Child Adolesc Psychiatry* 2003; **42**: 786–96.

23 Kessler RC, Avenevoli S, Green J et al.: National comorbidity survey replication adolescent supplement (NCS-A): III. Concordance of DSM-IV/CIDI diagnoses with clinical reassessments. *J Am Acad Child Adolesc Psychiatry* 2009; **48**: 386–99.

24 Lynch F, Mills C, Daly I et al.: Challenging times: prevalence of psychiatric disorders and suicidal behaviours in Irish adolescents. *J Adolesc* 2006; **29**: 555–73.

25 Verhulst FC, van der Ende J, Ferdinand RF et al.: The prevalence of DSM-III-R diagnoses in a national sample of Dutch adolescents. *Arch Gen Psychiatry* 1997; **54**: 329–36.

26 Lewinsohn PM, Klein DN, Seeley JR: Bipolar disorders in a community sample of older adolescents: prevalence, phenomenology, comorbidity, and course. *J Am Acad Child Adolesc Psychiatry* 1995; **34**: 454–63.

27 Costello EJ, Angold A, Burns BJ et al.: The Great Smoky Mountains Study of Youth. Goals, design, methods, and the prevalence of DSM-III-R disorders. *Arch Gen Psychiatry* 1996; **53**: 1129–36.

28 Harpaz-Rotem I, Rosenheck RA: Changes in outpatient psychiatric diagnosis in privately insured children and adolescents from 1995 to 2000. *Child Psychiatry Hum Dev* 2004; **34**: 329–40.

29 Harpaz-Rotem I, Leslie DL, Martin A et al.: Changes in child and adolescent inpatient psychiatric admission diagnoses between 1995 and 2000. *Soc Psychiatry Psychiatr Epidemiol* 2005; **40**: 642–7.

30 Blader JC, Carlson GA: Increased rates of bipolar disorder diagnoses among U.S. child, adolescent, and adult inpatients, 1996–2004. *Biol Psychiatry* 2007; **62**: 107–14.

31 Moreno C, Laje G, Blanco C et al.: National trends in the outpatient diagnosis and treatment of bipolar disorder in youth. *Arch Gen Psychiatry* 2007; **64**: 1032–9.

32 Pavuluri MN, Birmaher B, Naylor MW: Pediatric bipolar disorder: a review of the past 10 years. *J Am Acad Child Adolesc Psychiatry* 2005; **44**: 846–71.

33 Geller B, Zimerman B, Williams M et al.: Phenomenology of prepubertal and early adolescent bipolar disorder: examples of elated mood, grandiose behaviors, decreased need for sleep, racing thoughts and hypersexuality. *J Child Adolesc Psychopharmacol* 2002; **12**: 3–9.

34 Kowatch RA, Youngstrom EA, Danielyan A et al.: Review and meta-analysis of the phenomenology and clinical characteristics of mania in children and adolescents. *Bipolar Disord* 2005; **7**: 483–96.

35 Axelson D, Birmaher B, Strober M et al.: Phenomenology of children and adolescents with bipolar spectrum disorders. *Arch Gen Psychiatry* 2006; **63**: 1139–48.

36 Leibenluft E, Rich BA: Pediatric bipolar disorder. *Annu Rev Clin Psychol* 2008; **4**: 163–87.

37 Stringaris A, Baroni A, Haimm C et al.: Pediatric bipolar disorder versus severe mood dysregulation: risk for manic episodes on follow-up. *J Am Acad Child Adolesc Psychiatry* 2010; **49**: 397–405.

38 Geller B, Zimerman B, Williams M et al.: DSM-IV mania symptoms in a prepubertal and early adolescent bipolar disorder phenotype compared to attention-deficit hyperactive and normal controls. *J Child Adolesc Psychopharmacol* 2002; **12**: 11–25.

39 Chengappa KN, Kupfer DJ, Frank E et al.: Relationship of birth cohort and early age at onset of illness in a bipolar disorder case registry. *Am J Psychiatry* 2003; **160**: 1636–42.

40 Lish JD, Dime-Meenan S, Whybrow PC et al.: The National Depressive and Manic-depressive Association (DMDA) survey of bipolar members. *J Affect Disord* 1994; **31**: 281–94.

41 Biederman J, Faraone SV, Chu MP et al.: Further evidence of a bidirectional overlap between juvenile mania and conduct disorder in children. *J Am Acad Child Adolesc Psychiatry* 1999; **38**: 468–76.

42 Geller B, Tillman R, Craney JL et al.: Four-year prospective outcome and natural history of mania in children with a prepubertal and early adolescent bipolar disorder phenotype. *Arch Gen Psychiatry* 2004; **61**: 459–67.

43 Birmaher B, Axelson D, Strober M et al.: Clinical course of children and adolescents with bipolar spectrum disorders. *Arch Gen Psychiatry* 2006; **6**: 175–83.

44 Findling RL, Gracious BL, McNamara NK et al.: Rapid, continuous cycling and psychiatric co-morbidity in pediatric bipolar I disorder. *Bipolar Disord* 2001; **3**: 202–10.

45 Leibenluft E, Charney DS, Towbin KE et al.: Defining clinical phenotypes of juvenile mania. *Am J Psychiatry* 2003; **160**: 430–7.

46 Birmaher B, Axelson D, Goldstein B et al.: Four-year longitudinal course of children and adolescents with bipolar spectrum disorders: the Course and Outcome of Bipolar Youth (COBY) study. *Am J Psychiatry* 2009; **166**: 795–804.

47 McClellan J, Kowatch R, Findling RL et al.: Practice parameter for the assessment and treatment of children and adolescents with bipolar disorder. *J Am Acad Child Adolesc Psychiatry* 2007; **46**: 1071–25.

48 Goodwin FK, Jamison KR: *Manic-depressive Illness: Bipolar Disorders and Recurrent Depression*, 2nd edn. New York, NY: Oxford University Press, 2007.

49 Birmaher B, Axelson DA, Pavuluri MN: *Bipolar Disorder*, 4th ed. Philadelphia, PA: Lippincott Williams & Wilkins, 2007.

50 Neuman RJ, Geller B, Rice JP et al.: Increased prevalence and earlier onset of mood disorders among relatives of prepubertal versus adult probands. *J Am Acad Child Adolesc Psychiatry* 1997; **36:** 466–73.

51 Goodwin FK, Jamieson KR: *Manic-Depressive Illness*. New York, NY: Oxford University Press, 1990.

52 Tsuang MT, Faraone SV: *The Genetics of Mood Disorders*. Baltimore: Johns Hopkins University Press, 1990.

53 Birmaher B, Axelson D, Monk K et al.: Lifetime psychiatric disorders in school-aged offspring of parents with bipolar disorder: the Pittsburgh Bipolar Offspring study. *Arch Gen Psychiatry* 2009; **66:** 287–96.

54 Birmaher B, Ryan ND, Williamson D et al.: Childhood and adolescent depression: a review of the past 10 years—Part I. *J Am Acad Child Adolesc Psychiatry* 1996; **35:** 1427–39.

55 Geller B, Zimerman B, Williams M et al.: Bipolar disorder at prospective follow-up of adults who had prepubertal major depressive disorder. *Am J Psychiatry* 2001; **158:** 125–7.

56 Kovacs M: Presentation and course of major depressive disorder during childhood and later years of the life span. *J Am Acad Child Adolesc Psychiatry* 1996; **35:** 705–15.

57 Strober M, Carlson G: Bipolar illness in adolescents with major depression: Clinical, genetic, and psychopharmacologic predictors in a three- to four-year prospective follow-up investigation. *Arch Gen Psychiatry* 1982; **39:** 549–55.

58 Weissman MM, Wolk S, Goldstein RB et al.: Depressed adolescents grown up. *JAMA* 1999; **281:** 1707–13.

59 Geller B, Cooper TB, Zimerman B et al.: Lithium for prepubertal depressed children with family history predictors of future bipolarity: a double-blind, placebo-controlled study. *J Affect Disord* 1998; **51:** 165–75.

60 DelBello MP, Adler CM, Whitsel RM et al.: A 12-week single-blind trial of quetiapine for the treatment of mood symptoms in adolescents at high risk for developing bipolar I disorder. *J Clin Psychiatry* 2007; **68:** 789–95.

61 Chang KD, Dienes K, Blasey C et al.: Divalproex monotherapy in the treatment of bipolar offspring with mood and behavioral disorders and at least mild affective symptoms. *J Clin Psychiatry* 2003; **64:** 936–42.

62 Findling RL, Frazier TW, Youngstrom EA et al.: Double-blind, placebo-controlled trial of divalproex monotherapy in the treatment of symptomatic youth at high risk for developing bipolar disorder. *J Clin Psychiatry* 2007; **68:** 781–8.

63 Tandon R, Nasrallah HA, Keshavan M: Schizophrenia, "just the facts" 5. Treatment and prevention. Past, present, and future. *Schizophr Res* 2010; **122:** 1–23.

64 See comment in *Evid Based Ment Health* 2004 **7**(3): 72.

65 Muzina DJ, Calabrese JR: Maintenance therapies in bipolar disorder: focus on randomized controlled trials. *Aust N Z J Psychiatry* 2005; **39:** 652–61.

66 Kowatch RA, Fristad M, Birmaher B et al.: Treatment guidelines for children and adolescents with bipolar disorder. *J Am Acad Child Adolesc Psychiatry* 2005; **44:** 213–35.

67 Youngerman J, Canino IA: Lithium carbonate use in children and adolescents. A survey of the literature. *Arch Gen Psychiatry* 1978; **35:** 216–24.

68 DeLong GR, Aldershof AL: Long-term experience with lithium treatment in child-hood: correlation with clinical diagnosis. *J Am Acad Child Adolesc Psychiatry* 1987; **26:** 389–94.

69 Gram LF, Rafaelsen OJ: Lithium treatment of psychotic children and adolescents. A controlled clinical trial. *Acta Psychiatr Scand* 1972; **48:** 253–60.

70 Lena B, Surtrees SJ, Maggs R: *The efficacy of Lithium in the Treatment of Emotional Disturbances in Children and Adolescents.* Baltimore: University Park Press, 1978.

71 McKnew DH, Cytryn L, Buchsbaum MD et al.: Lithium in children of lithium-responding parents. *Psychiatry Res* 1981; **4:** 171–80.

72 DeLong GR, Nieman GW: Lithium-induced behavior changes in children with symptoms suggesting manic-depressive illness. *Psychopharmacol Bull* 1983; **19:** 258–65.

73 Schou M, Juel-Nielsen N, Stromgren E et al.: The treatment of manic psychoses by the administration of lithium salts. *J Neurol Neurosurg Psychiatry* 1954; **17:** 250–60.

74 Bowden CL, Brugger AM, Swann AC et al.: Efficacy of divalproex vs. lithium and placebo in the treatment of mania. The Depakote Mania Study Group. *JAMA* 1994; **271:** 918–24.

75 Bowden CL: Key treatment studies of lithium in manic-depressive illness: efficacy and side effects. *J Clin Psychiatry* 1998; **59:** 13–20.

76 Perlis RH, Welge JA, Vornik LA et al.: Atypical antipsychotics in the treatment of mania: a meta-analysis of randomized, placebo-controlled trials. *J Clin Psychiatry* 2006; **67:** 509–16.

77 Biederman J, Mick E, Bostic JQ et al.: The naturalistic course of pharmacologic treatment of children with maniclike symptoms: A systematic chart review. *J Clin Psychiatry* 1998; **59:** 628–37.

78 Geller B, Cooper TB, Sun K et al.: Double-blind and placebo-controlled study of lithium for adolescent bipolar disorders with secondary substance dependency. *J Am Acad Child Adolesc Psychiatry* 1998; **37:** 171–8.

79 Kowatch RA, Suppes T, Carmody TJ et al.: Effect size of lithium, divalproex sodium, and carbamazepine in children and adolescents with bipolar disorder. *J Am Acad Child Adolesc Psychiatry* 2000; **39:** 713–20.

80 Kafantaris V, Coletti DJ, Dicker R et al.: Lithium treatment of acute mania in ado-lescents: a large open trial. *J Am Acad Child Adolesc Psychiatry* 2003; **42:** 1038–45.

81 Kafantaris V, Coletti DJ, Dicker R et al.: Lithium treatment of acute mania in adoles-cents: a placebo-controlled discontinuation study. *J Am Acad Child Adolesc Psychiatry* 2004; **43:** 984–93.

82 Findling RL, McNamara NK, Gracious BL et al.: Combination lithium and dival-proex sodium in pediatric bipolarity. *J Am Acad Child Adolesc Psychiatry* 2003; **42:** 895–901.

83 Findling RL, McNamara NK, Youngstrom EA et al.: Double-blind 18-month trial of lithium versus divalproex maintenance treatment in pediatric bipolar disorder. *J Am Acad Child Adolesc Psychiatry* 2005; **44:** 409–17.

84 Findling RL, McNamara NK, Stansbrey R et al.: Combination lithium and dival-proex sodium in pediatric bipolar symptom re-stabilization. *J Am Acad Child Adolesc Psychiatry* 2006; **45:** 142–8.

85 Grof P, Duffy A, Cavazzoni P et al.: Is response to prophylactic lithium a familial trait? *J Clin Psychiatry* 2003; **63:** 942–7.

86 Duffy A, Alda M, Kutcher S et al.: A prospective study of the offspring of bipolar parents responsive and nonresponsive to lithium treatment. *J Clin Psychiatry* 2002; **63:** 1171–8.

87 Duffy A, Alda M, Milin R et al.: A consecutive series of treated affected offspring of parents with bipolar disorder: is response associated with the clinical profile? *Can J Psychiatry* 2007; **52**: 369–76.

88 Calabrese JR, Shelton MD, Rapport DJ et al.: A 20-month, double-blind, maintenance trial of lithium versus divalproex in rapid-cycling bipolar disorder. *Am J Psychiatry* 2005; **162**: 2152–61.

89 Masi G, Perugi G, Millepiedi S et al.: Pharmacological response in juvenile bipolar disorder subtypes: A naturalistic retrospective examination. *Psychiatry Res* 2010; **177**: 192–8.

90 Pavuluri MN, Henry DB, Carbray JA et al.: A one-year open-label trial of risperidone augmentation in lithium nonresponder youth with preschool-onset bipolar disorder. *J Child Adolesc Psychopharmacol* 2006; **16**: 336–50.

91 Strober M, DeAntonio M, Schmidt-Lackner S et al.: Early childhood attention deficit hyperactivity disorder predicts poorer response to acute lithium therapy in adolescent mania. *J Affect Disord* 1998; **51**: 145–51.

92 Strober M, Morrell W, Burroughs J et al.: A family study of bipolar I disorder in adolescence. Early onset of symptoms linked to increased familial loading and lithium resistance. *J Affect Disord* 1988; **15**: 255–68.

93 Correll CU, Sheridan EM, DelBello MP: Antipsychotic and mood stabilizer efficacy and tolerability in pediatric and adult patients with bipolar I mania: a comparative analysis of acute, randomized, placebo-controlled trials. *Bipolar Disord* 2010; **12**: 116–41.

94 Sachs GS, Grossman F, Ghaemi SN et al.: Combination of a mood stabilizer with risperidone or haloperidol for treatment of acute mania: a double-blind, placebo-controlled comparison of efficacy and safety. *Am J Psychiatry* 2002; **159**: 1146–54.

95 Yatham LN, Grossman F, Augustyns I et al.: Mood stabilisers plus risperidone or placebo in the treatment of acute mania. International, double-blind, randomised controlled trial. *Br J Psychiatry* 2003; **182**: 141–7.

96 Tohen M, Chengappa KN, Suppes T et al.: Efficacy of olanzapine in combination with valproate or lithium in the treatment of mania in patients partially nonresponsive to valproate or lithium monotherapy.[see comment]. *Arch Gen Psychiatry* 2002; **59**: 62–9.

97 Sachs G, Chengappa KN, Suppes T et al.: Quetiapine with lithium or divalproex for the treatment of bipolar mania: a randomized, double-blind, placebo-controlled study. *Bipolar Disord* 2004; **6**: 213–23.

98 Yatham LN, Vieta EY, Young AH et al.: A double blind, randomized, placebo-controlled trial of quetiapine as an add-on therapy to lithium or divalproex for the treatment of bipolar mania. *Int Clin Psychopharmacol* 2007; **22**: 212–20.

99 Vieta E, T'joen C, McQuade RD et al.: Efficacy of adjunctive aripiprazole to either valproate or lithium in bipolar mania patients partially nonresponsive to valproate/lithium monotherapy: a placebo-controlled study. *Am J Psychiatry* 2008; **165**: 1316–25.

100 Citrome L: Ziprasidone HCl capsules for the adjunctive maintenance treatment of bipolar disorder in adults. *Expert Rev Neurother* 2010; **10**: 1031–7.

101 Compton MT, Nemeroff CB: The treatment of bipolar depression. *J Clin Psychiatry* 2000; **61**: 57–67.

102 Zornberg GL, Pope HG: Treatment of depression in bipolar disorder: new directions for research. *J Clin Psychopharmacol* 1993; **13**: 397–408.

103 Biederman J, Mick E, Spencer TJ et al.: Therapeutic dilemmas in the pharmacotherapy of bipolar depression in the young. *J Child Adolesc Psychopharmacol* 2000; **10:** 185–92.

104 Patel NC, DelBello MP, Bryan HS et al.: Open-label lithium for the treatment of adolescents with bipolar depression. *Journal of the American Academy of Child & Adolescent Psychiatry* 2006; **45:** 289–97.

105 Geddes JR, Goodwin GM, Rendell J et al.: Lithium plus valproate combination therapy versus monotherapy for relapse prevention in bipolar 1 disorder (BALANCE): a randomised open-label trial. *Lancet* 2010; **375:** 385–95.

106 Goodwin GM, Bowden CL, Calabrese JR et al.: A pooled analysis of 2 placebo-controlled 18-month trials of lamotrigine and lithium maintenance in bipolar I disorder. *J Clin Psychiatry* 2004; **65:** 432–41.

107 Tohen M, Chengappa KN, Suppes T et al.: Relapse prevention in bipolar I disorder: 18-month comparison of olanzapine plus mood stabiliser v. mood stabiliser alone. *Br J Psychiatry* 2004; **184:** 337–45.

108 Baldessarini RJ, Tondo L, Hennen J: Effects of lithium treatment and its discontinuation on suicidal behavior in bipolar manic-depressive disorders. *J Clin Psychiatry* 1999; **60:** 77–84.

109 Strober M, Morrell W, Lampert C et al.: Relapse following discontinuation of lithium maintenance therapy in adolescents with bipolar I illness: a naturalistic study. *Am J Psychiatry* 1990; **147:** 457–61.

110 Varanka TM, Weller RA, Weller EB et al.: Lithium treatment of manic episodes with psychotic features in prepubertal children. *Am J Psychiatry* 1988; **145:** 1557–9.

111 Kafantaris V, Coletti DJ, Dicker R et al.: Adjunctive antipsychotic treatment of adolescents with bipolar psychosis. *J Am Acad Child Adolesc Psychiatry* 2001; **40:** 1448–56.

112 Crossley NA, Bauer M: Acceleration and augmentation of antidepressants with lithium for depressive disorders: two meta-analyses of randomized, placebo-controlled trials. *J Clin Psychiatry* 2007; **68:** 935–40.

113 Bauer M, Adli M, Bschor T et al.: Lithium's emerging role in the treatment of refractory major depressive episodes: augmentation of antidepressants. *Neuropsychobiology* 2010; **62:** 36–42.

114 Nierenberg AA, Fava M, Trivedi MH et al.: A comparison of lithium and T(3) augmentation following two failed medication treatments for depression: a STAR*D report. *Am J Psychiatry* 2006; **163:** 1519–30.

115 Geller B, Fox LW, Cooper TB et al.: Baseline and 2- to 3-year follow-up characteristics of placebo-washout responders from the nortriptyline study of depressed 6- to 12-year-olds. *J Am Acad Child Adolesc Psychiatry* 1992; **31:** 622–8.

116 Ryan N, Meyer V, Dachille S et al.: Lithium antidepressant augmentation in TCA-refractory depression in adolescents. *J Am Acad Child Adolesc Psychiatry* 1988; **27:** 371–6.

117 Strober M, Freeman R, Rigali J et al.: The pharmacotherapy of depressive illness in adolescence: II. Effects of lithium augmentation in nonresponders to imipramine. *J Am Acad Child Adolesc Psychiatry* 1992; **31:** 16–20.

118 Dickstein DP, Towbin KE, Van der Veen JW et al.: Randomized double-blind placebo-controlled trial of lithium in youths with severe mood dysregulation. *J Child Adolesc Psychopharmacol* 2009; **19:** 61–73.

119 Sheard MH: Lithium in the treatment of aggression. *J Nerv Ment Dis* 1975; **160:** 108–18.

120 Connor DF, Carlson GA, Chang KD et al.: Juvenile maladaptive aggression: a review of prevention, treatment, and service configuration and a proposed research agenda. *J Clin Psychiatry* 2006; **67**: 808–20.

121 Vetró A, Szentistványi I, Pallag L et al.: Therapeutic experience with lithium in childhood aggressivity. *Neuropsychobiology* 1985; **14**: 121–7.

122 Campbell P, Perry R, Green WH: Use of lithium in children and adolescents. *Psychosomatics* 1984; **25**: 95–106.

123 Campbell M, Small AM, Green WH et al.: Behavioral efficacy of haloperidol and lithium carbonate. a comparison in hospitalized aggressive children with conduct disorder. *Arch Gen Psychiatry* 1984; **41**: 650–6.

124 Campbell M, Adams PB, Small AM et al.: Lithium in hospitalized aggressive children with conduct disorder: a double-blind and placebo-controlled study. *J Am Acad Child Adolesc Psychiatry* 1995; **34**: 445–53.

125 Rifkin A, Karajgi B, Dicker R et al.: Lithium treatment of conduct disorders in adolescents. *Am J Psychiatry* 1997; **154**: 554–5.

126 Malone RP, Delaney MA, Luebbert JF et al.: A double-blind placebo-controlled study of lithium in hospitalized aggressive children and adolescents with conduct disorder. *Arch Gen Psychiatry* 2000; **57**: 649–54.

127 Findling RL, Frazier JA, Kafantaris V et al.: The Collaborative Lithium Trials (CoLT): specific aims, methods, and implementation. *Child Adolesc Psychiatry Ment Health* 2008; **2**: 21.

128 Malone RP, Delaney MA, Luebbert JF et al.: The lithium test dose prediction method in aggressive children. *Psychopharmacol Bull* 1995; **31**: 379–82.

129 Schou M, Amdisen A, Thomsen K et al.: Lithium treatment regimen and renal water handling: the significance of dosage pattern and tablet type examined through comparison of results from two clinics with different treatment regimens. *Psychopharmacology* 1982; **77**: 387–90.

130 Hetmar O, Rafaelsen OJ: Lithium: long-term effects on the kidney. IV. Renal lithium clearance. *Acta Psychiatr Scand* 1987; **76**: 193–8.

131 Hetmar O, Brun C, Ladefoged J et al.: Long-term effects of lithium on the kidney: functional-morphological correlations. *J Psychiatr Res* 1989; **23**: 285– 97.

132 Spencer EK, Campbell M, Adams P et al.: Saliva and serum lithium monitoring in hospitalized children. *Psychopharmacol Bull* 1990; **26**: 239–43.

133 InstaRead Lithium System: *Med Lett Drugs Ther* 2005; **47**: 82–3.

134 Morriss R, Benjamin B: Lithium and eGFR: a new routinely available tool for the prevention of chronic kidney disease. *Br J Psychiatry* 2008; **193**: 93–4.

135 Tredget J, Kirov A, Kirov G: Effects of chronic lithium treatment on renal function. *J Affect Disord* 2010; **126**: 436–40.

136 Schwartz GJ, Muñoz A, Schneider MF et al.: New equations to estimate GFR in children with CKD. *J Am Soc Nephrol* 2009; **20**: 629–37.

137 Ragheb M, Ban TA, Buchanan D et al.: Interaction of indomethacin and ibuprofen with lithium in manic patients under a steady-state lithium level. *J Clin Psychiatry* 1980; **41**: 397–8.

138 Ragheb MA, Powell AL: Failure of sulindac to increase serum lithium levels. *J Clin Psychiatry* 1986; **47**: 33–4.

139 Teicher MH, Altesman RI, Cole JO et al.: Possible nephrotoxic interaction of lithium and metronidazole. *JAMA* 1987; **257**: 3365–6.

140 Giles JJ, Bannigan JG: Teratogenic and developmental effects of lithium. *Curr Pharm Des* 2006; **12**: 1531–41.

141 Yacobi S, Ornoy A: Is lithium a real teratogen? What can we conclude from the prospective versus retrospective studies? A review. *Isr J Psychiatry Relat Sci* 2008; **45:** 95–106.

142 Campbell M, Silva RR, Kafantaris V et al.: Predictors of side effects associated with lithium administration in children. *Psychopharmacol Bull* 1991; **27:** 373–80.

143 Hagino OR, Weller EB, Weller RA et al.: Untoward effects of lithium treatment in children aged four through six years. *J Am Acad Child Adolesc Psychiatry* 1995; **34:** 1584–90.

144 Labbate LA, Fava M, Rosenbaum JF et al.: Drugs for the treatment of bipolar disorders. *Handbook of Psychiatric Drug Therapy*, 6th edn. Philadelphia, PA: Lippincott Williams & Wilkins, 2010.

145 Jefferson JW, Griest JH: Lithium. *Kaplan and Sadock's Comprehensive Textbook of Psychiatry*, 9th ed. Philadelphia, PA: Lippincott Williams & Wilkins, 2009.

146 Platt JE, Campbell M, Green WH et al.: Cognitive effects of lithium carbonate and haloperidol in treatment-resistant aggressive children. *Arch Gen Psychiatry* 1984; **41:** 657–62.

147 Pavuluri MN, Schenkel LS, Aryal S et al.: Neurocognitive function in unmedicated manic and medicated euthymic pediatric bipolar patients. *Am J Psychiatry* 2006; **163:** 286–93.

148 Henin A, Mick E, Biederman J et al.: Is psychopharmacologic treatment associated with neuropsychological deficits in bipolar youth? *J Clin Psychiatry* 2009; **70:** 1178–85.

149 Saul RF, Hamburger HA, Selhorst JB: Pseudotumor cerebri secondary to lithium carbonate. *JAMA* 1985; **253:** 2869–70.

150 Stone KA: Lithium-induced nephrogenic diabetes insipidus. *J Am Board Fam Pract* 1999; **12:** 43–7.

151 Boton R, Gaviria M, Batlle DC: Prevalence, pathogenesis, and treatment of renal dysfunction associated with chronic lithium therapy. *Am J Kidney Dis* 1987; **10:** 329–45.

152 Bendz H, Sjödin I, Aurell M: Renal function on and off lithium in patients treated with lithium for 15 years or more. A controlled, prospective lithium-withdrawal study. *Nephrol Dial Transplant* 1996; **11:** 457–60.

153 Presne C, Fakhouri F, Noël LH et al.: Lithium-induced nephropathy: rate of progression and prognostic factors. *Kidney Int* 2003; **64:** 585–92.

154 Hestbech J, Hansen HE, Amdisen A et al.: Chronic renal lesions following long-term treatment with lithium. *Kidney Int* 1977; **12:** 205–13.

155 Grünfeld JP, Rossier BC: Lithium nephrotoxicity revisited. *Nat Rev Nephrol* 2009; **5:** 270–6.

156 Bedford JJ, Weggery S, Ellis G et al.: Lithium-induced nephrogenic diabetes insipidus: renal effects of amiloride. *Clin J Am Soc Nephrol* 2008; **3:** 1324–31.

157 Barbesino G: Drugs affecting thyroid function. *Thyroid* 2010; **20:** 763–70.

158 Bocchetta A, Cocco F, Velluzzi F et al.: Fifteen-year follow-up of thyroid function in lithium patients. *J Endocrinol Invest* 2007; **30:** 363–6.

159 Kirov G, Tredget J, John R et al.: A cross-sectional and a prospective study of thyroid disorders in lithium-treated patients. *J Affect Disord* 2005; **87:** 313–17.

160 Gracious BL, Findling RL, Seman C et al.: Elevated thyrotropin in bipolar youths prescribed both lithium and divalproex sodium. *J Am Acad Child Adolesc Psychiatry* 2004; **43:** 215–20.

161 Lazarus JH, McGregor AM, Ludgate M et al.: Effect of lithium carbonate therapy on thyroid immune status in manic depressive patients: a prospective study. *J Affect Disord* 1986; **11**: 155–60.

162 Berens SC, Bernstein RS, Robbins J et al.: Antithyroid effects of lithium. *J Clin Invest* 1970; **49**: 1357–67.

163 Burrow GN, Burke WR, Himmelhoch JM et al.: Effect of lithium on thyroid function. *J Clin Endocrinol Metab* 1971; **32**: 647–52.

164 Spaulding SW, Burrow GN, Bermudez F et al.: The inhibitory effect of lithium on thyroid hormone release in both euthyroid and thyrotoxic patients. *J Clin Endocrinol Metab* 1972; **35**(6): 905–11.

165 Myers DH, Carter RA, Burns BH et al.: A prospective study of the effects of lithium on thyroid function and on the prevalence of antithyroid antibodies. *Psychol Med* 1985; **15**(1): 55–61.

166 Hundley JC, Woodrum DT, Saunders BD et al.: Revisiting lithium-associated hyperparathyroidism in the era of intraoperative parathyroid hormone monitoring. *Surgery* 2005; **138**(6): 1027–31.

167 Chan HH, Wing Y, Su R et al.: A control study of the cutaneous side effects of chronic lithium therapy. *J Affect Disord* 2000; **57**(1–3): 107–13.

168 Wagner KD, Teicher MH: Lithium and hair loss in childhood. *Psychosomatics* 1991; **32**(3): 355–6.

CHAPTER 12

Anticonvulsants Used in Child and Adolescent Psychiatric Disorders

Mani Pavuluri & Tushita Mayanil
Pediatric Brain Research and Intervention Center, University of Illinois at Chicago, Chicago, USA

Introduction

A number of antiepileptic drugs have gained popularity since the early 2000s for treatment of pediatric epilepsy. Research has shown the efficacy of these drugs for off-label indications like migraines, movement disorders and psychiatric disorders in children. Common biological mechanisms underlying epilepsy and psychiatric disorders, specifically mood disorders, including bipolar disorder, have led to the widespread use of anti-epileptics for the treatment of psychiatric conditions. The increased frequency of diagnosis and treatment of pediatric bipolar disorder and emphasis on early pharmacotherapeutic interventions has led to more research and clinical experience with anti-epileptics. Clinical trials of anticonvulsants illustrated promising results towards their use in child and adolescent psychiatric disorders. This chapter aims to review commonly used antiepileptic medications used in this population.

The pharmacokinetic profile and recommendations for monitoring each anticonvulsant have been listed in Tables 12.1 and 12.2 respectively.

Divalproex sodium

Chemical property and mechanism of action

Divalproex sodium is a simple branched-chain carboxylic acid (n-dipropylacetic acid), which was serendipitously discovered in 1963, and has since then been used widely for its broad spectrum antiepileptic and mood stabilizing properties [1]. Divalproex sodium, a compound containing an equal proportion, on a molar basis, of sodium divalproex

Pharmacotherapy of Child and Adolescent Psychiatric Disorders, Third Edition.
Edited by David R. Rosenberg and Samuel Gershon.

Table 12.1 Pharmacokinetics of anticonvulsants

Drug	Bioavailability and peak levels	Volume of distribution	Half life (hours)	Clearance (l/hr/kg)	Plasma protein binding	Site of metabolism and metabolites	Comments
divalproex	– divalproex capsule 93%; peak levels one to two hours. – divalproex enteric-coated (ER) 90% peak levels four hours of dosing [6]	0.26 L/kg in children and 0.19 L/kg in adults	children 7.2 ± 2.3 hours; adults 13.9 ± 3.4 hours [5]	children 0.027 l/hr/kg; adults 0.0066 l/hr/kg	90%; concentration dependent (increases linearly)	Liver	– Peak time for both formulations is delayed by food intake – Steady state plasma level attained in 2–4 days [4] – ER preparation has a hydrophilic polymer matrix controlled-release tablet system, allowing slow release of drug in the gastrointestinal tract over an 18 to 24 hour period
carbamazepine	unpredictable absorption and 80% bioavailability	0.8 to 2 L/kg	– Before autoinduction 24 hours – After autoinduction 8 hours (2–4 weeks after initiation of carbamazepine).	1.3 to 1.7 L/hr/kg	76%	– Liver – Mainly CYP3A4 to 10, 11–epoxide – Minor CYP1A2, CYP2B6, CYP2C8/9 and CYP2E1 to – Both carbamazepine and epoxide metabolite are clinically active – Epoxide metabolite broken down by epoxide hydroxylase which is induces CYP3A4 and hence leads to auto-induction	– Due to auto induction, dose needs to be increased in order maintain therapeutic blood levels – Large inter-individual variability in the levels and the corresponding clinical response and adverse effects – Epoxide metabolite responsible for both clinical response and adverse effect profile – ER preparation-lesser variability in absorption and plasma concentration fluctuations and allows twice daily administration

Table 12.1 (*Continued*)

Drug	Bioavailability and peak levels	Volume of distribution	Half life (hours)	Clearance (l/hr/kg)	Plasma protein binding	Site of metabolism and metabolites	Comments
oxcarbazepine	– Bioavailability is >95% – peak plasma concentrations oxcarbazepine 1–3 hours; MHD 4–12 h after a single oral dose	3.93 ± 2.22 L/kg	oxcarbazepine 1–5 hours; MHD 7–20h	– 13–20 ml/min	– 40% MHD is plasma bound	– clinically active monohydroxy derivative (MHD) i.e.10, 11-dihydro-10-hydroxy-carbazepine by UDP-glucuronosyl transferases (UGT) in liver – eliminated by kidneys	– highly lipophilic and first order kinetics – no auto-induction – weight normalized clearance higher in children
lamotrigine	– 100% – no effect of food on bioavailability – no first pass metabolism	1.25 and 1.47 l/kg	24–35 hours	0.64 ± 0.26 ml/min/kg	55%.	glucuronidation by UGT	– in children and adolescents, the concentration to dose decreases with age, which may require higher dosing among older children and adolescents to achieve the same concentration
gabapentin	– peak 2–3 hours after administration	High 50–60 L	6–8 hours	120–130 ml/min	no protein binding	– renally excreted – no metabolites	– the plasma levels do not exhibit a linear relationship with the dose administered because of an active L-amino acid transport carrier which is saturable – renal dosing for renal failure
topiramate	81–95% bioavailability – no effect of food – peak levels between 1.4 and 4.3 hours	0.6–0.8 L/kg	19–25h	10–20 ml/min	15% minimal protein binding	– 20% metabolized in the liver – major renal elimination	– the plasma levels increase linearly with dose – saturable binding of the drug to erythrocytes

CYP = cytochrome.

Table 12.2 Monitoring for specific anticonvulsants

Drug	Parameters for monitoring and frequency
divalproex	**1** Obtain plasma level 5–7 days after the initial dose. Therapeutic levels in the range of 50–125 µg/ml should be targeted **2** Liver enzymes and complete blood counts (CBC) should be measured at baseline, every three months during the first 6 months, and every 6 months thereafter
carbamazepine	**1** Obtain plasma level 2–3 weeks after the initial dose **2** Liver enzymes should be measured at baseline, every 3 months during the first 6 months, and every 6 months thereafter **3** CBC at baseline and as clinically warranted
oxcarbazepine	**1** No plasma levels monitoring required except in renal failure **2** Liver enzymes at baseline and as clinically warranted; sodium at baseline and at 1 month and thereafter as clinically warranted
lamotrigine	Monitor for rash every visit
gabapentin	No monitoring required
topiramate	Baseline and periodic bicarbonate levels

µg = micro grams.

and valproic acid, dissociates to the divalproex ion in the gastrointestinal tract. In spite of its widespread clinical use, the exact mechanism of action of divalproex is still not determined. Given its structural similarity to gamma amino butyric acid (GABA), it has been postulated to have GABAergic action through stimulation of GABA-secreting enzyme glutamic acid decarboxylase and inhibition of GABA-degrading enzymes GABA transaminase. Another proposed mechanism includes membrane stabilization through effect on voltage gated sodium (Na^+) channels and modulation of N-Methyl-D-aspartic acid (NMDA) receptors. Recent epigenetic data from transgenic animal and preliminary human research has shown that divalproex is a histone deacetylase (HDAC) inhibitor. It enables open chromatin structure facilitating RNA polymerase binding and transcription and hence may exert a direct effect on the epigenome [2, 3].

Drug interactions

Valproate, being highly protein bound, can precipitate toxicity of other highly protein bound drugs at high serum concentration. It inhibits hepatic microsomal P450 enzymes. As a result, it can increase serum concentrations of several drugs like phenobarbital, carbamazepine, phenytoin, tricyclics, and lamotrigine metabolized by the P450 enzymes. Further, divalproex levels are increased by drugs like erythromycin, fluoxetine and cimetidine, which inhibit microsomal enzymes like CYP 3A4.

Indications

Bipolar disorder

Several new studies are now available in pediatric bipolar disorder (PBD) [4–15], although a larger and more informative body of evidence is available through adult studies [16]. The most recent adult study showed that both combination therapy with lithium plus valproate (hazard ratio = 0.59, 95% CI 0.42–0.83, p = 0.0023) and lithium monotherapy (hazard ratio = 0.71, 0.51–1.00, p = 0.0472) are more likely to prevent relapse than is valproate monotherapy [17]. Most studies for pediatric bipolar patients both suffer from small sample size or differences in diagnostic methodologies and must be interpreted carefully.

Prospective open trials have demonstrated more optimistic results in the efficacy of divalproex in children and adolescents with bipolar disorder [5, 10, 11, 14, 15]. Case studies have shown efficacy of intravenous divalproex in the treatment of adolescents with acute mania but more rigorous trials are needed to address this treatment option [18]. A study in severely ill patients with manic or mixed episodes that examined combination therapy of divalproex with risperidone and lithium with risperidone in a six-month trial (Young Mania Rating Scale (YMRS) yielded effect sizes at 4.36 and 2.82, respectively) [14]. Risperidone could have been just as effective as monotherapy, without the combination treatment. Given the often noted tolerance to monotherapy of second-generation antipsychotics after an initial phase of improvement, these results illustrate a positive outcome over a longer follow-up period of six months with combination treatment of two types of medications often required in severely ill patients.

There are only four published, randomized trials in acute mania using divalproex treatment in this population [7, 13]. The first study compared divalproex with lithium and carbamazepine in acute mania and hypomania in 8 to 18 year olds and showed response rates of around 50% with all three agents [13]. The second study was a double-blind randomized controlled trial (DBRCT) comparing divalproex and quetiapine for an acute manic episode in 12–18 year-old patients [7]. There was no significant difference on the YMRS with a drop of 23 points on quetiapine and 19 points on divalproex. Remission rate, however, was significantly higher with quetiapine relative to divalproex. The slope of reduction in symptoms was also steeper in the quetiapine versus divalproex group. Within the group of bipolar adolescents with psychosis, quetiapine was significantly more effective than divalproex. Results from these two studies coupled with findings from open trials in pediatric mania showing that divalproex is useful are in sharp contrast to those from the DBRCT of divalproex extended release (ER) showing no benefit relative to placebo [19].

Results from this trial reported an YMRS score reduction of 8.8 points with divalproex relative to 7.9 points on placebo [19]. The fourth study, a DBRCT, compared divalproex with risperidone. The response rate on YMRS was 78.1% for risperidone and 45.5% for divalproex. The remission rate for risperidone was 62.5%, compared with 33.3% for divalproex [12]. Of note is the fact that antipsychotics usually achieve behavioral control faster than traditional mood stabilizers like lithium or divalproex, and this may not equate to more efficacy.

Aggression

Post hoc analysis of two trials of divalproex has shown significant reductions in aggression and irritability subscales of YMRS [20] and Positive and Negative Syndrome Scale-Excited Component scales in children with comorbid bipolar and disruptive behavior [21] respectively. It is still unclear if divalproex independently improves aggression or if these effects are secondary to the improvement in mania.

Attention deficit hyperactivity disorder (ADHD)

A retrospective chart review of subjects (treated with lithium and divalproex) with comorbid PBD and ADHD showed a response rate of 57.1% in patients with comorbid ADHD when compared to 92.6% in patients without ADHD (p = 0.007) with no significant differences in response rates for lithium or divalproex sodium [22]. An eight-week open-label trial [23] of divalproex sodium to control manic symptoms was conducted, followed by a four-week randomized, double-blind, placebo-controlled crossover trial (mixed amphetamine salts vs. placebo while still on divalproex sodium). Divalproex sodium showed improvement in YMRS scores, but not in ADHD symptoms. In the crossover phase of the study, when compared to placebo, ADHD symptoms greatly improved with mixed amphetamine salts. Chronic aggressive behavior refractory to optimized stimulant treatment in children with a primary diagnosis of ADHD may respond to the addition of divalproex [24].

Autism/pervasive developmental disorder

In a 12-week DBRCT of divalproex sodium for irritability/aggression in children and adolescents with autism spectrum disorder, 62.5% of subjects on divalproex vs. 9% of subjects on placebo responded with improvement shown on Aberrant Behavior Checklist-Irritability subscale scores (p = 0.048) and CGI-irritability score (Odds Ratio = 16.7, Fisher's exact p = 0.008) [25]. However, no statistical difference was observed between divalproex and placebo in another DBRCT for treating aggression in children and adolescents with pervasive developmental disorders [26].

Conduct disorder and posttraumatic stress disorder (PTSD)

Adolescent males with at least one crime conviction diagnosed with conduct disorder (n = 71) were enrolled in a randomized, controlled, seven-week clinical trial of high-dose vs. low-dose divalproex. Significant associations between divalproex treatment and ratings on the CGI-S (p = 0.02), CGI-I (p = 0.0008) and self-reported impulse control (p < 0.05) were observed. *Post hoc* analysis of the same study for 12 youths with PTSD and conduct disorder showed significantly greater improvement in CGI-S scores and core PTSD symptoms (intrusion and avoidance with hyperarousal) [27].

Adverse effects

The most common adverse effects such as tremors, thrombocytopenia, alopecia, asthenia, diarrhea, vomiting, and anorexia are mostly dose dependent. In a multicenter trial of divalproex monotherapy in patients with poorly controlled partial epilepsy randomly assigned to a "high" (80 to 150 µg/mL) versus a "low" (25 to 50 µg/mL) valproate plasma level groups, these adverse effects were significantly more frequent in the "high" serum level group compared to the "low" serum level group [28].

Overall, divalproex was commonly associated with adverse effects such as gastrointestinal symptoms (for example, abdominal pain, nausea, vomiting and diarrhea), tremors and sedation [5, 10, 11, 14, 15].

Gastrointestinal

The most common gastrointestinal adverse effects in the pediatric age group include nausea, increased appetite, and vomiting. Usually seen during initiation of treatment, these adverse effects are dose dependent and transient [29]. They are less commonly experienced with ER and enteric coated preparations than with immediate release preparation.

Hepatic toxicity

The four main subtypes of liver injury associated with divalproex are: transient and reversible elevation in hepatic transaminases, toxic hepatitis, hyperammonemia, and Reye-like syndrome. Asymptomatic and reversible abnormalities in the form of elevated hepatic transaminases are seen in 44% of patients. Elevation of transaminases 2–3 times the normal reference range warrants immediate discontinuation of the drug and further investigation. Clinically significant hepatotoxicity requiring discontinuation is seen in 1 in 15 000 adult cases and 1 in 800 cases in children less than two years of age [30]. Hyperammonemia, which presents with confusion and waxing and waning of consciousness [31], may or may not present with elevated liver enzymes. No relationship has been found between either serum divalproex levels and serum ammonia levels or serum ammonia levels and clinical severity of hyperammonemia. An underlying ornithine carbamoyltransferase deficiency may be suspected in children with divalproex associated hyperammonemia. Concomitant treatment with topiramate poses another risk factor due to its carbonic anhydrase inhibitory action [32]. Reye's-syndrome-like liver toxicity is associated with risk factors such as young age (<2 years), polytherapy, developmental delay, and coincident metabolic disorders [32]. Cases of children and adolescents with liver failure have been reported [32–35]. Carnitine deficiency has been implicated as one of the mechanisms for divalproex induced hepatotoxicity [36, 37].

Central nervous system adverse effects

Sedation is one of the most common adverse effects noticed during treatment initiation. It is usually transient and dose related. It may be minimized by dosage reduction, slow titration, use of extended-release formulations, and taking all of the medication at bedtime. The other adverse effect (tremors) may respond to a reduction in dosage or treatment with propranolol. Extended-release or enteric-coated formulations may lessen the frequency of tremor [38, 39]. Serious neurotoxicity with divalproex is usually consequent to the hyperammonemia (discussed above) and is postulated to be consequent to increased glutamine uptake, and resultant astrocyte swelling and edema. Dose-dependent cognitive impairment has been studied for divalproex with more impairment seen with higher doses [40].

Metabolic effects and weight gain

Weight gain is a common adverse effect of valproate therapy averaging 3–24 pounds over 3–12 months [16] with levels >125 µg/mL more likely to cause weight gain. Significant increases in ghrelin levels in prepubertal patients on valproate [41, 42] may be the mechanism implicated in weight gain. However some studies have shown that valproate does not lead to weight gain in the prepubertal age group [43]. A three year Italian study demonstrated that the weight gain in prepubertal children leveled off after 16 months of therapy [44]. Concentration of insulin and serum Insulin like Growth Factor (IGF-1) was found to be normal in valproate-treated girls with epilepsy on valproate for a shorter length of years, suggesting that insulin resistance and hyperinsulinemia are a consequence rather than a cause of valproate-related weight gain [45].

Alopecia

Valproate administration results in alopecia in up to 12% of patients in a dose-dependent manner and alopecia [16] is seen in almost 28% of patients with high valproate level exposure [46]. Depleted serum zinc and low serum biotinidase activity may be responsible for the alopecia [47].

Lipid and cardiovascular changes

Meta-analysis [48] of many studies in children and adolescents on valproate demonstrates significant elevation in serum lipoprotein levels while no significant differences were seen in serum apo A1, apo B levels, and high-density lipoprotein (HDL-C) levels. Significant reduction was seen in HDL2-C/HDL3-C ratio. Serum LDL-C levels were either shown to be unchanged or significantly lower in valproate monotherapy compared to pretreatment and control groups. The same meta-analysis demonstrated that children on valproate showed significant increase in homocysteine levels and decrease in B6 levels compared to baseline values. Though valproate carries a lower, long-term cardiovascular risk than carbamazepine the increased homocysteine levels and low HDL2-C/HDL3-C ratio may be a risk factor for microvascular enthothelial injury [49, 50].

Bone density changes

Studies show that children on valproate for >18 months have a 14% and 10% reduction in bone density at the axial and appendicular sites, respectively, thus increasing the likelihood of osteoporotic fractures. The mechanisms of this bone loss have been postulated to be reversible Fanconi-like syndrome [51] leading to electrolyte loss in urine and a direct osteoclastic effect on bones [52].

Reproductive and sexual issues

Multiple studies [53–55] show that up to 45–60% of women on divalproex monotherapy experienced menstrual disorders and 70–90% of these women had polycystic ovarian syndrome (PCOS) and/or hyperandrogenism and increased serum mean androgen levels. The increase in serum testosterone and androstenedione levels can be seen in approximately 50% of women within three months after starting divalproex. In a prospective study [56] comparing the endocrine effects of divalproex and lamotrigine, women with epilepsy beginning treatment with divalproex at age <26 years were at highest risk for developing PCOS whereas those women beginning treatment with divalproex at age ≥26 years had no higher risk than women with epilepsy receiving lamotrigine. Though obesity and related hyperinsulinemia may not cause menstrual problems, they may exacerbate the divalproex-related endocrine disorders. Hence, women younger than 26 years old should be carefully monitored for menstrual disturbances, weight gain and symptoms of hyperandrogenism.

Teratogenicity

Incidence of neural tube defects (NTD) is 1–2% with valproate exposure during pregnancy which is 10–20 times that of the general population. Anomalies with the highest increase in incidence were NTD [57–59], cardiovascular anomalies [60, 61], limb defects—especially radial limb reduction defects [62–64], and hypospadias [65].

Spontaneous abortions and premature births have been reported with valproate in utero exposure [66]. Dose related effects were seen in a prospective study where exposure to >1000 mg/day of valproate was associated with a 5.4% incidence of NTDs, which is higher than the general population [67]. Hence, valproate should be used in pregnancy only if absolutely essential and the dose should be kept below 1000 mg/day in three divided doses [68]. Folic acid deficiency and histone deacetylase inhibition have been postulated to be mechanisms for defective neural tube closure [69].

Hematological Adverse Effects

Serum levels greater than 100 μg/ml are usually associated with hematological toxicities like thrombocytopenia and leukopenia in children, which can usually be reversed with dose reduction or drug discontinuation [70]. A prospective German study with children on valproate followed for six months showed an asymptomatic but statistically significant decrease in von Willebrand's factor, factor XIII; hypofibrinogenemia and prolonged activated partial thromboplastin time [71].

Valproate toxicity

Though divalproex is rapidly absorbed from the GI tract, delayed peak levels may be seen from 1 to 18 hours postingestion. This warrants serial monitoring of divalproex levels in cases of acute toxic doses. The free fraction of the drug increases with peak levels of divalproex due to saturation of protein binding sites, which contributes to the toxic effects. Central nervous system depression is the most common manifestation in acute overdose. Acute cerebral edema, which is often associated with hyperammonemia from hepatic failure, presents 48–72 hours after ingestion. Although acute pancreatitis occurs in settings of both acute and chronic toxicity, hepatic failure is rarely a presentation of acute toxicity. Hypotension, electrolyte imbalance, thrombocytopenia and hyperammonemia are the other manifestations [72]. Extracorporeal elimination is viable at supratherapeutic doses because of increased, unbound fraction and both conventional hemodialysis and high-flux hemodiafiltration have been shown to be effective in pediatric patients [73, 74]. L-carnitine has been used with some success, but controlled, randomized and

Table 12.3 Dose for divalproex

Initiation dose for mania	Maintenance dose
15 mg/kg/day in B.I.D doses	increase every three days by 10 mg/kg/day and titrate based on clinical response and side effects the maximum daily dose is 60 mg/kg/day in B.I.D doses

B.I.D = twice daily.

multicentric trials are needed to further investigate its role [36, 75]. There is some evidence for use of naloxone in reversing the acute toxicity [76].

Dose and dosage forms
See Tables 12.3 and 12.4 respectively.

Carbamazepine

Carbamazepine was synthesized in the 1950s and approved in 1974 for the treatment of epilepsy in adults and in 1987 for the treatment of

Table 12.4 Dosage forms of anticonvulsants

Drug	Dosage form	Strength available
divalproex	valproic acid	250 mg
	softgel capsules (Depakene)	250 mg/5 ml
	syrup (Depakene)	
	divalproex sodium	
	– sprinkles	125 mg,
	– delayed release tablets (Depakote)	125 mg, 250 mg, 500 mg
	– extended release tablets (Depakote ER)	250 mg, 500 mg
	valproate injection (Depacon)	100 mg/ml
carbamazepine	chewable tablets	100 mg
	regular tablets	200 mg
	XR (extended release)	100, 200 and 400 mg
	suspension	100 mg/5 ml
oxcarbazepine	tablets	150 mg, 300 mg and 600 mg
	suspension	300 mg/5 ml (60 mg/ml)
lamotrigine	tablets	25, 100, 150, 200 mg
	chewable dispersible tablets	2, 5, 25 mg
	orally disintegrating tablets	25, 50, 100, 200 mg
gabapentin	capsules	100, 300, 400 mg
	tablets	600, 800 mg
	oral solution	250 mg/5 mL
topiramate	tablets	25, 50, 100, 200 mg
	sprinkle capsules	15, 25 mg

children. The seminal work by Ballenger and Post [77], drawing parallels between progression of affective episodes and the amygdala kindled seizures, paved a path for off-label use of carbamazepine for mood disorder in the 1980s and 1990s. The extended release preparation of carbamazepine was approved by the U.S. FDA for acute manic and mixed episodes in patients with bipolar disorder in 2004. It is also approved by the FDA for use in partial seizures with complex symptomatology, generalized tonic clonic seizures, mixed seizures and trigeminal neuralgia.

Chemical property and mechanism of action

Carbamazepine is an iminostilbine derivative with a tricylic nucleus similar to imipramine. Carbamazepine controls amygdala kindled seizures and hence believed to prevent and treat affective dysregulation in bipolar disorder resulting from a hyperexcitable limbic system [77–79]. Carbamazepine, like phenytoin, stabilizes inactive forms of sodium channels (Na^+) and retards its recovery from inactivation; thus preventing repetitive sustained firing. It is also shown to decrease cyclic AMP (adenosine monophosphate) by inhibiting the adenylyl cyclase. Inhibition of calcium intake in glial cells and interaction with GABA receptors are other putative mechanisms of action [80].

Indications

Bipolar disorder

In adult studies, carbamazepine immediate release preparation has shown efficacy in both manic [77, 81–83] and depressive phases [84] of illness along with the maintenance treatment [85]. However, these studies are limited by small sample size and lack of consistency between study designs. Unlike lithium, which is known for its efficacy in "classical" bipolar illness, carbamazepine has shown to be more effective in "nonclassical" forms such as bipolar II disorder, bipolar not otherwise specified (NOS), bipolar disorder with mood incongruent delusions, mixed states and co-morbid anxiety or substance abuse [86, 87]. Double blind placebo controlled multi-center trials with carbamazepine ER forms in adults with mania and mixed (including depressed) states led to its FDA approval for this patient population in 2005 [88, 89].

Studies in bipolar disorder (BPD) with immediate release preparation have shown efficacy in bipolar manic and mixed states [90–92]. Specifically, using a ≥50% change from baseline to exit in the YMRS scores to define response; the effect size was 1.63 for divalproex sodium, 1.06 for lithium, and 1.00 for carbamazepine. Using this same response measure with the intent-to-treat sample, the response rates were as follows: sodium divalproex, 53%; lithium, 38%; and carbamazepine, 38%

(chi 2(2) = 0.85, p = 0.60). A recent trial with carbamazepine ER preparation in BPD showed improvement in depressive, ADHD, and psychotic symptoms along with manic symptoms [93].

Aggression and conduct disorder

Improvement in emotional lability, impulsivity and aggression was observed with carbamazepine in a review of non epileptic children with behavioral problems [94]. Similarly, Kafantaris found significant reduction in explosive behavior and severe aggression in an open-label trial of carbamazepine for children with conduct disorder [95]. However, this was not replicated in a double-blind placebo controlled trial [96]. Hence, more studies are needed to determine the role of carbamazepine in the treatment of aggression in conduct disorder.

ADHD

A meta-analysis [97] of seven open-label and three double-blind placebo-controlled studies showed results favoring carbamazepine for use in ADHD. However, carbamazepine has not been directly compared to first- or second-line agents in the treatment of ADHD.

Adverse effects

Central nervous system effects

Sedation, ataxia, diplopia, and nystagmus are early and dose dependent adverse effects, and usually resolve after auto-induction. It may be beneficial to switch to ER preparation at bedtime.

Dermatological effects

Benign maculopapular rash, commonly seen with immediate release preparations, is usually idiosyncratic, widespread, and nonprogressive; it resolves with discontinuation of the drug and a trial of antihistamines and/or steroids. The patient may be rechallenged with carbamazepine under steroid cover or switched to an alternative agent. Cross sensitivity to oxcarbazapine is seen in a third of subjects.

Less frequently seen are more serious rashes like Stevens–Johnson syndrome (SJS) and toxic epidermal necrolysis. Rechallenging with carbamazepine is not recommended. Highest incidence is seen during the first 8–10 weeks after initiation of the carbamazepine treatment, but the overall risk is low (1.4 cases per 10 000 new carbamazepine users) [98]. HLA-B*1502 allele is strongly linked with a higher risk of serious dermatological adverse effects especially in Asian populations, and a screening for these alleles is recommended in patients of Asian descent [99]. Carbamazepine should be avoided in patients positive for this allele.

The frequency of this allele is between 1–15% in different ethnic sub-groups of the Asian population. HLA-B*5901 is another allele that is being investigated to ascertain its association with serious dermatological adverse effects [100].

Hematological effects

Benign leucopenia, which is seen in approximately 2.1% of carbamazepine-treated patients, is not predictive of risk of serious blood dyscrasias [101]. Treatment options include decreasing the dose of carbamazepine and adding lithium or granulocyte-colony stimulating factor (G-CSF) to counter the inhibitory effect of carbamazepine. The risk of aplastic anemia and agranulocytosis with carbamazepine is five to eight times that of the general population [102].

Gastrointestinal and hepatic effects

Mild gastritis and nausea may accompany carbamazepine administration during early treatment. However, presence of severe nausea, icterus and abdominal pain may be indicative of fatal hepatoxicity.

Metabolic effects

Hyponatremia has been reported to occur in 13% of carbamazepine-treated patients compared to 30% of oxcarbazapine treated patients [102]. Older age and a higher dose of carbamazepine are risk factors for development of hyponatremia.

Endocrine effects

Carbamazepine was found to be associated with low-serum thyroxine and free thyroxine concentrations but normal triiodothyronine and thyrotropin levels in clinically euthyroid subjects [103, 104].

Reproductive issues

Pregnancy registries have reported a malformation rate of between 2.2–5.4% with carbamazepine monotherapy exposure [105, 106]. Carbamazepine has been placed in pregnancy category D and is associated with low birth weight, craniofacial deformities, digital hypoplasia, and neural tube defects. Recent meta-analysis of epilepsy studies showed that children with *in utero* carbamazepine exposure had significantly lower PIQ (performance intelligence quotient) but similar FSIQ (full scale intelligence quotient) and VIQ (verbal intelligence quotient) as compared to unexposed children [105, 106].

Toxicity

Carbamazepine displays delayed peak levels with resultant delayed clinical effects due to its lipophilic nature, erratic absorption and slowed gut transition time (anticholinergic action). Production of clinically active epoxide metabolite and slow sustained release of carbamazepine due to delayed gut motility may lead to a cyclical worsening of the clinical scenario. Immediate release and controlled release preparations may lead to peak serum concentrations up to 72 hours and 96 hours respectively, after consumption [107–110]. Symptoms of toxicity include a combination of central effects like coma, respiratory failure, ataxia, nystagmus, hyper-reflexia and peripheral effects like pupillary dilatation, ileus and other anticholinergic effects. Cardiac arrthymias and left ventricular dysfunction have been reported in children [109]. Serum levels more than 40mcg/mL are thought to be predictive of a severe overdose in adults. Children generally show a more severe clinical picture at even lower serum levels [107–110].

Dose and dosage forms
See Tables 12.5 and 12.4 respectively.

Drug interactions
See Table 12.6.

Oxcarbazepine

Oxcarbazepine is a relatively new drug that has gained worldwide popularity for the treatment of partial seizures. Oxcarbazepine is FDA approved as a monotherapy for partial seizures in adults and in children four years of age and older, and as an adjunctive therapy for adults and for children two years of age and older.

Chemical properties and mechanism of action
Oxcarbazepine is a 10 keto-analogue of carbamazepine. It is a prodrug, which is rapidly metabolized by hepatic cytosolic enzymes through keto

Table 12.5 Dose for carbamazepine

Dose	Initiation dose	Maintenance dose
<6 years of age	initiate with 10–20 mg/kg/day in B.I.D–Q.I.D doses	up to <35 mg/kg/day in B.I.D–Q.I.D doses
6–12 years of age	initiate with 100 mg B.I.D	increase by 100 mg per week to maximum of 400–800 mg daily in B.I.D–T.I.D doses
>12 years of age	initiate with 200 mg B.I.D	increase by 200 mg per week to maximum of 800–1200 mg daily in B.I.D–T.I.D doses

BID = twice per day; QID = four times; TID = three times; BID-QID = two to four times.

Table 12.6 Drug interactions for carbamazepine

Effect of drugs on carbamazepine levels	Central nervous system active agents	Other agents
increase carbamazepine levels (CYP 3A4 inhibitors)	fluoxetine, divalproex	cimetidine, danazol, diltiazem, macrolides, erythromycin, clarithromycin, terfenadine, isoniazid, niacinamide, nicotinamide, propoxyphene, ketaconazole, itraconazole, verapamil
decrease carbamazepine levels (CYP 3A4 inducers)	felbamate, phenobarbital, phenytoin, primidone	cisplatin, doxorubicin, rifampin, theophylline
effect of carbamazepine on drug levels		
increased drug levels	clomipramine HCl, phenytoin, primidone	
decreased drug levels	alprazolam, clonazepam, clozapine, olanzapine, risperidone, quetiapine, aripripazole, haloperidol, divalproex, lamotrigine, carbamazepine, oxcarbazapine, phenytoin, theophylline, tiagabine, topiramate, divalproex, ethosuximide, zonisamide, methylphenidate, modafinil	acetaminophen, dicumarol, doxycycline, oral contraceptives, warfarin, nimodipine, nifedipine

CYP = cytochrome.

reduction to a clinically active monohydroxy derivative (MHD) 10, 11-dihydro-10-hydroxy-carbazepine.

Though the exact mechanism of action is unclear, like carbamazepine, oxcarbazepine inhibits voltage-activated sodium (Na^+) channels repetitively firing at high frequencies and consequently inhibits excitatory neurotransmission. This, along with the recently postulated suppressive effect on delayed rectifier potassium (K^+) currents, may exert a synergistic blocking effect on excitatory neuronal pathways [111]. There is some preliminary evidence of possible neuroprotective effects modulated through the intracellular signaling pathways like the phosphoinositide-3-kinase pathway [112]. In animal studies, MHD inhibits glutamatergic excitatory postsynaptic potentials in corticostriatal pathways through reversible inhibition of high voltage calcium currents in the cortical pyramidal cells [113].

Indications

Bipolar disorder

Oxcarbazepine monotherapy has been shown to be more effective than placebo and as effective as divalproex or haloperidol in acute episodes of bipolar disorder in adult subjects [114–120]. The Cochrane review [121] pointed out that there was insufficient evidence for its role in maintenance treatment in bipolar disorder but a recent randomized, controlled trial [122] showed that oxcarbazepine was as efficacious as carbamazepine for maintenance.

Pediatric studies are limited in number. Though oxcarbazepine monotherapy in youth with epilepsy and bipolar disorder showed improved CGI-I scores [123], oxcarbazepine was shown to be less effective than divalproex for bipolar disorder with aggression [124]. Similarly in a multicentric DBRCT conducted in 116 subjects between the ages of seven and 18 years old with bipolar I disorder, with either manic or mixed episodes, oxcarbazepine (mean dose = 1515 mg/day) did not significantly improve YMRS scores at endpoint compared with placebo [adjusted mean change: oxcarbazepine, -10.90 (n = 55); placebo, -9.79 (n = 55)] [125].

Drug interactions

In contrast to carbamazepine, oxcarbazepine has significantly fewer drug interactions because of (a) limited interaction with hepatic isoenzyme systems; (b) no auto-induction properties; (c) lesser susceptibility to interference of concomitantly administered drugs with metabolism of oxcarbazepine to MHD, and (d) no significant interactions or toxic effects of MHD unlike the epoxide metabolite of carbamazepine.

Effects of oxcarbazepine on other drugs: (a) Moderate induction of the CYP 3A group of enzymes may lead to decreased concentrations of felodipine, benzodiazepines (alprazolam, clonazepam), buprenorphine and oral contraceptive pills. Oral contraceptives with higher hormonal doses and use of additional contraceptive measures are recommended. (b) Mild to moderate inhibition of the CYP 2C19 enzyme may or may not produce a clinically significant change in phenytoin levels. (c) Mild UDP-GT enzyme induction may produce decreases in lamotrigine concentrations. Topiramate and leviteracetam concentrations may be decreased by oxcarbazepine. No significant interactions are seen with divalproex.

Effects of other drugs on oxcarbazepine: (a) Decrease in MHD levels may be seen because of concomitant administration of other antiepiletics like phenytoin, carbamazepine and phenobarbital. (b) No clinically significant effects were produced on MHD concentrations by divalproex, clobazam, lamotrigine or clonazepam. (c) Erthromcyin, a commonly prescribed antibiotic in the pediatric age group, can be safely co-administered with oxcarbazepine because of minimal interaction (unlike carbamazepine).

Adverse effects

Extensive pediatric safety and tolerability data is available from the Novartis oxcarbazepine safety database. The most common adverse effects reported during epilepsy clinical trials are headaches, somnolence, vomiting and dizziness (20–35% patients). More than 10% of the subjects experience nausea, fatigue, ataxia and diplopia. Around 4% of subjects withdrew because of rash. No association between adverse effects and MHD levels was found. No long-term, cognitive adverse effects in the pediatric population have been reported [126, 127].

Hyponatremia

An effect on Na^+ channels has been implicated in oxcarbazepine induced hyponatremia. The prevalence in adult studies is estimated to be 30% compared to 13% for carbamazepine. Pre-treatment hyponatremia and advancing age have been identified as the risk factors for developing hyponatremia on oxcarbazepine [128, 129]. In a pediatric sample with normal baseline sodium levels (sodium levels <135 mmol/l), no clinical symptoms were observed in 26.6% of the patients. In a pediatric sample with sodium levels below 125 mmol/l, clinical symptoms were observed in 2.6%, and clinically symptomatic hyponatremia occurred in one girl (1.3%). A case report of oxcarbazepine induced hyponatremic coma (sodium levels 113 mmol/l) in a seven-year-old boy has been reported [130]; as a result, monitoring is warranted.

Rare adverse effects

Giant hepatic adenoma has been reported in a 16 year old on oxcarbazepine [131]. Oxcarbazapine has been reported to cause parkinsonian symptoms [132], Stevens–Johnson syndrome [133], leukopenia [134], and thrombocytopenia [135].

Reproductive issues

Both oxcarbazepine and MHD cross the placenta substantially (umbilical cord/plasma = 0.92–1.0) and the breast milk concentration of oxcarbazepine and MHD is approximately half of that found in the maternal plasma (milk/plasma = 0.5–0.65). No acute side-effects have been noted in these neonates. Although the American Academy of Pediatrics has not made any recommendations in this regard, mothers on oxcarbazepine need to be warned about the possible effects on neonates. Data on pregnancy outcomes with oxcarbazepine is scarce, with four major malformations reported in 291 pregnancies with oxcarbazepine monotherapy (malformation rate 4/291 = 1.3%), which does not seem to be elevated from the malformation rate of 2–4% in the general population [136].

Toxicity

Oxcarbazapine is believed to be less toxic in overdoses than carbamazepine. An overdose with 100 tablets of oxcarbazepine (300 mg each) in a 37-year-old male led to a tenfold higher level of oxcarbazepine, but only twofold higher MHD peak levels [137]. The conversion of oxcarbazepine, which is a prodrug for active compound MHD, is the rate-limiting step and hence may prevent toxic clinical effects [138–140]. Similarly in other reported adult cases, acute central nervous system depression followed by rapid recovery was noted. In a single pediatric case report of overdose with 15 g of oxcarbazepine in a 13-year-old autistic boy, no metabolic or clinical effects were reported except for somnolence [141].

Dose and dosage forms

See Tables 12.7 and 12.4 respectively.

Lamotrigine

Synthesized in the 1980s, lamotrigine was approved for treatment of epilepsy in Europe in the early 1990s and by the FDA in 1994. Today, FDA approves it as (a) an adjunct for partial seizures with or without secondary generalization in ages two and above, and (b) an adjunct for Lennox–Gastaut syndrome in both pediatric and adult patients, and (c) monotherapy for treatment of partial seizures in adults. Its psychiatric indications include maintenance treatment of bipolar disorder.

Chemical property and mechanism of action

Lamotrigine is structurally a phenyltriazine derivative [142] but its mechanism of action is not completely understood. It has been postulated that its mood-stabilizing and anti-epileptic effect is exerted through blockage of repetitive sustained firing in voltage-gated sodium channels [143].

Table 12.7 Dose for oxcarbazapine

Body weight	Initiation dose	Maintenance dose (achieved in two weeks)
20–29 kg	10 mg/kg not to exceed 600 mg/day in a B.I.D dose	900 mg/day in a B.I.D dose
29.1–39 kg		1200 mg/day in a B.I.D dose
>39 kg		1800 mg/day in a B.I.D dose

B.I.D = twice per day.

Involvement of postsynaptic serotonin (5-HT 1A) receptors as demonstrated in animal models may be responsible for its antidepressant action [144]. Preliminary fMRI studies show decreased amygdalar activation when compared to baseline activation ($r = 0.91$, $p = 0.002$) after eight weeks of lamotrigine treatment in adolescents with bipolar depression [145, 146]. fMRI studies in lamotrigine-treated subjects with adolescent bipolar disorder shows enhanced prefrontal activity during a response inhibition task, demonstrating action on brain circuitry [147].

Indications

Bipolar disorder

A forty-eight week open label prospective trial of lamotrigine in seventy five treatment refractory adult bipolar patients as monotherapy ($n = 15$) or as an adjunct ($n = 60$) found broad therapeutic activity with response in both manic and depressed patients. Despite many limitations, this study showed broad therapeutic efficacy of lamotrigine in this population [148]. A four-week DBRCT in hospitalized manic patients randomized to lamotrigine, olanzapine and lithium showed statistically significant and similar improvement from baseline on Mania Rating Scale scores ($P < 0.0002$, Wilcoxon Sign Rank Test) in all three groups [149]. However, efficacy in mania is not well founded [150].

A twelve-week open label prospective trial on 39 pediatric subjects (age 6–17 years) with manic or mixed symptoms showed improvement over baseline in manic (decrease in mean YMRS score 14.9 ± 9.7, $P < 0.001$), depressive (CDRS score 40.1 ± 12.9 vs. 31.8 ± 13.7, $p = 0.0002$), attention-deficit/hyperactivity disorder (ADHD-RS 35.6 ± 11.2 vs. 22.5 ± 15.7, $P < 0.0001$), and psychotic symptoms (BPRS: 41.0 ± 7.9 vs. 29.9 ± 9.2, $P < 0.0001$) [151].

Bipolar depression

In a seven-week randomized control trial comparing 66 bipolar subjects, lamotrigine 200 mg showed statistically significant improvement ($p < 0.005$) on MADRS, CGI-S and CGI-I over baseline at the endpoint [148, 149]. In a meta-analysis of five randomized controlled trials with 1072 subjects comparing lamotrigine (100–400 mg/day) monotherapy to placebo over a seven-to-ten-week period in bipolar depressed subjects, more individuals treated with lamotrigine than placebo responded to treatment on both the Hamilton Rating Scale for Depression (HRSD) (relative risk (RR) = 1.27, 95% CI 1.09–1.47, $p = 0.002$) and Montgomery–Asberg Depression Rating Scale (MADRS) (RR=1.22, 95% CI 1.06-1.41, $p = 0.005$) [152]. These studies demonstrate the modest benefit of using lamotrigine for acute depression in bipolar subjects [152].

In a retrospective chart review, half of the 42 adolescents with mood disorders treated with lamotrigine showed improvement with mean CGI-S score decreasing from 4.9 ± 1.0 at baseline to 3.5 ± 1.4 at endpoint ($z = 3.204$, $p < 0.002$) [153]. In an eight-week open-label trial of lamotrigine with 20 adolescents ages 12–17 years with diagnoses of bipolar disorder I, II, or not otherwise specified, experiencing a depressive episode, 84% responded with a response of 1 or 2 on the CGI-I scale at week 8 [146].

Bipolar disorder—maintenance

Efficacy and safety of lamotrigine has been demonstrated in many trials outlined below. In a 52-week continuation study [154] of the seven-week double-blind, placebo-controlled study [155], the lamotrigine subjects ($n = 77/124$) were continued on the same dose and the placebo group ($n = 47/124$) switched to lamotrigine in the fourth week. All subjects maintained their improved MADRS scores throughout the continuation phase ($p < 0.05$). Two similarly designed studies [156, 157] and pooled analysis of these studies [158] showed that lamotrigine and lithium were superior to placebo for time to intervention for any mood episode (median survival: placebo, 86 days [95% CI $= 58$ to 121]; lithium, 184 days [95% CI $=119$ to not calculable]; lamotrigine, 197 days [95% CI $= 144$ to 388]). Lithium and lamotrigine were superior to placebo for time to intervention for mania and lamotrigine was superior to placebo for time to intervention for depression (median survival: placebo, 270 days [95% CI $= 138$ to not calculable). None of the active treatments caused an affective switch. In a secondary analysis of this study, hazard ratio for the emergence of mania symptoms with lamotrigine was not significantly different from placebo (hazard ratio $= 0.79$;95% CI, 0.53 to 1.16) [159].

In an open-label prospective trial, 46 children and adolescents (8–18 years) with manic or hypomanic symptoms were treated in an eight-week acute phase with second generation antipsychotics while slowly titrating up lamotrigine. This was followed by a six-week lamotrigine monotherapy phase for stabilized patients. The response rate on manic symptoms (YMRS <12) was 72%, on depressive symptoms was 82% (Children's Depression Rating Scale-Revised [CDRS-R] <40), and the remission rate was 56% at the 14-week end point [160].

Drug interactions

Lamotrigine undergoes glucoronidation by 1A4 isoform of UGT. This isoform is induced by phenobarbital, phenytoin and carbamazepine, which decrease the plasma levels of lamotrigine by almost 50%. Oxcarbazepine exerts half the enzyme inducing effect on lamotrigine metabolism as compared to carbamazepine. Divalproex competitively inhibits the UGT isoform and increases the half-life of lamotrigine to almost 70 hours requiring clinical dose reduction [161–163].

UGT1A4 isoform is induced by the estrogenic component of oral contraceptive pills, thus decreasing levels of concomitantly administered lamotrigine. The progestogen-only compounds do not influence lamotrigine levels, regardless of whether administered by the oral, intramuscular, subdermal, or intrauterine modes [164].

Adverse effects

Most data on pediatric tolerability of lamotrigine is available from pediatric and adult epilepsy studies, and some adult and pediatric bipolar studies. Messenheimer [165] reported somnolence (8%), asthenia (16%), dizziness (8%), ataxia (<1%), insomnia (6%), headache (20%), nausea (10%), tremors (2%) and rashes (12%) in epilepsy studies involving 4000 epileptic patients greater than 12 years old. Rash was the only adverse effect that led to withdrawal of more than 5% of patients; 0.9% experienced serious rash with 0.3% requiring hospitalization for the rash, of which four patients were diagnosed with Stevens–Johnson syndrome (0.1%). Pediatric epilepsy data has shown that rash is the most common adverse effect and incidence of serious rash is higher in children (0.8%) compared with adults (0.3%) [166].

Bowden [167] analyzed eight placebo controlled trials of lamotrigine for both acute episodes and maintenance treatment of adult bipolar patients. The results, comparable to the epilepsy studies, showed that the adverse effects are somnolence (9%), dizziness (9%), insomnia (7%), headache (25%), nausea (14%), tremors (5%) and rashes (9%). Compared to lithium, lamotrigine has lower incidence of tremor and diarrhea and higher incidence of headache and rash. A serious adverse effect is defined as any untoward experience, regardless of its suspected cause, which is fatal, life-threatening or permanently disabling, a congenital anomaly or cancer; or that requires inpatient hospitalization. This was seen in 8% for both lamotrigine and lithium and in 7% for placebo. The serious adverse effects leading to discontinuation of lamotrigine were mania (2%) and rash (3%). No statistically significant difference in suicide rates was found between lamotrigine (1.8% per year) and placebo (1.1% per year). Neither sexual adverse effects nor weight fluctuations were found to be significantly different from placebo. Serious rash was seen in 0.1% of patients in open label trials of lamotrigine but was determined not to be Stevens–Johnson syndrome. Incidence of rash with lamotrigine (9%) was comparable to placebo (8%). Pediatric and adolescent studies reported data comparable to adult bipolar studies without any serious dermatological adverse effects.

Lamotrigine has been associated with cases of aspetic meningitis [168], hallucinosis [169], frank psychosis [170], chorea [171], blepharospasm, tourettism and obsessive-compulsive symptoms [172], and fulminant hepatitis [173, 174].

Dermatological effects

Lamotrigine-associated rash could range from simple morbilliform rash, urticaria (hives) and erythema multiforme to more severe reactions such as hypersensitivity syndrome, Stevens-Johnson syndrome, and toxic epidermal necrolysis. A history of rash after another antiepileptic (13.9% versus 4.6%; OR = 3.62; p < 0.001) and age less than 13 years (10.7% versus. 4.3%; OR = 2.77; p < 0.001) are found to be the strongest predictors of lamotrigine-induced rash [175]. Other risk factors for rash include exceeding recommended initial doses and titration schedule and co-administration of divalproex. In children, the etiology of rash may be difficult to pinpoint because of other causative agents like bacterial and viral infections (pharyngeal and dermatological) and reactions to antibiotics used to treat these (beta lactams) [176].

Rashes seen in the first five days of initiation of treatment are unlikely to be lamotrigine related. Benign rashes are nonconfluent and nontender, without systemic involvement. They disappear within a few days and may be treated symptomatically. Discontinuation of lamotrigine may be required depending on the characteristics of the rash and dependability of the patient. Rash occurring in the first eight weeks of treatment, confluent and widespread, purpuric and tender, involving the face, neck or upper trunk or mucosal surfaces along with laboratory and/or systemic involvement, needs immediate discontinuation of lamotrigine along with concomitant medications (if any) like divalproex or carbamazepine [177]. Though rechallenging the patient with lamotrigine is not recommended, 39 cases of successful lamotrigine rechallenge after a rash have been reported [178]. Dermatological precautions (avoiding new medicines, foods, cosmetics, conditioners, deodorants, detergents, and fabric softeners, as well as sunburn and exposure to poison ivy/oak; not starting lamotrigine within two weeks of a rash, viral syndrome, or vaccination) have not shown any statistical difference in the incidence of rash on lamotrigine (8.8%) when compared to placebo (8.6%) [179].

Toxicity

Retrospective analysis [180] of 493 cases reported to The American Association of Poison Control Centers in 2000 and 2001 showed that more than half the patients (52%) with lamotrigine toxicity experienced no major adverse effects. The most common clinical effects reported in overdose were drowsiness/lethargy (20.9%), vomiting (11%), nausea (5.1%),

Table 12.8 Dose for lamotrigine

	Lamotrigine	Lamotrigine + divalproex	Lamotrigine + carbamazpine
Week 1 and 2	0.3 mg/kg/day in 1–2 divided doses	0.15 mg/kg/day in 1–2 divided doses	0.6 mg/kg/day in 1–2 divided doses
Week 3 and 4	0.6 mg/kg/day in 1–2 divided doses; increase by 0.6 mg/kg/day every 1–2 weeks	0.3 mg/kg/day in 1–2 divided doses; increase by 0.3 mg/kg/day every 1–2 weeks	1.2 mg/kg/day in 1–2 divided doses; increase by 1.2 mg/kg/day every 1–2 weeks

ataxia (4.9%), dizziness/vertigo (4.5%), and tachycardia (4.3%). Major clinical effects included coma (n = 6), seizures (n = 8), and respiratory depression (n = 3). The pediatric population may be more paradoxically prone to seizures in overdose [181, 182].

Dose and dosage forms
See Tables 12.8 and 12.4 respectively.

Gabapentin

Gabapentin is a novel antiepileptic drug which is approved by U.S. FDA for adjunctive therapy for partial seizures with or without secondary generalization and neuropathic pain associated with post herpetic neuralgia.

Chemical property and mechanism of action

In spite of its structural similarity to the inhibitory neurotransmitter GABA (gamma amino butyric acid), gabapentin is not a GABA precursor, agonist, or antagonist. Multiple mechanisms of actions have been postulated including increased activity of glutamic acid decarboxylase responsible for converting glutamate to GABA and decreased activity of GABA-transaminase responsible for breakdown of GABA; subsequently increasing synaptic GABA levels [183]. It is also implicated in modulation of GAT-1(GABA transporter-1), increased N-methyl-d-aspartate (NMDA)-evoked currents in rat brains and regulation of voltage gated sodium and potassium channels [184]. It inhibits presynaptic high voltage activated calcium channels containing the alpha-2 delta subunit which subsequently leads to reduced neurotransmitter release and attenuation of postsynaptic excitability [185, 186].

Indications

There is a dearth of studies defining the role of gabapentin in pediatric psychiatric disorders. Controlled adult studies demonstrate limited efficacy as monotherapy, but some benefit as an adjunct for bipolar disorder

[187, 188]. Gabapentin has also shown promising results in placebo controlled trials for treatment of social anxiety and panic disorder [189, 190]. Controlled studies are lacking in children but gabapentin may be used as an adjunct in pediatric bipolar disorder with comorbid anxiety. There is a case report of decreased self-mutilatory behavior in a child with Lesch Nyhan syndrome [191]. Caution must, however, be exercised because of the reported increase in aggression and tantrums when gabapentin was used as an adjunct for pediatric seizure disorder in children with baseline attention deficit hyperactivity disorder and developmental delays [192].

Drug interactions
No clinically significant drug interactions are known.

Adverse effects
Gabapentin is generally well tolerated and the most common adverse effects are somnolence and dizziness. Other reported adverse effects are ataxia, tremor, nausea, diplopia, headache and weight gain. Most overdoses with gapapentin are not lethal. Clinical effects, which include drowsiness and ataxia, develop early and resolve within ten hours.

Dosage
Dose: initiation 10 mg/kg/day. Maintenance: 30–40 mg/kg/day.

Dosage forms
See Table 12.4.

Topiramate

Topiramate is approved by FDA for monotherapy in patients 10 years of age and older with partial onset or primary generalized tonic-clonic seizures and in adults for the prophylaxis of migraine headache. Its role in pediatric psychiatric disorders is largely unclear due to dearth of RCTs.

Mechanism of action and chemical structure
Topiramate is a derivative of the naturally occurring monosaccharide D-fructose with the sulfamate moiety responsible for its antiepileptic activity. It is believed to exert its therapeutic efficacy through voltage-activated sodium channels, (GABA) type A receptors, glutamate receptors, and high-voltage-activated calcium channels [193].

Indications

Bipolar disorder
Adult studies have largely shown that topiramate has poor efficacy as both monotherapy and adjunctive medication [194, 195]. The pediatric

bipolar trial was prematurely terminated after negative results from the adult studies [196]. There is some evidence that topiramate may be useful in bipolar disorder with psychiatric co-morbidities like alcohol abuse and eating disorders, such as bulimia and binge eating disorder and with medical co-morbidities like obesity, psychotropic induced weight gain and migraine [197, 198].

Eating disorder
Two RCTs of 99 subjects with bulimia showed significant reduction in the frequency of binge and purge days (p = 0.004) and led to significant weight loss (1.8 kg mean weight loss for topiramate versus 0.2 kg mean weight increase for placebo; p = 0.004) [199–201]. Three RCTs of binge eating disorder showed significant therapeutic efficacy in terms of weight loss and binge frequency [202–204].

Psychotropic associated weight gain
Topiramate has shown promising results in adult subjects with psychotropic associated weight gain [201, 205, 206] but there are no trials to demonstrate efficacy and safety in pediatric groups.

Drug interactions
Hepatic enzyme-inducing drugs such as carbamazepine may decrease topiramate levels. Topiramate induces metabolism of ethinyl estradiol at doses >200 mg/day.

Adverse effects
Paresthesias, decreased appetite, dry mouth, and weight loss were the most common side-effects in adult bipolar trials, and decreased appetite, nausea, diarrhea, paresthesias, somnolence, insomnia, and rash were the most commonly seen side-effects in PBD trials [194–196]. Central adverse effects such as sedation, fatigue and cognitive impairment have been noted. Rare adverse effects like renal stones, acute myopia with secondary angle-closure glaucoma and metabolic acidosis have been reported, which may be related to its mild carbonic anhydrase inhibitory activity [197].

Dose
Initiation: 25 mg twice daily. Maintenance: 100–200 mg/day titrated over 3–4 weeks.

Dosage forms
See Table 12.4. See Table 12.9 for anticonvulsant profiles.

Table 12.9 Profiles for specific anticonvulsants

Specific profile of mood stabilizer

Mood stabilizer	Advantages	Disadvantages
divalproex	1 Broad range efficacy 2 Extended release form enabling once a day dosing 3 Multiple mechanisms of action 4 Rapid titration to reach therapeutic doses	1 Interactions with CYP system of hepatic enzymes leading to drug interactions 2 Weight gain potential and sedation 3 Need for monitoring blood levels 4 Teratogenicity, hepatoxicity and risk of pancreatitis
carbamazepine	1 Multiple mechanisms of action	1 Widespread interaction (induction or inhibition) with CYP system of hepatic enzymes leading to multitude of drug interactions 2 Auto induction and production of clinically active epoxide metabolite 3 Adverse effect profile including dermatological and hematological reactions 4 Need for monitoring serum drug concentrations and poor correlation between drug levels and clinical effects 5 Endocrine, reproductive and teratogenic effects
oxcarbazepine	1 Additional action on calcium channels 2 Minimal interaction with P450 system of microsomal enzymes 3 Lesser incidence of adverse effects including dermatological effects than carbamazepine 4 No toxic metabolite (unlike the epoxide metabolite for carbamazepine) and no auto-induction 5 Routine therapeutic drug monitoring not required	1 Risk of hyponatremia
lamotrigine	1 No first pass metabolism or interaction with hepatic CYP enzymes; hence minimal drug interactions except interaction with divalproex and carbamazepine	1 Rare but serious risk of rash especially in pediatric age group (<13 years of age) 2 Slow titration required to reach therapeutic dose

(continued)

Table 12.9 (*Continued*)

Specific profile of mood stabilizer		
Mood stabilizer	Advantages	Disadvantages
gabapentin	1 Tolerable adverse effects including minimal weight gain potential 2 No significant drug interactions due to negligible protein binding, no active metabolite and minimal effect on hepatic enzymes	1 Less evidence for use given paucity of clinical trials
topiramate	1 Minimal protein binding, no hepatic metabolism and negligible drug interactions 2 Weight loss	1 Less evidence for use given paucity of clinical trials

CYP = cytochrome.

Conclusion

Further research is required in order to understand the neurobiological basis of the pathology of childhood psychiatric disorders. Meanwhile, clinicians need to exercise caution while using these drugs given the lack of evidence in the form of large-sized double-blinded placebo-controlled trials. A careful review of the risks and benefits of using these medications will enable clinicians to judiciously choose one agent over the other. It is, therefore, critical to interpret the preliminary data presented above, in the light of emergent and definitive future discoveries yet to add value to the continued and thoughtful use of these medications across all pertinent childhood disorders.

References

1 Peterson GM, Naunton M: Valproate: a simple chemical with so much to offer. *J Clin Pharm Ther* 2005; **30**: 417–21.
2 Sharma RP, Rosen C, Kartan S et al.: Valproic acid and chromatin remodeling in schizophrenia and bipolar disorder: preliminary results from a clinical population. *Schizophr Res* 2006; **88**: 227–31.
3 Machado-Vieira R, Ibrahim L, Zarate CA Jr.: Histone deacetylases and mood disorders: epigenetic programming in gene-environment interactions. *CNS Neurosci Ther* 2010; doi: 10.1111/j.1755-5949.2010.00203.x.
4 Azorin JM, Findling RL: Valproate use in children and adolescents with bipolar disorder. *CNS Drugs* **21**: 2007; 1019–33.
5 Wagner KD, Weller EB, Carlson GA et al.: An open-label trial of divalproex in children and adolescents with bipolar disorder. *J Am Acad Child Adolesc Psychiatry* 2002; **41**: 1224–30.

6 Findling RL, Frazier TW, Youngstrom EA et al.: Double-blind, placebo-controlled trial of divalproex monotherapy in the treatment of symptomatic youth at high risk for developing bipolar disorder. *J Clin Psychiatry* 2007; **68:** 781–8.

7 DelBello MP, Kowatch RA, Adler CM et al.: A double-blind randomized pilot study comparing quetiapine and divalproex for adolescent mania. *J Am Acad Child Adolesc Psychiatry* 2006; **45:** 305–13.

8 Delbello MP, Schwiers ML, Rosenberg HL et al.: A double-blind, randomized, placebo-controlled study of quetiapine as adjunctive treatment for adolescent mania. *J Am Acad Child Adolesc Psychiatry* 2002; **41:** 1216–23.

9 Calabrese JR, Shelton MD, Rapport DJ et al.: A 20-month, double-blind, maintenance trial of lithium versus divalproex in rapid-cycling bipolar disorder. *Am J Psychiatry* 2005; **162:** 2152–61.

10 Deltito JA, Levitan J, Damore J et al.: Naturalistic experience with the use of divalproex sodium on an in-patient unit for adolescent psychiatric patients. *Acta Psychiatr Scand* 1998; **97:** 236–40.

11 Papatheodorou G, Kutcher SP, Katic M et al.: The efficacy and safety of divalproex sodium in the treatment of acute mania in adolescents and young adults: an open clinical trial. *J Clin Psychopharmacol* 1995; **15:** 110–16.

12 Pavuluri MN, Henry DB, Findling RL et al.: Double-blind randomized trial of risperidone versus divalproex in pediatric bipolar disorder. *Bipolar Disord* 2010; **12:** 593–605.

13 Kowatch RA, Suppes T, Carmody TJ et al.: Effect size of lithium, divalproex sodium, and carbamazepine in children and adolescents with bipolar disorder. *J Am Acad Child Adolesc Psychiatry* 2000; **39:** 713–20.

14 Pavuluri MN, Henry DB, Carbray JA et al.: Open-label prospective trial of risperidone in combination with lithium or divalproex sodium in pediatric mania. *J Affect Disord* 2004; **82**(Suppl 1): S103–111.

15 Pavuluri MN, Henry DB, Carbray JA et al.: Divalproex sodium for pediatric mixed mania: a 6-month prospective trial. *Bipolar Disord* 2005; **7:** 266–73.

16 Bowden CL: Valproate. *Bipolar Disord* 2003; **5:** 189–202.

17 BALANCE investigators and collaborators, Geddes JR, Goodwin GM, Rendell J et al.: Lithium plus valproate combination therapy versus monotherapy for relapse prevention in bipolar I disorder (BALANCE): a randomised open-label trial. *Lancet* 2010; **375**(3712): 385–95.

18 Thakur A, Dutta S, Sinha VK: Intravenous valproate in acute adolescent mania: a preliminary report. *Eur Child Adolesc Psychiatry* 2004; **13:** 258–61.

19 Segal S: A double-blind, placebo-controlled trial to evaluate the safety and efficacy of depakote ER for the treatment of mania associated with bipolar disorder in children and adolescents, 2006. Available at: http://www.clinicalstudyresults .org/drugdetail.

20 DelBello MP, Adler C, Strakowski SM: Divalproex for the treatment of aggression associated with adolescent mania. *J Child Adolesc Psychopharmacol* 2004; **14:** 325–8.

21 Barzman DH, DelBello MP, Adler CM et al.: The efficacy and tolerability of quetiapine versus divalproex for the treatment of impulsivity and reactive aggression in adolescents with co-occurring bipolar disorder and disruptive behavior disorder(s). *J Child Adolesc Psychopharmacol* 2006; **16:** 665–70.

22 State RC, Frye MA, Altshuler LL et al.: Chart review of the impact of attention-deficit/hyperactivity disorder comorbidity on response to lithium or divalproex sodium in adolescent mania. *J Clin Psychiatry* 2004; **65:** 1057–63.

23 Scheffer RE, Kowatch RA, Carmody T et al.: Randomized, placebo-controlled trial of mixed amphetamine salts for symptoms of comorbid ADHD in pediatric bipolar disorder after mood stabilization with divalproex sodium. *Am J Psychiatry* **162:** 2005; 58–64.

24 Blader JC, Schooler NR, Jensen PS et al.: Adjunctive divalproex versus placebo for children with ADHD and aggression refractory to stimulant monotherapy. *Am J Psychiatry* 2009; **166:** 1392–401.

25 Hollander E, Chaplin W, Soorya L et al.: Divalproex sodium vs. placebo for the treatment of irritability in children and adolescents with autism spectrum disorders. *Neuropsychopharmacology* 2010; **35:** 990–8.

26 Hellings JA, Weckbaugh M, Nickel EJ et al.: A double-blind, placebo-controlled study of valproate for aggression in youth with pervasive developmental disorders. *J Child Adolesc Psychopharmacol* 2005; **15:** 682–92.

27 Steiner H, Saxena KS, Carrion V et al.: Divalproex sodium for the treatment of PTSD and conduct disordered youth: a pilot randomized controlled clinical trial. *Child Psychiatry Hum Dev* 2007; **38:** 183–93.

28 Beydoun A, Sackellares JC, Shu V: Safety and efficacy of divalproex sodium monotherapy in partial epilepsy: a double-blind, concentration-response design clinical trial. Depakote Monotherapy for Partial Seizures Study Group. *Neurology* 1997; **48:** 182–8.

29 DeVane CL: Pharmacokinetics, drug interactions, and tolerability of valproate. *Psychopharmacol Bull* 2003; **37**(Suppl 2): 25–42.

30 Bryant AE 3rd, Dreifuss FE: Valproic acid hepatic fatalities. III. U.S. experience since 1986. *Neurology* 1996; **46:** 465–9.

31 Koenig SA, Buesing D, Longin E et al.: Valproic acid-induced hepatopathy: nine new fatalities in Germany from 1994 to 2003. *Epilepsia* 2006; **47:** 2027–31.

32 Segura-Bruna N, Rodriguez-Campello A, Puente V et al.: Valproate-induced hyperammonemic encephalopathy. *Acta Neurol Scand* 2006; **114:** 1–7.

33 Koenig SA, Buesing D, Longin E et al.: Valproic acid-induced hepatopathy: nine new fatalities in Germany from 1994 to 2003. *Epilepsia* 2006; **47:** 2027–31.

34 Saneto RP, Lee IC, Koenig MK et al.: POLG DNA testing as an emerging standard of care before instituting valproic acid therapy for pediatric seizure disorders. *Seizure* 2010; **19:** 140–6.

35 Gerstner T, Buesing D, Longin E et al.: Valproic acid induced encephalopathy—19 new cases in Germany from 1994 to 2003—a side effect associated to VPA-therapy not only in young children. *Seizure* 2006; **15:** 443–8.

36 Lheureux PE, Hantson P: Carnitine in the treatment of valproic acid-induced toxicity. *Clin Toxicol (Phila)* 2009; **47:** 101–11.

37 Lheureux PE, Penaloza A, Zahir S et al.: Science review: carnitine in the treatment of valproic acid-induced toxicity—what is the evidence? *Crit Care* 2005; **9:** 431–40.

38 Karas BJ, Wilder BJ, Hammond EJ et al.: Treatment of valproate tremors. *Neurology* 1983; **33:** 1380–2.

39 Zarate CA Jr, Tohen M, Narendran R et al.: The adverse effect profile and efficacy of divalproex sodium compared with valproic acid: a pharmacoepidemiology study. *J Clin Psychiatry* 1999; **60:** 232–6.

40 Loring DW, Meador KJ: Cognitive side effects of antiepileptic drugs in children. *Neurology* 2004; **62:** 872–7.

41 Gungor S, Yucel G, Akinci A et al.: The role of ghrelin in weight gain and growth in epileptic children using valproate. *J Child Neurol* 2007; **22:** 1384–8.

42 Prodam F, Bellone S, Casara G et al.: Ghrelin levels are reduced in prepubertal epileptic children under treatment with carbamazepine or valproic acid. *Epilepsia* 2010; **51:** 312–15.

43 Espinosa PS, Salazar JC, Yu L et al.: Lack of valproic acid-associated weight gain in prepubertal children. *Pediatr Neurol* 2008; **39:** 177–80.

44 Grosso S, Mostardini R, Piccini B et al.: Body mass index and serum lipid changes during treatment with valproic acid in children with epilepsy. *Ann Pharmacother* 2009; **43:** 45–50.

45 Rattya J, Vainionpaa L, Knip M et al.: The effects of valproate, carbamazepine, and oxcarbazepine on growth and sexual maturation in girls with epilepsy. *Pediatrics* 1999; **103:** 588–93.

46 Mercke Y, Sheng H, Khan T et al.: Hair loss in psychopharmacology. *Ann Clin Psychiatry* 2000; **12:** 35–42.

47 Yilmaz Y, Tasdemir HA, Paksu MS: The influence of valproic acid treatment on hair and serum zinc levels and serum biotinidase activity. *Eur J Paediatr Neurol* 2009; **13:** 439–43.

48 Cheng LS, Prasad AN, Rieder MJ: Relationship between antiepileptic drugs and biological markers affecting long-term cardiovascular function in children and adolescents. *Can J Clin Pharmacol* 2010; **17:** e5–46.

49 Castro-Gago M, Novo-Rodriguez MI, Blanco-Barca MO et al.: Evolution of serum lipids and lipoprotein (a) levels in epileptic children treated with carbamazepine, valproic acid, and phenobarbital. *J Child Neurol* 2006; **21:** 48–53.

50 Gerstner T, Woelfing C, Witsch M et al.: Capillary microscopy and hemorheology in children during antiepileptic monotherapy with carbamazepine and valproate. *Seizure* 2006; **15:** 606–9.

51 Lande MB, Kim MS, Bartlett C et al.: Reversible Fanconi syndrome associated with valproate therapy. *J Pediatr* 1993; **123:** 320–2.

52 Sato Y, Kondo I, Ishida S et al.: Decreased bone mass and increased bone turnover with valproate therapy in adults with epilepsy. *Neurology* 2001; **14:** 445–9.

53 Isojarvi J: Disorders of reproduction in patients with epilepsy: antiepileptic drug related mechanisms. *Seizure* 2008; **17:** 111–19.

54 Isojarvi JI, Laatikainen TJ, Pakarinen AJ et al.: Polycystic ovaries and hyperandrogenism in women taking valproate for epilepsy. *N Engl J Med* 1993; **329:** 1383–8.

55 Isojarvi JI, Tauboll E, Herzog AG: Effect of antiepileptic drugs on reproductive endocrine function in individuals with epilepsy. *CNS Drugs* 2005; **19:** 207–23.

56 Morrell MJ, Hayes FJ, Sluss PM et al.: Hyperandrogenism, ovulatory dysfunction, and polycystic ovary syndrome with valproate versus lamotrigine. *Ann Neurol* 2008; **64:** 200–11.

57 Robert E, Guibaud P: Maternal valproic acid and congenital neural tube defects. *Lancet* 1982; **2:** 937.

58 Robert E, Robert JM, Lapras C: Is valproic acid teratogenic? *Rev Neurol (Paris)* 1983; **139:** 445–7.

59 Bjerkedal T, Czeizel A, Goujard J et al.: Valproic acid and spina bifida. *Lancet* 1982; **2:** 1096.

60 Lindhout D, Omtzigt JG, Cornel MC: Spectrum of neural-tube defects in 34 infants prenatally exposed to antiepileptic drugs. *Neurology* **42**(4 Suppl 5): 1992; 111–18.

61 Wyszynski DF, Nambisan M, Surve T et al.: Increased rate of major malformations in offspring exposed to valproate during pregnancy. *Neurology* 2005; **64:** 961–5.

62 Diav-Citrin O, Shechtman S, Bar-Oz B et al.: Pregnancy outcome after in utero exposure to valproate : evidence of dose relationship in teratogenic effect. *CNS Drugs* 2008; **22**: 325–34.

63 Langer B, Haddad J, Gasser B et al.: Isolated fetal bilateral radial ray reduction associated with valproic acid usage. *Fetal Diagn Ther* 1994; **9**: 155–8.

64 Okada T, Tomoda T, Hisakawa H et al.: Valproate syndrome with reduction deformity of limb. *Acta Paediatr Jpn* 1995; **37**: 58–60.

65 Yerby MS: Management issues for women with epilepsy: neural tube defects and folic acid supplementation. *Neurology* 2003; **61**(6 Suppl 2): S23–6.

66 Pittschieler S, Brezinka C, Jahn B et al.: Spontaneous abortion and the prophylactic effect of folic acid supplementation in epileptic women undergoing antiepileptic therapy. *J Neurol* 2008; **255**: 1926–31.

67 Omtzigt JG, Los FJ, Grobbee DE et al.: The risk of spina bifida aperta after first-trimester exposure to valproate in a prenatal cohort. *Neurology* 1992; **42**(4 Suppl 5): 119–25.

68 Eadie MJ, Vajda FJ: Should valproate be taken during pregnancy? *Ther Clin Risk Manag* 2005; **1**: 21–6.

69 Rasalam AD, Hailey H, Williams JH et al.: Characteristics of fetal anticonvulsant syndrome associated autistic disorder. *Dev Med Child Neurol* 2005; **47**: 551–5.

70 Acharya S, Bussel JB: Hematologic toxicity of sodium valproate. *J Pediatr Hematol Oncol* 2000; **22**: 62–5.

71 Koenig S, Gerstner T, Keller A et al.: High incidence of vaproate-induced coagulation disorders in children receiving valproic acid: a prospective study. *Blood Coagul Fibrinolysis* 2008; **19**: 375–82.

72 Sztajnkrycer MD: Valproic acid toxicity: overview and management. *J Toxicol Clin Toxicol* 2002; **40**: 789–801.

73 Dharnidharka VR, Fennell RS,3rd, Richard GA: Extracorporeal removal of toxic valproic acid levels in children. *Pediatr Nephrol* 2002; **17**: 312–15.

74 Thanacoody RH: Extracorporeal elimination in acute valproic acid poisoning. *Clin Toxicol (Phila)* 2009; **47**: 609–16.

75 Houghton BL, Bowers JB: Valproic acid overdose: a case report and review of therapy. *MedGenMed* 2003; **5**: 5.

76 Alberto G, Erickson T, Popiel R et al.: Central nervous system manifestations of a valproic acid overdose responsive to naloxone. *Ann Emerg Med* 1989; **18**: 889–91.

77 Ballenger JC, Post RM: Therapeutic effects of carbamazepine in affective illness: a preliminary report. *Commun Psychopharmacol* 1978; **2**: 159–75.

78 Albright PS: Effects of carbamazepine, clonazepam, and phenytoin on seizure threshold in amygdala and cortex. *Exp Neurol* 1983; **79**: 11–17.

79 Albright PS, Burnham WM: Effects of phenytoin, carbamazepine, and clonazepam on cortex—and amygdala—evoked potentials. *Exp Neurol* 1983; **81**: 308–19.

80 White HS: Clinical significance of animal seizure models and mechanism of action studies of potential antiepileptic drugs. *Epilepsia* 1997; **38**(Suppl 1): S9–17.

81 Okuma T, Inanaga K, Otsuki S et al.: Comparison of the antimanic efficacy of carbamazepine and chlorpromazine: a double-blind controlled study. *Psychopharmacology (Berl)* 1979; **66**: 211–17.

82 Okuma T, Yamashita I, Takahashi R et al.: Clinical efficacy of carbamazepine in affective, schizoaffective, and schizophrenic disorders. *Pharmacopsychiatry* 1989; **22**: 47–53.

83 Brown D, Silverstone T, Cookson J: Carbamazepine compared to haloperidol in acute mania. *Int Clin Psychopharmacol* 1989; **4**: 229–38.

84 Dilsaver SC, Swann SC, Chen YW et al.: Treatment of bipolar depression with carbamazepine: results of an open study. *Biol Psychiatry* 1996; **40:** 935–7.

85 Davis JM, Janicak PG, Hogan DM: Mood stabilizers in the prevention of recurrent affective disorders: a meta-analysis. *Acta Psychiatr Scand* 1999; **100:** 406–17.

86 Greil W, Kleindienst N, Erazo N et al.: Differential response to lithium and carbamazepine in the prophylaxis of bipolar disorder. *J Clin Psychopharmacol* 1998; **18:** 455–60.

87 Kleindienst N, Greil W: Differential efficacy of lithium and carbamazepine in the prophylaxis of bipolar disorder: results of the MAP study. *Neuropsychobiology* 2000; **42**(Suppl 1): 2–10.

88 Weisler RH, Kalali AH, Ketter TA, SPD417 Study Group: A multicenter, randomized, double-blind, placebo-controlled trial of extended-release carbamazepine capsules as monotherapy for bipolar disorder patients with manic or mixed episodes. *J Clin Psychiatry* 2004; **65:** 478–84.

89 Weisler RH, Keck PE Jr, Swann AC et al.: Extended-release carbamazepine capsules as monotherapy for acute mania in bipolar disorder: a multicenter, randomized, double-blind, placebo-controlled trial. *J Clin Psychiatry* 2005; **66:** 323–30.

90 Woolston JL: Case study: carbamazepine treatment of juvenile-onset bipolar disorder. *J Am Acad Child Adolesc Psychiatry* 1999; **38:** 335–8.

91 Kowatch RA, Suppes T, Carmody TJ et al.: Effect size of lithium, divalproex sodium, and carbamazepine in children and adolescents with bipolar disorder. *J Am Acad Child Adolesc Psychiatry* 2000; **39:** 713–20.

92 Wozniak J, Biederman J, Richards JA: Diagnostic and therapeutic dilemmas in the management of pediatric-onset bipolar disorder. *J Clin Psychiatry* 2001; **62**(Suppl 14): 10–15.

93 Joshi G, Wozniak J, Mick E et al.: A prospective open-label trial of extended-release carbamazepine monotherapy in children with bipolar disorder. *J Child Adolesc Psychopharmacol* 2010; **20:** 7–14.

94 Remschmidt H: Recent results of research on juvenile delinquency. *Prax Kinderpsychol Kinderpsychiatr* 1978; **27:** 29–40.

95 Kafantaris V, Campbell M, Padron-Gayol MV et al.: Carbamazepine in hospitalized aggressive conduct disorder children: an open pilot study. *Psychopharmacol Bull* 1992; **28:** 193–9.

96 Cueva JE, Overall JE, Small AM et al.: Carbamazepine in aggressive children with conduct disorder: a double-blind and placebo-controlled study. *J Am Acad Child Adolesc Psychiatry* 1996; **35:** 480–90.

97 Silva RR, Munoz DM, Alpert M: Carbamazepine use in children and adolescents with features of attention-deficit hyperactivity disorder: a meta-analysis. *J Am Acad Child Adolesc Psychiatry* 1996; **35:** 352–8.

98 Mockenhaupt M, Messenheimer J, Tennis P et al.: Risk of Stevens–Johnson syndrome and toxic epidermal necrolysis in new users of antiepileptics. *Neurology* 2005; **64:** 1134–8.

99 Chung WH, Hung SI: Genetic markers and danger signals in Stevens–Johnson syndrome and toxic epidermal necrolysis. *Allergol Int* 2010; **59:** 325–32.

100 Hung SI, Chung WH, Jee SH et al.: Genetic susceptibility to carbamazepine-induced cutaneous adverse drug reactions. *Pharmacogenet Genomics* 2006; **16:** 297–306.

101 Tohen M, Castillo J, Baldessarini RJ et al.: Blood dyscrasias with carbamazepine and valproate: a pharmacoepidemiological study of 2228 patients at risk. *Am J Psychiatry* 1995; **152:** 413–18.

102 Dong X, Leppik IE, White J et al.: Hyponatremia from oxcarbazepine and carbamazepine. *Neurology* 2005; **65:** 1976–8.

103 Isojarvi JI, Turkka J, Pakarinen AJ et al.: Thyroid function in men taking carbamazepine, oxcarbazepine, or valproate for epilepsy. *Epilepsia* 2001; **42:** 930–4.

104 Vainionpaa LK, Mikkonen K, Rattya J et al.: Thyroid function in girls with epilepsy with carbamazepine, oxcarbazepine, or valproate monotherapy and after withdrawal of medication. *Epilepsia* 2004; **45:** 197–203.

105 Banach R, Boskovic R, Einarson T et al.: Long-term developmental outcome of children of women with epilepsy, unexposed or exposed prenatally to antiepileptic drugs: a meta-analysis of cohort studies. *Drug Saf* 2010; **33:** 73–9.

106 Tomson T, Battino D: Teratogenic effects of antiepileptic medications. *Neurol Clin* 2009; **27:** 993–1002.

107 Graudins A, Peden G, Dowsett RP: Massive overdose with controlled-release carbamazepine resulting in delayed peak serum concentrations and life-threatening toxicity. *Emerg Med (Fremantle)* 2002; **14:** 89–94.

108 Winnicka RI, Topacinski B, Szymczak WM et al.: Carbamazepine poisoning: elimination kinetics and quantitative relationship with carbamazepine 10,11-epoxide. *J Toxicol Clin Toxicol* 2002; **40:** 759–65.

109 Seymour JF: Carbamazepine overdose. Features of 33 cases. *Drug Saf* 1993; **8:** 81–8.

110 Stremski ES, Brady WB, Prasad K et al.: Pediatric carbamazepine intoxication. *Ann Emerg Med* 1995; **25:** 624–30.

111 Huang CW, Huang CC, Lin MW et al.: The synergistic inhibitory actions of oxcarbazepine on voltage-gated sodium and potassium currents in differentiated NG108-15 neuronal cells and model neurons. *Int J Neuropsychopharmacol* 2008; **11:** 597–610.

112 Simao F, Zamin LL, Frozza R et al.: Protective profile of oxcarbazepine against oxygen-glucose deprivation in organotypic hippocampal slice culture could involve PI3K cell signaling pathway. *Neurol Res* 2009; **31:** 1044–8.

113 Stefani A, Pisani A, De Murtas M et al.: Action of GP 47779, the active metabolite of oxcarbazepine, on the corticostriatal system. II. Modulation of high-voltage-activated calcium currents. *Epilepsia* 1995; **36:** 997–1002.

114 Emrich HM, Gunther R, Dose M: Current perspectives in the pharmacopsychiatry of depression and mania. *Neuropharmacology* 1983; **22:** 385–8.

115 Emrich HM, Altmann H, Dose M et al.: Therapeutic effects of GABA-ergic drugs in affective disorders. A preliminary report. *Pharmacol Biochem Behav* 1983; **19:** 369–72.

116 Emrich HM, Dose M, von Zerssen D: The use of sodium valproate, carbamazepine and oxcarbazepine in patients with affective disorders. *J Affect Disord* 1985; **8:** 243–50.

117 Hummel B, Walden J, Stampfer R et al.: Acute antimanic efficacy and safety of oxcarbazepine in an open trial with an on-off-on design. *Bipolar Disord* 2002; **4:** 412–17.

118 Muller M, Marson AG, Williamson PR: Oxcarbazepine versus phenytoin monotherapy for epilepsy. *Cochrane Database Syst Rev* 19 April, 2006 (2): CD003615.

119 Suppes T, Kelly DI, Hynan LS et al.: Comparison of two anticonvulsants in a randomized, single-blind treatment of hypomanic symptoms in patients with bipolar disorder. *Aust N Z J Psychiatry* 2007; **41:** 397–402.

120 Kakkar AK, Rehan HS, Unni KE et al.: Comparative efficacy and safety of oxcarbazepine versus divalproex sodium in the treatment of acute mania: a pilot study. *Eur Psychiatry* 2009; **24:** 178–82.

121 Vasudev A, Macritchie K, Watson S et al.: Oxcarbazepine in the maintenance treatment of bipolar disorder. *Cochrane Database Syst Rev* 23 January, 2008 (1): CD005171.

122 Mosolov SN, Kostiukova EG, Ladyzhenskii MI: Comparative efficacy and tolerability of carbamazepine and oxcarbazepine during long therapy of patients with bipolar and schizoaffective disorders. *Zh Nevrol Psikhiatr Im S S Korsakova* 2009; **109**: 36–41.

123 Salpekar JA, Conry JA, Doss W et al.: Clinical experience with anticonvulsant medication in pediatric epilepsy and comorbid bipolar spectrum disorder. *Epilepsy Behav* 2006; **9**: 327–34.

124 MacMillan CM, Korndorfer SR, Rao S et al.: A comparison of divalproex and oxcarbazepine in aggressive youth with bipolar disorder. *J Psychiatr Pract* 2006; **12**: 214–22.

125 Wagner KD, Kowatch RA, Emslie GJ et al.: A double-blind, randomized, placebo-controlled trial of oxcarbazepine in the treatment of bipolar disorder in children and adolescents. *Am J Psychiatry* 2006; **163**: 1179–86.

126 Glauser T, Ben-Menachem E, Bourgeois B et al.: ILAE treatment guidelines: evidence-based analysis of antiepileptic drug efficacy and effectiveness as initial monotherapy for epileptic seizures and syndromes. *Epilepsia* 2006; **47**: 1094–120.

127 Chung AM, Eiland LS: Use of second-generation antiepileptic drugs in the pediatric population. *Paediatr Drugs* 2008; **10**: 217–54.

128 Dong X, Leppik IE, White J et al.: Hyponatremia from oxcarbazepine and carbamazepine. *Neurology* 2005; **65**: 1976–8.

129 Leppik IE: Three new drugs for epilepsy: levetiracetam, oxcarbazepine, and zonisamide. *J Child Neurol* 2002; **17**(Suppl 1): S53–57.

130 Paliwal V, Garg RK, Kar AM et al.: Oxcarbazepine induced hyponatremic coma. *Neurol India* 2006; **54**: 214–15.

131 Lautz TB, Finegold MJ, Chin AC et al.: Giant hepatic adenoma with atypical features in a patient on oxcarbazepine therapy. *J Pediatr Surg* 2008; **43**: 751–4.

132 Okuyucu EE, Duman T, Akcin E: Reversible parkinsonism with oxcarbazepine use. *Parkinsonism Relat Disord* 2009; **15**: 787–8.

133 Lin CH, Lu CH, Wang FJ et al.: Risk factors of oxcarbazepine-induced hyponatremia in patients with epilepsy. *Clin Neuropharmacol* 2010; **33**: 293–6.

134 Milia A, Pilia G, Mascia MG et al.: Oxcarbazepine-induced leukopenia. *J Neuropsychiatry Clin Neurosci* 2008; **20**: 502–3.

135 Mahmud J, Mathews M, Verma S et al.: Oxcarbazepine-induced thrombocytopenia. *Psychosomatics* 2006; **47**: 73–4.

136 Montouris G: Safety of the newer antiepileptic drug oxcarbazepine during pregnancy. *Curr Med Res Opin* 2005; **21**: 693–701.

137 van Opstal JM, Janknegt R, Cilissen J et al.: Severe overdosage with the antiepileptic drug oxcarbazepine. *Br J Clin Pharmacol* 2004; **58**: 329–31.

138 Barker MJ, Benitez JG, Ternullo S et al.: Acute oxcarbazepine and atomoxetine overdose with quetiapine. *Vet Hum Toxicol* 2004; **46**: 130–2.

139 Furlanut M, Franceschi L, Poz D et al.: Acute oxcarbazepine, benazepril, and hydrochlorothiazide overdose with alcohol. *Ther Drug Monit* 2006; **28**: 267–8.

140 Raja M, Azzoni A: Oxcarbazepine, risperidone and atenolol overdose with benign outcome. *Int J Neuropsychopharmacol* 2003; **6**: 309–10.

141 Pedrini M, Noguera A, Vinent J et al.: Acute oxcarbazepine overdose in an autistic boy. *Br J Clin Pharmacol* 2009; **67**: 579–81.

142 Goa KL, Ross SR, Chrisp P: Lamotrigine. A review of its pharmacological properties and clinical efficacy in epilepsy. *Drugs* 1993; **46**: 152–76.

143 Xie X, Hagan RM: Cellular and molecular actions of lamotrigine: Possible mechanisms of efficacy in bipolar disorder. *Neuropsychobiology* 1998; **38**: 119–30.

144 Bourin M, Masse F, Hascoet M: Evidence for the activity of lamotrigine at 5-HT(1A) receptors in the mouse forced swimming test. *J Psychiatry Neurosci* 2005; **30**: 275–82.

145 Chang KD, Wagner C, Garrett A et al.: A preliminary functional magnetic resonance imaging study of prefrontal-amygdalar activation changes in adolescents with bipolar depression treated with lamotrigine. *Bipolar Disord* 2008; **10**: 426–31.

146 Chang K, Saxena K, Howe M: An open-label study of lamotrigine adjunct or monotherapy for the treatment of adolescents with bipolar depression. *J Am Acad Child Adolesc Psychiatry* 2006; **45**: 298–304.

147 Pavuluri MN, Passarotti AM, Harral EM et al.: Enhanced prefrontal function with pharmacotherapy on a response inhibition task in adolescent bipolar disorder. *J Clin Psychiatry* 2010; **71**: 1526–34.

148 Calabrese JR, Bowden CL, McElroy SL et al.: Spectrum of activity of lamotrigine in treatment-refractory bipolar disorder. *Am J Psychiatry* 1999; **156**: 1019–23.

149 Berk M: Lamotrigine and the treatment of mania in bipolar disorder. *Eur Neuropsychopharmacol* 1999; **9**(Suppl 4): S119–23.

150 Yatham LN, Kusumakar V, Calabrese JR et al.: Third generation anticonvulsants in bipolar disorder: a review of efficacy and summary of clinical recommendations. *J Clin Psychiatry* 2002; **63**: 275–83.

151 Biederman J, Joshi G, Mick E et al.: A prospective open-label trial of lamotrigine monotherapy in children and adolescents with bipolar disorder. *CNS Neurosci Ther* 2010; **16**: 91–102.

152 Geddes JR, Calabrese JR, Goodwin GM: Lamotrigine for treatment of bipolar depression: independent meta-analysis and meta-regression of individual patient data from five randomised trials. *Br J Psychiatry* 2009; **194**: 4–9.

153 Carandang C, Robbins D, Mullany E et al.: Lamotrigine in adolescent mood disorders: a retrospective chart review. *J Can Acad Child Adolesc Psychiatry* 2007; **16**: 1–8.

154 McElroy SL, Zarate CA, Cookson J et al.: A 52-week, open-label continuation study of lamotrigine in the treatment of bipolar depression. *J Clin Psychiatry* 2004; **65**: 204–10.

155 Calabrese JR, Bowden CL, Sachs GS et al.: A double-blind placebo-controlled study of lamotrigine monotherapy in outpatients with bipolar I depression. Lamictal 602 Study Group. *J Clin Psychiatry* 1999; **60**: 79–88.

156 Calabrese JR, Bowden CL, Sachs G et al.: A placebo-controlled 18-month trial of lamotrigine and lithium maintenance treatment in recently depressed patients with bipolar I disorder. *J Clin Psychiatry* 2003; **64**: 1013–24.

157 Bowden CL, Calabrese JR, Sachs G et al.: A placebo-controlled 18-month trial of lamotrigine and lithium maintenance treatment in recently manic or hypomanic patients with bipolar I disorder. *Arch Gen Psychiatry* 2003; **60**: 392–400.

158 Goodwin GM, Bowden CL, Calabrese JR et al.: A pooled analysis of 2 placebo-controlled 18-month trials of lamotrigine and lithium maintenance in bipolar I disorder. *J Clin Psychiatry* 2004; **65**: 432–41.

159 Goldberg JF, Calabrese JR, Saville BR et al.: Mood stabilization and destabilization during acute and continuation phase treatment for bipolar I disorder with lamotrigine or placebo. *J Clin Psychiatry* 2009; **70**: 1273–80.

160 Pavuluri MN, Henry DB, Moss M et al.: Effectiveness of lamotrigine in maintaining symptom control in pediatric bipolar disorder. *J Child Adolesc Psychopharmacol* 2009; **19**: 75–82.

161 Goldsmith DR, Wagstaff AJ, Ibbotson T et al.: Spotlight on lamotrigine in bipolar disorder. *CNS Drugs* 2004; **18**: 63–7.

162 Bialer M: The pharmacokinetics and interactions of new antiepileptic drugs: an overview. *Ther Drug Monit* 2005; **27**: 722–6.

163 Hahn CG, Gyulai L, Baldassano CF et al.: The current understanding of lamotrigine as a mood stabilizer. *J Clin Psychiatry* 2004; **65**: 791–804.

164 Reimers A, Helde G, Brodtkorb E: Ethinyl estradiol, not progestogens, reduces lamotrigine serum concentrations. *Epilepsia* 2005; **46**: 1414–17.

165 Messenheimer J, Mullens EL, Giorgi L et al.: Safety review of adult clinical trial experience with lamotrigine. *Drug Saf* 1998; **18**: 281–96.

166 Chung AM, Eiland LS: Use of second-generation antiepileptic drugs in the pediatric population. *Paediatr Drugs* 2008; **10**: 217–54.

167 Bowden CL, Asnis GM, Ginsberg LD et al.: Safety and tolerability of lamotrigine for bipolar disorder. *Drug Saf* 2004; **27**: 173–84.

168 Lam GM, Edelson DP, Whelan CT: Lamotrigine: an unusual etiology for aseptic meningitis. *Neurologist* 2010; **16**: 35–6.

169 Huber B, Hilgemann C: Hallucinosis using lamotrigine. *Nervenarzt* 2009; **80**: 202–3.

170 Brandt C, Fueratsch N, Boehme V et al.: Development of psychosis in patients with epilepsy treated with lamotrigine: report of six cases and review of the literature. *Epilepsy Behav* 2007; **11**: 133–9.

171 Zaatreh M, Tennison M, D'Cruz O et al.: Anticonvulsants-induced chorea: a role for pharmacodynamic drug interaction? *Seizure* 2001; **10**: 596–9.

172 Alkin T, Onur E, Ozerdem A: Co-occurence of blepharospasm, tourettism and obsessive-compulsive symptoms during lamotrigine treatment. *Prog Neuropsychopharmacol Biol Psychiatry* 2007; **31**: 1339–40.

173 Ouellet G, Tremblay L, Marleau D: Fulminant hepatitis induced by lamotrigine. *South Med J* 2009; **102**: 82–4.

174 Amante MF, Filippini AV, Cejas N et al.: Dress syndrome and fulminant hepatic failure induced by lamotrigine. *Ann Hepatol* 2009; **8**: 75–7.

175 Hirsch LJ, Weintraub DB, Buchsbaum R et al.: Predictors of Lamotrigine-associated rash. *Epilepsia* 2006; **47**: 318–22.

176 Guberman AH, Besag FM, Brodie MJ et al.: Lamotrigine-associated rash: risk/benefit considerations in adults and children. *Epilepsia* 1999; **40**: 985–91.

177 Calabrese JR, Sullivan JR, Bowden CL et al.: Rash in multicenter trials of lamotrigine in mood disorders: clinical relevance and management. *J Clin Psychiatry* 2002; **63**: 1012–19.

178 Lorberg B, Youssef NA, Bhagwagar Z: Lamotrigine-associated rash: to rechallenge or not to rechallenge? *Int J Neuropsychopharmacol* 2009; **12**: 257–65.

179 Ketter TA, Greist JH, Graham JA et al.: The effect of dermatologic precautions on the incidence of rash with addition of lamotrigine in the treatment of bipolar I disorder: a randomized trial. *J Clin Psychiatry* 2006; **67**: 400–6.

180 Lofton AL, Klein-Schwartz W: Evaluation of lamotrigine toxicity reported to poison centers. *Ann Pharmacother* 2004; **38**: 1811–15.

181 Thundiyil JG, Anderson IB, Stewart PJ et al.: Lamotrigine-induced seizures in a child: case report and literature review. *Clin Toxicol (Phila)* 2007; **45**: 169–72.

182 Briassoulis G, Kalabalikis P, Tamiolaki M et al.: Lamotrigine childhood overdose. *Pediatr Neurol* 1998; **19**: 239–42.

183 Taylor CP: Emerging perspectives on the mechanism of action of gabapentin. *Neurology* 1994; **44**(6 Suppl 5): S10-6; discussion S31–2.

184 Loscher W, Honack D, Taylor CP: Gabapentin increases aminooxyacetic acid-induced GABA accumulation in several regions of rat brain. *Neurosci Lett* 1991; **128:** 150–4.

185 Maneuf YP, Luo ZD, Lee K: Alpha2delta and the Mechanism of Action of Gabapentin in the Treatment of Pain. *Semin Cell Dev Biol* 2006; **17:** 565–70.

186 Sills GJ: The mechanisms of action of gabapentin and pregabalin. *Curr Opin Pharmacol* 2006; **6:** 108–13.

187 Frye MA, Ketter TA, Kimbrell TA et al.: A placebo-controlled study of lamotrigine and gabapentin monotherapy in refractory mood disorders. *J Clin Psychopharmacol* 2000; **20:** 607–14.

188 Pande AC, Crockatt JG, Janney CA et al.: Gabapentin in bipolar disorder: a placebo-controlled trial of adjunctive therapy. Gabapentin Bipolar Disorder Study Group. *Bipolar Disord* 2000; **2:** 249–55.

189 Pande AC, Pollack MH, Crockatt J et al.: Placebo-controlled study of gabapentin treatment of panic disorder. *J Clin Psychopharmacol* 2000; **20:** 467–71.

190 Pande AC, Davidson JR, Jefferson JW et al.: Treatment of social phobia with gabapentin: a placebo-controlled study. *J Clin Psychopharmacol* 1999; **19:** 341–8.

191 McManaman J, Tam DA: Gabapentin for self-injurious behavior in Lesch-Nyhan syndrome. *Pediatr Neurol* 1999; **20:** 381–2.

192 Lee DO, Steingard RJ, Cesena M et al.: Behavioral side effects of gabapentin in children. *Epilepsia* 1996; **37:** 87–90.

193 Shank RP, Gardocki JF, Streeter AJ et al.: An overview of the preclinical aspects of topiramate: pharmacology, pharmacokinetics, and mechanism of action. *Epilepsia* 2000; **41**(Suppl 1): S3–9.

194 Kushner SF, Khan A, Lane R, Olson WH: Topiramate monotherapy in the management of acute mania: results of four double-blind placebo-controlled trials. *Bipolar Disord* 2006; **8:** 15–27.

195 Chengappa KN, Rathore D, Levine J: et al. Topiramate as add-on treatment for patients with bipolar mania. *Bipolar Disord* 1999; **1:** 42–53.

196 Delbello MP, Findling RL, Kushner S et al.: A pilot controlled trial of topiramate for mania in children and adolescents with bipolar disorder. *J Am Acad Child Adolesc Psychiatry* 2005; **44:** 539–47.

197 Guille C, Sachs G: Clinical outcome of adjunctive topiramate treatment in a sample of refractory bipolar patients with comorbid conditions. Prog Neuropsychopharmacol *Biol Psychiatry* 2002; **26:** 1035–9.

198 Shapira NA, Goldsmith TD, McElroy SL: Treatment of binge-eating disorder with topiramate: a clinical case series. *J Clin Psychiatry* 2000; **61:** 368–72.

199 Hedges DW, Reimherr FW, Hoopes SP et al.: Treatment of bulimia nervosa with topiramate in a randomized, double-blind, placebo-controlled trial, part 2: improvement in psychiatric measures. *J Clin Psychiatry* 2003; **64:** 1449–54.

200 Hoopes SP, Reimherr FW, Hedges DW et al.: Treatment of bulimia nervosa with topiramate in a randomized, double-blind, placebo-controlled trial, part 1: improvement in binge and purge measures. *J Clin Psychiatry* 2003; **64:** 1335–41.

201 Nickel C, Tritt K, Muehlbacher M et al.: Topiramate treatment in bulimia nervosa patients: a randomized, double-blind, placebo-controlled trial. *Int J Eat Disord* 2005; **38:** 295–300.

202 McElroy SL, Arnold LM, Shapira NA et al.: Topiramate in the treatment of binge eating disorder associated with obesity: a randomized, placebo-controlled trial. *Am J Psychiatry* 2003; **160:** 255–61.

203 McElroy SL, Hudson JI, Capece JA et al.: Topiramate for the treatment of binge eating disorder associated with obesity: a placebo-controlled study. *Biol Psychiatry* 2007; **61**: 1039–48.

204 Claudino AM, de Oliveira IR, Appolinario JC et al.: Double-blind, randomized, placebo-controlled trial of topiramate plus cognitive-behavior therapy in binge-eating disorder. *J Clin Psychiatry* 2007; **68**: 1324–32.

205 Ko YH, Joe SH, Jung IK et al.: Topiramate as an adjuvant treatment with atypical antipsychotics in schizophrenic patients experiencing weight gain. *Clin Neuropharmacol* 2005; **28**: 169–75.

206 Egger C, Muehlbacher M, Schatz M et al.: Influence of topiramate on olanzapine-related weight gain in women: an 18-month follow-up observation. *J Clin Psychopharmacol* 2007; **27**: 475–78.

CHAPTER 13

Anxiolytics

Barbara J. Coffey[1] & Amanda L. Zwilling[2]

[1] New York University Langone School of Medicine and Nathan Kline Institute
for Psychiatric Research, New York, USA
[2] New York University Langone School of Medicine, New York, USA

Anxiolytic and sedative-hypnotic agents are frequently prescribed in medical and psychiatric practice. Although the current standard of clinical care is to use the selective serotonin reuptake inhibitors for treatment of childhood onset anxiety disorders, other anxiolytics, including the benzodiazepines, antihistamines and azapirones, are also used to treat anxiety and sleep disorders in youth, and will be reviewed in this chapter.

Chemical properties

Benzodiazepines

Mechanism of action

Benzodiazepine receptors appear to be part of membrane complexes involving chloride channels and gamma amino butyric acid (GABA) receptors, the principal inhibitory neurotransmitter in the brain. At these sites, benzodiazepines bind to large protein complexes located on the receptor, and facilitate GABA-A transmission, leading to increased chloride conductance and increased inhibition of the central nervous system (CNS). Benzodiazepines have also been found to reduce serotonin turnover and activity [1,2], to decrease the spontaneous firing of noradrenergic neurons in the locus coeruleus [3], and to decrease dopaminergic function [4].

Benzodiazepines have diffuse inhibitory effects on the central nervous system. The benzodiazepine receptors appear to have their highest density in the limbic system; however, they are also found in the cerebral cortex, hippocampus, and the substantia nigra. It is thought that impact upon specific areas of the brain determine the clinical effect; cortical and limbic effects produce reduction in anxiety, striatal effects are associated with anticonvulsant actions, and spinal cord effects result in muscle relaxation.

Pharmacotherapy of Child and Adolescent Psychiatric Disorders, Third Edition.
Edited by David R. Rosenberg and Samuel Gershon.
© 2012 John Wiley & Sons, Ltd. Published 2012 by John Wiley & Sons, Ltd.

Diffuse inhibitory effects of benzodiazepines are also mediated through inhibition of polysynaptic reflexes at the spinal cord. Benzodiazepines can cause mild decreases in respiration, and, in animals, may slightly reduce blood pressure and left ventricular function.

There are numerous studies of the effects of benzodiazepines on animal behavior. In conflict-producing procedures, benzodiazepines greatly reduce the behavior-suppressing effects of punishment in animals—an effect that has been hypothesized to parallel the alleviation of behavioral results of conflict in humans [5].

The facilitation of GABAergic transmission and inhibition of CNS functions is believed to produce directly the anxiolytic, sedative, hypnotic, anticonvulsant, and muscle-relaxant properties. Tics and behavior disorders might improve indirectly, in response to the decrease in anxiety.

Absorption and metabolism

Disposition of the various benzodiazepines have been extensively studied in adults, and provides a basis for understanding certain effects of this class of drugs in adolescents and children.

Absorption in adults is highly variable, but is generally slow after oral administration for most benzodiazepine compounds, except diazepam. Peak concentrations are usually reached within several hours, and in about 1 hour for diazepam. Most agents are highly bound to plasma proteins (85–98%). The apparent volumes of distribution are relatively high (1–3 L/kg). Elimination and distribution phase kinetics are complicated and depend on the route of administration. Most studies indicate a half-life in the range of 20–50 h for benzodiazepines, though one of diazepam's primary metabolic products (desmethyldiazepam) appears to have a half-life of 51–120 h.

The benzodiazepines are generally converted to active metabolic products by hepatic microsomal enzymes. The parent compounds and certain products are metabolically active. Hydroxylation and demethylation are the two primary metabolic processes involved in the biotransformation of these drugs. Most of the benzodiazepines are excreted as glucuronide or sulfate conjugates, whose higher water solubility permits excretion.

Experimental data on the pharmacokinetics of benzodiazepines in children are rather limited, and even more limited in adolescents. The few studies that compare the metabolic capacity of children and adults indicate an increased ability to metabolize and eliminate diazepam in children, consistent with the typical findings of faster hepatic biotransformation and renal clearance in children [6]. There are essentially no data in adolescents, but the usual developmental pharmacokinetic principles would suggest that adolescents probably have slower metabolism and clearance than younger children, and that adult pharmacokinetic patterns are attained by late adolescence.

Interestingly, there is more data on benzodiazepine metabolism in infants, based on maternal usage during pregnancy. Maternal metabolism and the role of maternal-fetal transfer can be complicating factors but it appears that newborn and premature infants have a limited capacity for metabolism and elimination of diazepam. Compared with older children and adults, infants show longer half-lives of parent compounds and lower rates of drug biotransformation, particularly in glucuronide conjugation [7].

Therapeutic blood levels have not been established in children, adolescents, or adults. A study of alprazolam in the treatment of panic disorder in adults indicates that an average serum level of 6 ng/ml correlates with a 100% blockage of panic attacks [8].

Antihistamines

Many antihistamines are available, and are used to treat a wide variety of medical problems including allergic and dermatological reactions, motion sickness, vertigo, nausea and vomiting, coughing, parkinsonism and drug-induced extrapyramidal symptoms, among others. However, for the treatment of anxiety, agitation and behavioral problems in children and adolescents, the two most commonly used antihistamines are diphenhydramine and hydroxyzine.

Mechanism of action

Diphenhydramine is an ethanolamine derivative with two attached benzene rings, but other antihistamines have alkylamine (chlorpheniramine), piperazine (cyproheptadine), phenothiazine (promethazine), or butyrophenone (terfenadine) structures. Hydroxyzine is a diethylenediamine derivative. The mechanism of action of antihistamines in the CNS is not known. There are histamine-releasing neurons in the brain (especially the cerebral cortex), and H1 histamine receptor blockers can depress, and at times, stimulate CNS functions. These agents also block muscarinic acetylcholine receptors, and some actions result from the anticholinergic effects.

The anti-motion-sickness properties are probably mediated by a central blockade of muscarinic acetylcholine receptors in the vestibular cerebellar midbrain vomiting center and medullary chemoreceptive trigger zone. There is no clear correlation between peripheral and central histamine blocking activity.

Absorption and metabolism

In general, antihistamines are well absorbed and reach maximum concentration between 1 and 4 hours after ingestion. In adults, oral diphenhydramine reaches peak plasma concentration at 2 hours, is widely distributed throughout the body, is 98–99% protein bound, and has a plasma elimination half-life of 1–4 h. Breakdown products are excreted unchanged in the urine. Most antihistamines are metabolized in the liver by the P450 cytochrome enzyme system.

There are very few studies of pharmacokinetics in children. One study of diphenhydramine in a group of seven children (mean age 8.9 ± 1.7 years) reported that after a single dose of diphenhydramine, (1.25 mg/kg in mean doses of 39.5 ± 8.4 mg,) the mean serum elimination half-life was 5.4 ± 1.8 hours. Clearance rate was 49.2 ± 22.8 mL/min/kg [9]. For hydrox-yzine, at a dose of 0.7 mg/kg, in 12 children (mean age 6.1± 4.6,) mean serum half-life was 7.1 ± 2.3 hours and time to peak plasma concentration was 2.0 ± 0.9 h [10].

Another study of a single 5 mg dose of levocetirizine, the active enan-tiomer of cetirizine, in 14 children, ages 6–11 years, (mean age 8.6 ± 0.4 years) reported peak serum concentration of 450 + 37 ng/ml 1.2 ± 0.2 hours after ingestion. Terminal elimination half-life was 5.7 ± 0.2 hours; oral clearance was 0.83 ± 0.05 mL/min/kg, and volume of distribution was 0.4 ± 0.02 L/kg [11].

Buspirone

Buspirone is a more recently introduced anxiolytic agent that is generally reported to be associated with less sedation than the benzodiazepines, and has less potential for risk of abuse or physical dependence. In early studies, buspirone was reported to have neuroleptic effects in animals, and was subsequently thought to have antipsychotic properties. However, even in very high doses (up to 2400 mg/day) in patients with schizophrenia, buspirone was not effective. Additional, older clinical trials demonstrated anxiolytic efficacy similar to diazepam. Since then, studies have reported buspirone's unique "anxioselective" properties, in that it did not induce hypomotility and ataxia characteristic of diazepam [12]. Buspirone's ability to produce an anti-anxiety effect with relatively less sedation demonstrates that anxiety reduction can be achieved with fewer seda-tive side-effects that impair cognition and performance. However, there is a limited scientific evidence base for buspirone's utility in treatment of childhood onset anxiety disorders.

Mechanism of action

Buspirone, an azaspirodecanedione, has a novel structure. It is not a derivative of benzodiazepines, barbiturates, or neuroleptics.

The mechanism of action of buspirone is not well defined, but the anti-anxiety effect appears to be pharmacologically unique because it has fewer sedative properties than other anxiolytics. Buspirone binds to central sero-tonin (5HT1A) and dopamine (D2) receptors. Unlike benzodiazepines, it does not interact with benzodiazepine receptors, influence GABA binding, or have anticonvulsant or muscle relaxation properties, and does not impair tests of psychomotor or cognitive skills. In contrast to other anxiolytics, buspirone increases rather than decreases the basal firing rate of noradrenergic neurons in the locus coeruleus.

Absorption and metabolism

In healthy adult volunteers, buspirone is completely and rapidly absorbed, does not show reduced bioavailability when ingested with food, and undergoes extensive first-pass hepatic removal. Buspirone is highly protein bound (95%), reaches peak plasma levels at 60 to 90 minutes, and shows a mean elimination half-life of 2–3 h [13]. There are no active metabolites. Hepatic and renal clearance in adolescents, and especially in children, is expected to be faster than in adults.

In a 21-day open label multisite dose escalation study, which included 13 children and 12 adolescents, buspirone was rapidly absorbed, reaching peak plasma level at about one hour after ingestion. Peak plasma concentration was highest in children (1.96 ng/ml at 15 mg) and higher than in adults (0.93) and adolescents (1.44 ng/m). Buspirone is metabolized into 1-pyrimidinylpiperazine, and mean plasma concentration was also higher in children (13.13 at 15 mg) and adolescents (7.83) than adults (6.62). Mean half-life was 3.13 h at 15 mg in children, 3.44 h in adolescents and 3.5 h in adults [14].

Indications

Anxiety disorders are highly prevalent in youth; between 6 and 20% of children meet lifetime criteria for at least one anxiety disorder [15]. Anxiety disorders may become chronic, and may be predictive of other psychiatric disorders in adolescence or young adulthood, including major depression, substance abuse and suicidal behavior [16]. In a recent review, Witek et al. [17] reported that over the previous decade, benzodiazepine use in the pediatric population had nearly tripled. Nevertheless, the number of controlled studies of benzodiazepines in children and adolescents remains small. Early studies were often characterized by methodological problems, such as very small sample size, mixed anxiety disorders and inclusion of children with depression, and inadequate dosing [18]. Although rates of use in adults are thought to be around 25–30%, Zito et al. [19] report rates of use in pediatric samples up to about 6%. There is currently no established psychiatric indication for the use of benzodiazepines in children and adolescents, although they have been prescribed for treatment of anxiety, sleep disorders, psychosis and aggressive behavior [20,21].

Antihistamines are frequently prescribed in pediatric practice. Established indications for antihistamines include sleep induction, preoperative sedation, allergic pruritus, motion sickness, agitation, and drug-induced extrapyramidal reactions in adults and adolescents. Probable indications include anxiety, insomnia in children and adolescents, drug-induced extrapyramidal reactions in children, and emergency management of impulsivity, agitation, and anxiety (PRN use) in children. Antihistamines have also been used conjecturally in the treatment of behavior disorders in children and adolescents.

The established indication for use of buspirone in adults is generalized anxiety disorder (GAD). There are no established uses of buspirone for children or adolescents, although generalized anxiety disorder and other anxiety disorders may be expected to respond.

Anxiety disorders

Generalized anxiety disorder

In recent years, there has been increased recognition that generalized anxiety disorder (GAD), formerly described as overanxious disorder in DSM-III, is a severe, highly prevalent and often chronically disabling illness. Lifetime prevalence was reported to be 3.7% in epidemiologic catchment area studies of 5596 nonreferred adolescents 14 to 17 years of age [22], 2.4% in 1869 12-to-16 year old children [23], and nearly 3% for 792 children 11 years of age [24]. Keller et al. [25] reported that the median age of onset of GAD was 10 years of age in children. In a study of 300 children, ages 7 to 11 years, in a pediatric primary care setting, the prevalence of anxiety disorders was greater than 15%; the most common disorders were simple phobia, separation anxiety disorder and GAD [26].

Simeon and Ferguson [27] conducted a single-blind trial of alprazolam in 12 children with overanxious disorder (now GAD), and reported at least moderate improvement in seven (58%). Simeon et al. [28] went on to conduct a four-week, double-blind, placebo-controlled study of alprazolam in 30 children and adolescents with avoidant disorder or overanxious disorder. Mean alprazolam doses were 1.6 mg/day (range 0.5–3.5 mg/day); 88% of patients on alprazolam who completed the study showed improvement in anxiety, as compared to 62% of patients treated with placebo, although these differences were not statistically significant. Virtually all other trials of benzodiazepines in general childhood anxiety have been diagnostically nonspecific.

Buspirone has been reported to be effective for GAD in adults in double-blind comparisons with diazepam, oxazepam, alprazolam, and lorazepam [29–33]. Other azapirone partial 5HT1a agonists not currently available in the United States such as ipsapirone [34] appear to be effective in treating GAD.

There are no controlled studies in children and adolescents. Buspirone is probably used fairly often for children with GAD [35–38]. A single case study described a 13-year-old boy with overanxious disorder, school refusal, and physiological symptoms. A trial of desipramine 125 mg had been beneficial but adverse effects of constipation and tachycardia limited continued use. The patient was subsequently treated with buspirone 5 mg bid [39].

Simeon et al. [40] reported an open trial of buspirone in 15 patients, age 6–14 years, with anxiety disorders; mean maximum daily dose was 19 mg. Design was a two-week placebo washout followed by a four-week open trial. Results indicated that clinical global improvement was marked in three patients, moderate in ten, and minimal in two. Adverse effects were mild and transient, and included nausea, headaches and drowsiness [40]. Using a different diagnostic target, an open trial of buspirone, dose range 15–30 mg/day, was reported in 12 children, ages 6–12, (mean age 8–2 years) with attention deficit hyperactivity disorder; results indicated that all 12 subjects showed significant improvement in hyperactivity, impulsivity, inattention and disruptive behavior over the six-week study period. Adverse effects were minimal [41].

Hydroxyzine, diphenhydramine, and promethazine have been used for nonspecific anxiety symptoms in children, adolescents, and adults but have not been systematically studied. One early controlled study reported decreased physiological and psychological signs of anxiety in a mixed group of adult psychiatric patients after a single intramuscular dose of hydroxyzine [42] but no data were available on children and adolescents. Although anxiety is an approved indication for hydroxyzine, there is no evidence supporting the long-term benefit of antihistamines in the treatment of anxiety disorders. They are often used and may be effective for anticipatory or situational anxiety, such as a child might experience prior to an office procedure, but this, too, has a limited scientific evidence base [21].

Several studies in adults have compared buspirone to diazepam [43], buspirone to diazepam and placebo [32, 33, 44–46], and buspirone to alprazolam and orazepam [30], and have demonstrated comparable effectiveness of buspirone and these benzodiazepines. Diazepam is reported to be more effective in the reduction of somatic symptoms of anxiety, but buspirone is reported to be more effective in reduction of anger and hostility.

Panic disorder

Though panic attacks were at one time considered to occur only in adults, current evidence suggests that they do occur in children. An Australian survey reported that 43% of adolescents experienced at least one episode during their lives [47]. Whereas panic disorder is very uncommon before puberty [48, 49], retrospective investigation of adults with panic disorder suggests that panic disorder frequently has onset in adolescence and young adulthood [50]. Von Korff et al. [51] reported that peak age of onset of panic disorder was age 15 to 19 years. Hayward et al. [52] found 5.3% of 754 sixth-and seventh-grade pubertal girls in the United States had experienced at least one panic attack. Pubertal stage was strongly associated with panic attacks. Panic attack rates of 8% were observed in females who were sexually mature (Tanner Stage 5) but none of sexually immature girls (Tanner Stages 1 or 2) [52]. Bernstein et al. [53] reported that the increased rate of panic attacks associated with increased Tanner Stage was not due to differences in chronologic age, and suggested that sexual hormones could play a significant role in the development of panic attacks.

The prevalence rate of panic disorder in children and adolescents has not been well established [54]. More than half of 194 adult patients with panic disorder were reported to have had childhood anxiety disorders [55]. In addition, adult patients with panic disorder with a history of childhood anxiety disorder had significantly increased rates of comorbid mood disorders. More than 60% of adult patients suffering from panic disorder had two or more anxiety disorders during childhood [21].

The short-term efficacy of benzodiazepines in adult panic disorder is well documented [30, 56–60]. Alprazolam has received FDA approval for the treatment of panic disorder in patients 18 years of age and older. Treatment of childhood onset panic disorder includes case reports of clonazepam [61, 62] and the combination of alprazolam with imipramine [21, 63]. Taken together, there is very little data; although it seems likely that short-term efficacy of benzodiazepines in youth would be similar to that in adults, long-term studies are needed.

Antidepressants, particularly the selective serotonin reuptake inhibitors (SSRIs,) are currently the first-line pharmacotherapy of choice for panic disorder in children and adolescents. However, judicious use of alprazolam or clonazepam may be indicated in panic disorder in youth, as it is in adults [63]. Since the response to benzodiazepines is rapid and response to antidepressants (for example, SSRIs) may be delayed, this combination provides treatment without delay and with minimal risk of dependence or withdrawal symptoms from the benzodiazepine. In adults, benzodiazepine augmentation of antidepressant treatment may accelerate both antidepressant and anxiolytic response. As a result, this combination is often used in children and adolescents despite the lack of controlled studies [21].

Woods et al. [64], in adult patients, compared imipramine alone with combination treatment imipramine and alprazolam; they reported that, although combined treatment produced a more rapid response, it was also associated with intolerance of alprazolam discontinuation. Patients were treated with alprazolam for up to six weeks before attempting to taper, suggesting that if combined treatment is used it should be limited to the first few weeks of treatment. Caution in use of alprazolam is advised in youth with a history of substance abuse or dependence, or a strong family history of substance abuse or dependence.

Buspirone has been studied in adult panic disorder, but the results do not support its efficacy. Controlled trials have reported failed [65] or modestly successful [66] treatment of panic attacks. One case series suggested that it may be an effective adjunct to benzodiazepine treatment [67], but replication is needed. Unless further controlled trials support its use, buspirone is not recommended for childhood onset or adolescent onset panic disorder.

There is no data regarding the use of antihistamines for panic disorder in children and adolescents [21].

Separation anxiety disorder/school refusal

Separation anxiety and school refusal (often described as "school phobia") are closely related as they often coexist. Separation anxiety is a common problem in children and adolescents and has a lifetime prevalence of up to 84% in children diagnosed with any anxiety disorder [68]. Up to 80% of children with school refusal meet criteria for separation anxiety disorder [21, 69].

The evidence base for treatment of separation anxiety disorder is more extensive than other childhood anxiety disorders. Benzodiazepines have been used in several studies. D'Amato [70] reported an open trial of chlordiazepoxide in nine children with school phobia and, eight (89%) showed a good response. Kraft et al. [71] conducted an open trial of chlordiazepoxide with 130 diagnostically heterogeneous children ranging in age from two to 17 years. Of the 18 children with school phobia, ten were reported to be "excellent" responders and four were reported to be "good" responders (78%). Two children's (11%) symptoms worsened. In contrast, 38% of children with a primary behavioral disorder responded and 22% worsened.

Klein and Last [72] reported on a six-week open trial of alprazolam in 18 children, age 7–17 years, with separation anxiety; parents and clinicians reported an 80% improvement. In a study of 18 children and adolescents with separation anxiety disorder treated with clonazepam (0.5–0.6 mg/day), 64% were considered improved by their teachers, 65% by self-report, 82% by parents and 89% by their psychiatrists [72]. An eight-week double-blind, placebo-controlled study of alprazolam (mean dose 1.6 mg daily (range 0.5–3.5 mg/day) vs. imipramine in 24 children, ages 7–16, with school refusal and mixed depression and anxiety disorders, reported a trend toward improvement, but no statistically significant benefit [73]. These children were reported to have no significant improvement on imipramine. Graee et al. [74] conducted a double-blind, placebo-controlled crossover study of clonazepam in 15 children, ages seven to 13, with anxiety disorders, primarily separation anxiety disorder. Patients were treated with four weeks of clonazepam (0.5–2 mg/day) and four weeks of placebo. There was no significant difference observed between clonazepam and placebo treatment. However, notably, 50% of the subjects no longer met criteria for an anxiety disorder at the study conclusion [74].

The open trials, which reported a favorable response to benzodiazepines, were conducted using different diagnostic criteria from our current nomenclature, and undoubtedly represented a mixed sample of children with school refusal and anxiety. The controlled study by Bernstein and Borchardt [69] may have been less sensitive to a positive effect because the sample was selected for school refusal rather than for separation anxiety, and children with depressive disorders were included. Further controlled trials are necessary before short-term efficacy of benzodiazepines can be established for separation anxiety disorder. The long-term efficacy is unknown [21].

There have been, as yet, no controlled trials of buspirone for the treatment of separation anxiety disorder, although a case study reported success in a young boy [39]. Balon [75] also reported buspirone to be effective in the treatment of an adolescent boy with separation anxiety disorder. Additional controlled studies are needed.

There is no data regarding the use of antihistamines in the treatment of separation anxiety disorder.

Post traumatic stress disorder

Post traumatic stress disorder (PTSD) is common in children and adolescents, and may affect children exposed to single or repeated traumatic events, such as sexual abuse, kidnapping or a natural disaster [76–79]. Epidemiological studies have suggested that more than 6% of youth less than 18 years met lifetime diagnostic criteria for PTSD, in contrast to the adult population, in which 5–14% meet diagnostic criteria [80]. Antidepressants, particularly the selective serotonin reuptake inhibitors, are the pharmacologic treatment of choice for adults with PTSD and sertraline is approved for use in adults. Benzodiazepines and buspirone have also been evaluated, with mixed results [21]. Adult studies suggest that benzodiazepines may have little effect on central PTSD symptoms of re-experiencing and avoidance, and run the risk of inducing rebound anxiety and sleep disturbance [80].

For example, a double-blind, placebo-controlled study of alprazolam in 16 adults found no benefit [81]. Six (50%) of the patients (three were receiving alprazolam) dropped out of the study because of the drug's ineffectiveness, and those who completed showed a trend toward improvement of anxiety symptoms, but no effect on the major symptoms

of PTSD. Withdrawal effects increased anxiety in subjects receiving alprazolam [81]. Similar problems with withdrawal were observed in eight
combat veterans receiving long-term alprazolam treatment, including
severe sleep and anxiety problems, as well as an increase in the major
symptoms of PTSD [82]. The only favorable report is a letter by Feldman
[83], who saw improvement in 16 of 20 war veterans on alprazolam, but
increased aggressive outbursts in the remaining four. Based on this limited
data, benzodiazepines cannot be recommended for use in children with
PTSD. There are no data regarding the use of benzodiazepines in the management of children following sexual or physical abuse.

A single open trial of buspirone in three adult patients with PTSD reported improvement in anxiety, insomnia, depression, and flashbacks on
35–60 mg/day [84]. There are no controlled trials of buspirone for childhood and adolescent PTSD.

There are limited data regarding the use of antihistamines in the
treatment of PTSD in adults. Cyproheptadine has been reported to be
somewhat beneficial in the treatment of traumatic nightmares [80]. Since
it is generally well tolerated in children, and may be helpful as a sedative-
hypnotic, it may have limited utility in children. Controlled studies
are needed.

Obsessive compulsive disorder (OCD)

Benzodiazepines are not the treatment of choice for OCD [85], but they
are often used as adjuncts to antidepressants. Research has focused on
the anti-obsessive properties of the SSRIs and the tricyclic antidepressant,
clomipramine. Animal studies have demonstrated that clonazepam, in
particular, has an indirect effect on serotonergic transmission that is not
mediated by reuptake inhibition or receptor binding [86]. This effect provides a theoretical basis for clinical trials of clonazepam in OCD. In an
open trial, symptomatic improvement was observed in three adults with
OCD, and it persisted up to one year in two subjects [86]. However, one
subject was terminated for use of alcohol in conjunction with the medication. Benzodiazepines such as clonazepam are frequently used as
adjuncts in OCD, particularly when there are high levels of associated
anxiety, but at least one study suggests that they have little effect on primary OCD symptoms [87]. No controlled trials are available, and there is
no evidence supporting the use of benzodiazepines in childhood OCD. As
adjunctive treatment, these medications should be used cautiously, especially in patients with a personal or family history of substance abuse or
dependence [21].

As buspirone is an agonist at postsynaptic serotonergic receptors, benefit
in treatment of OCD might be expected. Although one open trial did not
support the efficacy of buspirone as a monotherapy [88] a double-blind,

placebo controlled trial in adults reported that buspirone 60 mg daily was as effective as clomipramine [89]. Open label studies have indicated some benefit in using buspirone in combination with other serotonergic agents; for example, a case of buspirone augmentation of fluoxetine in an 11-year old girl with OCD and depression was reported [90]. Markowitz et al. [91] reported the combination of buspirone and fluoxetine to be more effective than fluoxetine alone in an open trial for young adults with treatment-resistant OCD. On the other hand, placebo-controlled studies of SRI augmentation (clomipramine and fluoxetine) with buspirone [92,93] have not reported benefit of buspirone over placebo. No studies of buspirone in pediatric OCD are available [21].

There are no studies of antihistamine use in treatment of OCD.

Social anxiety disorder

Because of their sedative effects, benzodiazepines are usually not recommended for use in social anxiety disorder. There have been no controlled studies of these agents in children and adolescents.

Zwier and Rao [94] reported benefit of buspirone in an adolescent with social phobia. Additional controlled studies of this buspirone are necessary before it can be recommended for the treatment of this condition. There are no studies of antihistamines in the treatment of social anxiety disorder [21].

Anticipatory anxiety associated with medical procedures

Benzodiazepines have been reported to be beneficial for preoperative sedation to reduce anticipatory anxiety before surgery [95]. Small doses of diazepam might be useful in the treatment of anticipatory anxiety in imipramine-treated children with school refusal [96,97]. The most practical application of the use of benzodiazepines may be in the treatment of anticipatory anxiety prior to a painful procedure, as reported by Pfefferbaum et al. [98].

Alprazolam was reported to be beneficial in small doses as treatment for situational anxiety in 13 children with cancer undergoing painful procedures [98]. The investigators reported that open-label alprazolam treatment (0.125–1 mg/day) was effective in reducing anticipatory anxiety associated with bone marrow aspirations and lumbar punctures in 13 children with cancer. Single, small doses of benzodiazepines are likely to reduce the psychological trauma of such procedures and are unlikely to produce untoward effects. Hennes et al. [99] reported a double-blind, placebo-controlled study of the high-potency, short-acting benzodiazepine, midazolam (0.2 mg/kg, orally administered) in preschool-age children having surgical repair for lacerations. Midazolam was significantly more effective than placebo in reducing anxiety; 70% or 21 of

30 patients treated with midazolam improved, as compared to only 12% or three of 25 patients treated with placebo. The medication was well tolerated with no adverse events reported [99].

Oral midazolam was compared to hydroxyzine alone or in combination in a prospective, double blind, crossover study for dental procedures in 28 children ages 21 to 56 months (mean age 36.6 months). Results indicated that the combination of hydoxyzine (3.7 mg/kg) with midazolam (0.3 mg/kg) given 30 minutes before the procedures was both safe and effective; the combination resulted in less crying and movement during the first 30 and 20 minutes [100]. A study of melatonin versus midazolam premedication for elective surgery in 105 children ages 2–5 years reported that both drugs were equally effective in reduction of separation anxiety and preoperative anxiety. Melatonin was associated with a trend toward faster recovery and a lower incidence of postoperative excitement and sleep disturbance [101].

Triazolam, a short acting benzodiazepine, has also been used in pediatric dental patients as premedication for dental procedures, in both oral and sublingual forms [102, 103].

Administration of a benzodiazepine for anticipatory anxiety should probably be reserved for developmentally normal children, because two studies have reported that some children experience behavioral disinhibition with these medications; this effect appears to occur more frequently in children with developmental delays [104, 105]. If it is deemed necessary to use these agents in such populations, lower dosing and close monitoring is indicated. Behavioral disinhibition is the most significant risk of using these agents for anticipatory anxiety or as "as needed" sedatives (see "adverse reactions").

There are no data regarding the use of buspirone for anticipatory anxiety associated with medical procedures, since the anxiolytic effect is not acute [21].

Behavior disorders

A large study of 130 children and adolescents with various behavior disorders who were treated with chlordiazepoxide (up to 130 mg daily), reported that the improvement rate was 40%. However, of brain-damaged children, 50% worsened and 30% showed no change [71].

Quaison et al. [106] treated a hospitalized eight-year old boy with ADHD and conduct disorder with buspirone, up to 15 mg tid. The authors report that by day 10 there was a significant decrease in aggressive behavior, and elimination of the need for seclusion [106]. Ratey et al. [107, 108] reported reduction in anxiety, aggression and self-injurious behavior with buspirone in 20 developmentally disabled adults, age 18–63. Pfeffer et al. [109] reported an open study of 25 children (mean age eight years ± 1.8; range 5–11 years) with anxiety and aggressive behavior treated with buspirone. Of the 19 who completed the 11-week study, mean dose was 28 mg/day. The authors reported a significant reduction in depressive symptoms, as measured by the Children's Depression Inventory (CDI), and significant reduction in the number of restraints or use of seclusion. However, only three children were reported to have improved enough to remain on buspirone following the end of the study, and clinically significant aggression and anxiety remained [109].

Despite widespread clinical use in childhood and adolescence, there are virtually no controlled studies of antihistamines in the treatment of behavior disorders [21].

Tic disorders

There are no controlled data about the use of benzodiazepines in youth with tic disorders. Gonce and Barbeau [110] reported on seven cases of patients with Tourette syndrome who experienced partial reduction of symptoms with clonazepam. Steingard et al. [111] reported on the adjunctive use of clonazepam in combination with clonidine in children with comorbid ADHD and tic disorders. An open-label study of alprazolam or lorazepam in ten patients with tic and anxiety disorders showed three of five children and four of five adults with improvement in both tics and anxiety. There were no significant side-effects, apart from sedation [20].

Sleep disorders

Insomnia

Insomnia, which encompasses difficulty falling asleep, maintaining sleep or waking up too early, is a common problem in pediatric practice in general, and specifically in children and adolescents with psychiatric disorders. Insomnia is the most common problem for which sedatives and anxiolytics are prescribed. The term "hypnotic" refers to those sedatives and anxiolytics that are commonly prescribed for sleep induction, including antihistamines, short-acting benzodiazepines, and newer non-benzodiazepine sleep agents such as zolpidem tartrate and zaleplon.

In a recent survey of 671 pediatricians in the United States., 3–7% of visits were for insomnia. More than 75% of clinicians had recommended nonprescription medication, and more than 50% had prescribed a prescription sleep medication. Antihistamines were the most commonly prescribed nonprescription medications for sleep; alpha agonists were the most commonly prescribed sleep medication (31%) [112]. In another survey to assess prescribing practices of 222 pediatricians from Iowa, Oregon, Arizona and North Carolina, representing a cross section of the United States, 96% reported that they treated sleep disturbances.

Antihistamines were prescribed by 83%, followed by alpha adrenergic agonists (45.5%), melatonin (42%), tricyclic antidepressants (30.7%) and other antidepressants (29.5%); benzodiazepines were prescribed by 17%. More than one-third reported the use of clonidine for sleep onset, schedule, night and early morning awakening, and parasomnias. Clonidine was also frequently used by 142 (64%) for conditions other than sleep disturbance, including ADHD, behavior problems other than ADHD, and hypertension [113].

Insomnia is often a result of a primary psychiatric or clinical problem such as a mood or anxiety disorder, pain, or substance use (including caffeine, alcohol, nicotine, or drugs of abuse); management is best addressed through treatment of the primary disorder. Primary insomnia is an approved indication for hypnotic drugs; tolerance develops to the sedative properties of hypnotics, so they are only effective for a limited time [114]. Hypnotics are most appropriate for transient primary insomnia, in which symptoms last less than a month. Transient primary insomnia accounts for 15% of cases in adults [115] and is at least as common in children [21, 116].

Transient insomnia may be a consequence of an acute stressor such as a psychological or emotional problem or circadian phase shifts [114]. By definition, transient insomnia is self-limited, and pharmacologic treatment is often unnecessary. Behavioral intervention (improved sleep hygiene, regular sleep schedules and supportive measures) is usually effective [117, 118]. In children, mastery of sleep initiation and continuity represents a key developmental task, making behavioral approaches the clear treatment of choice, especially for younger children [113]. Nevertheless, hypnotic agents are sometimes indicated; in clinical practice they are probably quite frequently prescribed.

Benzodiazepines

Flurazepam, a long-acting benzodiazepine, first received approval as a hypnotic in 1974. Currently, there are several short acting benzodiazepines approved for use in adults for sleep induction, including nitrazepam and flunitrazepam.

Benzodiazepines induce changes in EEG sleep architecture by transiently suppressing slow-wave (Stage IV) sleep [119, 120], and reducing REM sleep and atypical sleep spindles [17].

Most short-acting benzodiazepines are approved for the short-term (up to 4–5 days) treatment of insomnia in adults when behavioral measures are ineffective. Placebo-controlled trials have demonstrated improvement in short term sleep quality for specific agents, including alprazolam [121], quazepam [122, 123], triazolam [124, 125], and temazepam [126]. The efficacy appears to attenuate after four to five days. For example, subjects treated with quazepam showed a significant improvement in sleep quality and latency during the first four days of treatment, but were not different from controls by day 5 [123].

Beyond short-term (five days) treatment, the effectiveness of benzodiazepines is less certain. Rebound insomnia occurs even after very limited use of hypnotics and may predispose to drug dependence [127]. Roehrs et al. [128] reported that significant rebound insomnia occurred in both patients and controls after six doses of triazolam 0.5 mg. The degree of rebound was similar for patients and controls but was more severe after abrupt discontinuation. The investigators reported that rebound increases the risk that patients will continue to self-administer hypnotics with the severity of the initial sleep problem, regardless of whether the subject received active drug or placebo [21, 129].

Studies suggest that rebound and dependence are of significant concern in patients with insomnia treated with benzodiazepines. In addition, next day carryover effects, such as reduction in alertness, may be experienced, particularly with long-acting agents (see "adverse reactions"). Taken together, it is recommended that benzodiazepines be used only when the immediate benefit of improved sleep outweighs both the immediate risk of residual daytime effects and the eventual risk of rebound insomnia or drug dependence.

Hishikawa [114] reviewed the use of benzodiazepine hypnotics for adult insomnia and recommended that patients be treated only when symptoms are severe, and not for more than three weeks. Additionally, the American Psychiatric Association has concluded that there is little evidence supporting the effectiveness of benzodiazepine hypnotics for more than 30 days of treatment [21, 130].

These data, unfortunately, are exclusively based on experience with adults. Benzodiazepine hypnotics have not been well studied in children. They are, however, widely prescribed despite the apparent clinical consensus that they are inferior to behavioral measures and low-dose antidepressants [116, 131]. The extant literature does not clearly answer the question of when to use benzodiazepine hypnotics but suggests that they will be most helpful for severe transient insomnia that is related to time-limited stressors. Clinical situations in which children and adolescents may be candidates for short-term pharmacotherapy for insomnia might include insomnia following trauma, or circadian shifts due to travel or work schedules. Since rebound insomnia may be a common adverse effect, worsened with abrupt discontinuation, the recommendation is for several days of a short-acting hypnotic followed by tapering the dose over several days. Potential therapeutic benefit needs to be weighed against potential adverse effects such as dependence, rebound sleep and anxiety symptoms, and cognitive effects on school performance [21].

Non-benzodiazepine agents

Zolpidem tartrate is effective in the short-term treatment of insomnia in adults [132, 133]. Chronic administration is not recommended. Despite a lack of controlled studies, zolpidem is being prescribed fairly often in children and adolescents with insomnia. Zaleplon is also indicated for the short-term treatment of insomnia in adults [134]. Zaleplon has not been demonstrated to reduce awakenings or increase total sleep time as compared to placebo. Both zolpidem and zaleplon have a rapid onset of action and reduce sleep latency. Zolpidem has a half-life of 2.5 hours, and zaleplon a half-life of one hour; given these differences, zolpidem may improve both sleep onset and duration, whereas zaleplon only improves sleep onset. Next-day sedation and carryover effects are minimal. Insomnia rebound is very uncommon. These agents are not recommended for use in children and adolescents, since there have been no controlled studies in pediatric samples [21].

Buspirone

The absence of significant sedative properties predicts that buspirone would be ineffective for primary insomnia. This was confirmed by Manfredi et al. [135], who tested the hypnotic effectiveness of buspirone in a manner similar to that for benzodiazepine hypnotic trials: four nights of placebo-baseline, seven nights of buspirone 10 mg, and five nights of placebo withdrawal. The six adults with chronic insomnia showed a significant *decrease* in total sleep, which was most prominent during the first three nights. Similarly, a three-week course of buspirone was tested by De Roeck et al. [136] in adult patients with anxiety and insomnia, and also yielded no hypnotic effect. There is no indication for buspirone in the treatment of primary insomnia in children and adolescents [21].

Antihistamines

Antihistamines have been used for decades to induce mild, rapid sedation. Diphenhydramine is available without prescription, so its use as a hypnotic agent undoubtedly exceeds physician prescriptions for that purpose. There are fewer controlled trials of antihistamines than benzodiazepines but those that are available support their short-term use for transient primary insomnia.

A 50 mg dose of diphenhydramine produces sedation roughly equivalent to that afforded by 100 mg of pentobarbital [137, 138]. In controlled clinical trials, diphenhydramine was reported to be superior to placebo in improving sleep latency, number of arousals, and total sleep time [139–141], while having few effects on the sleep of normal subjects [142]. Meulman et al. [143] reported that 50 mg of diphenhydramine was modestly superior to 15 mg of temazepam in improving total sleep time after five days of treatment (p < 0.05). The only placebo-controlled comparison of an antihistamine and a benzodiazepine, this trial was conducted on a small sample of elderly nursing-home residents and is, therefore, difficult to generalize to children. Promethazine is also superior to placebo in adults with insomnia [144]. Hydroxyzine has not been subjected to controlled trials but is probably effective [145]. Like the benzodiazepines, residual carry over daytime effects and a reduction in daytime performance tasks are reported (see "adverse effects"). Although tolerance to the sedative effects of diphenhydramine has been described [139], dependence and rebound insomnia have not been reported [21].

One controlled study in children reported that diphenhydramine 1 mg/kg was effective in decreasing sleep latency and mid-sleep awakenings in 50 children, ages 2–12 years, over the course of one week [146]. Adverse effects were minimal. Diphenhydramine did not prolong total sleep time in this study, probably due to the short (4–6 hours) duration of action.

Melatonin

Melatonin is the primary hormone secreted by the pituitary gland; it is synthesized from the precursor tryptophan, hydroxylated to 5-hydroxytryptophan, and decarboxylated to serotonin, and then n-acetylated and converted to melatonin. The pineal gland produces a circadian rhythm, which leads to low daytime and high night-time plasma levels. Melatonin is thought to have a phase-setting effect, as opposed to or in addition to a sedative-hypnotic effect. In adults, small doses of 0.1–0.3 mg are given in the evening, which produce serum concentrations in the normal nocturnal range. Most adult studies have been conducted with healthy volunteers, and thus efficacy in patient groups is more difficult to determine. There are few studies in children, particularly regarding dosing. In a case series of 15 neurologically impaired children, doses of 2–10 mg were reported to be effective [147].

Parasomnias

Parasomnias are defined as abnormal behaviors during sleep, including arousal disorders (sleepwalking, night terrors), sleep-wake transition disorders (sleep talking, leg movements), and REM-associated disorders (nightmares, REM behavior disorder). Several medications have been reported to exacerbate parasomnia symptoms, including neuroleptics, short-acting benzodiazepines, nonbenzodiazepine hypnotics, and tricyclic antidepressants [148, 149]. Case studies have reported success [150] and failure [151] with diazepam but no benzodiazepine has been systematically studied.

Benzodiazepines may be beneficial in treatment of disorders of Stage IV arousal such as night terrors (pavor nocturnus) and sleep-walking (somnambulism). Clonazepam has been recommended in low doses [147].

Generally, pharmacotherapy is not necessary for somnambulism in children. As the goal of treatment is to ensure the safety of the child, in most cases this can be achieved through the use of environmental controls, such as locking doors and windows, removing dangerous objects in the child's room, and placing the bed on the ground floor [152].

Night terrors

Night terrors, or pavor nocturnus, consist of the sudden onset of intense fear and autonomic discharge, usually taking place during slow-wave sleep. The child screams, is confused and inconsolable, and may cause injury by bolting from his or her bed. The prevalence is less than that of somnambulism (3-4% of preadolescents), and the manifestations are more distressing to parents. Environmental measures, supportive psychotherapy, and improved sleep habits are usually sufficient treatment, but short-term hypnotic therapy may be used in severe cases.

This use of benzodiazepines has been somewhat better studied in children than other sleep disorders. Diazepam was noted to be beneficial in one older study [153]. Popoviciu et al. [154] treated 15 children, ages six to 15 years with night terrors with 15 mg midazolam in a single-blind, placebo-controlled trial; results indicated an increase in total sleep time, a decrease in REM latency, changes in proportion of REM sleep and reduction in frequency of night-time awakening in the children. All but one child had a remission of symptoms. However, medication was administered for only two nights and thus longer term efficacy is unknown. It is likely that tolerance would develop as is the case with other benzodiazepines. Thus, pharmacotherapy of night terrors should be limited to short-term treatment. More studies with longer followups are required before this can be considered a standard treatment.

REM behavior disorder

REM behavior disorder, a rare and unusual syndrome that generally appears in adults [155], has been reported in children [156]. The syndrome is characterized by maintenance of muscle tone during REM sleep, causing elaborate, seemingly purposeful, behavior during sleep. Specific behaviors may include the acting out of dreams, self-injury, or violence. The majority of pharmacologic trials are uncontrolled adult case series from a single research center, where the syndrome has been successfully managed with clonazepam [157]. Tricyclic antidepressants and SSRIs may exacerbate or produce this disorder [158]. There is no consensus regarding treatment of its rare occurrence in children.

Summary: treatment of anxiety and sleep disorders

Anxiety disorders in children and adolescents are relatively common, and can be associated with significant reduction in quality of life, and impairment of social and academic functioning. Nonpharmacological treatment, such as cognitive behavioral therapy, is recommended, where possible, as the first-line intervention unless symptoms are severe.

Controlled studies of anxiolytics in youth with anxiety and sleep disorders are limited, and treatment recommendations are still drawn primarily from small controlled trials, open trials and adult studies. When pharmacologic treatment is necessary, selective serotonin reuptake inhibitor antidepressants are the recommended first-line treatment for panic disorder, separation anxiety disorder, GAD, PTSD, and OCD. Benzodiazepines may be beneficial for the treatment of anticipatory anxiety, anxiety associated with medical procedures, and for the first few weeks of panic disorder pharmacotherapy in children and adolescents, but appear to be of little benefit in separation anxiety disorder. There is little support for their use in OCD or the long-term treatment of GAD. There is no evidence for efficacy in childhood PTSD, and the possible exacerbation of symptoms upon withdrawal. Questions remain about optimal agents, dosage schedules and duration of treatment for any child or adolescent anxiety disorder. Controlled trials of benzodiazepines are most clearly needed for the treatment of separation anxiety disorder and panic disorder, for which both efficacy and the risks of long-term treatment in children must be established.

For sleep disorders in children and adolescents, behavioral measures are recommended as the first-line treatment for insomnia whenever possible. In cases when transient insomnia is severe and is related to time-limited stressors, both short-acting benzodiazepines and sedative antihistamines are effective in short-term improvement of sleep quality. Benzodiazepines may have limited short-term use in some parasomnias, such as pavor nocturnus. However, after four to seven days, tolerance may develop to both benzodiazepines and sedative antihistamines. If benzodiazepines are used, short-term (5–7 days) treatment is recommended, and medication should be tapered upon discontinuation to minimize rebound insomnia.

Contraindications

Benzodiazepines

Benzodiazepines are absolutely contraindicated only for patients with known hypersensitivity. Most of these agents are also contraindicated in narrow-angle glaucoma. Relative contraindications include a history of benzodiazepine dependence or abuse, substance or alcohol abuse, disinhibition, hepatic dysfunction (for agents that undergo hepatic metabolism),debilitated patients or patients at risk for aspiration; and patients with AIDS who are receiving zidovudine [20]. Due to muscle-relaxant properties of most benzodiazepines, these drugs should also be avoided for patients with symptomatic sleep apnea. Patients must be cautioned against driving or performing dangerous tasks while taking these agents, especially early in treatment [159].

Similar contraindications are recommended for the non-benzodiazepine sleep agents, zolpidem tartrate and zaleplon.

Buspirone

Buspirone is contraindicated for patients with known hypersensitivity to the drug. Because of the risk of hypertension and the so-called central excitatory syndrome, it should not be given concurrently with MAOIs. Buspirone is relatively contraindicated for patients with hepatic or renal dysfunction.

Antihistamines

Antihistamines are contraindicated in a variety of situations, depending on their degree of anti-cholinergic activity. Narrow-angle glaucoma, gastrointestinal or urinary obstructions, and mental-status changes that may be due to anticholinergic toxicity are contraindications to diphenhydramine and cyproheptadine. Most antihistamines potentiate other CNS depressants and analgesics, necessitating caution with these agents. Like benzodiazepines, these agents may cause impairment of driving or work performance, and patients must be cautioned against use accordingly.

Adverse effects

Benzodiazepines

Sedation, cognitive effects, and disinhibition are among the more common adverse effects of benzodiazepines [20, 160].

Sedation

Fatigue and drowsiness are common, but decreased cognitive function and motor coordination may be more problematic in children.

Cognitive and performance decrements

Psychomotor impairments, including short-term memory, are not well studied in children, but are potentially most problematic in young children. Although children and adolescents might be vulnerable to cumulative impairments in academic functioning, it is notable that interference with functioning has not actually been formally demonstrated in adolescents or children.

Behavioral disinhibition

Increased anxiety, agitation, or excitement may occur in younger patients. There are no systematic studies of disinhibition, but it appears to be more common in younger patients, perhaps more frequently in labile, impulse-ridden, or developmentally disabled individuals. In prepubertal children, behavioral features of disinhibition include overexcitement, hyperactivity, increased aggressive behavior, or explosive outbursts. It is difficult to predict which children or adolescents are at risk.

Rare but potentially serious adverse effects

Seizures

Benzodiazepine-induced seizures are observed primarily during drug withdrawal. They are more likely to occur after abrupt withdrawal of the agents with short half-lives.

Hallucinations

Hallucinations and perceptual disorganization can occur as a manifestation of CNS disinhibition.

Phlebitis at injection sites

With intravenous injections of diazepam, chlordiazepoxide, or lorazepam local irritation, swelling, or venous thrombosis may occur.

Leukopenia, thrombocytopenia, and agranulocytosis

These blood abnormalities are rare, but have been described in adults.

Suspected adverse effects not established

Teratogenicity

Pregnancy is always a possibility in sexually active female adolescents. Although older reports of an association of diazepam use in the first trimester with oral cleft abnormalities have not been substantiated, there are very few prospective data. Some reports have suggested that a "floppy baby syndrome" may occur during third trimester use [18]. Some more recent reports have indicated no specific increased risks [161], possible increased risks with alprazolam and clonazepam, but not diazepam and chlordiazepoxide [162], and possible increased risk of pylorostenosis or alimentary tract atresia [163]. Use of benzodiazepines during lactation may be associated with lethargy, sedation and weight loss in infants [162]. Overall, caution seems indicated.

Antihistamines

In general, antihistamines are quite safe and well tolerated. Sedation is the most common problem in children and adolescents. Interference with cognitive functioning is possible [20, 160].

Common adverse effects

Sedation
This is a very common effect, especially with diphenhydramine, during the first several hours after administration. For children receiving antihistamines at bedtime, a morning "hangover" effect may be seen. Sedative effects tend to increase with dose, but may be seen at any dose.

Anticholinergic effects
Antihistamines block muscarinic acetylcholine receptors, so anticholinergic symptoms may occur, including dryness of mouth, blurred vision, constipation, thickening of mucus, and postural hypotension. These effects are often dose dependent.

Uncommon but potentially serious adverse effects

Seizures
In patients with focal CNS lesions or a history of seizures, antihistamines may reduce seizure threshold.

Occasional adverse effects

Gastrointestinal effects
Gastrointestinal adverse effects are usually minimal but can include anorexia, nausea, vomiting, and epigastric discomfort.

Tics and dyskinesia
Involuntary movements are not common, and typically occur at the higher dose ranges, above 200 mg/daily.

Spaciness
Some children appear to be in a floating or dreamy state, neither sedated nor excited, which may be experienced as unpleasant.

Behavioral disinhibition
Increased behavioral impulsivity and agitation may occur occasionally.

Buspirone

Potential adverse effects of buspirone include dizziness, anxiety, nausea, headache, lightheadedness, restlessness, excitement, depression, or confusion. Although the sedative properties of buspirone appear to be about 30% of the sedation of benzodiazepines in adults, doses above 30 mg per day may be associated with sedation and dysphoria. Sedative effects are uncommonly a problem at lower doses [160].

Buspirone does not potentiate the sedative or impairing effects of alcohol [164].

Overdose

Benzodiazepines

Manifestations of benzodiazepine toxicity include somnolence, confusion, slurred speech, ataxia, trembling, decreased reflexes, slow pulse, shortness of breath, and coma. Respiratory depression is usually of minimal significance except in massive doses, poly-drug overdose, or concurrent disease. Benzodiazepines are relatively safe and generally nonlethal when taken alone in overdose but they can have additive effects when taken with other centrally depressant drugs, especially alcohol [160, 165].

Antihistamines

The most common manifestation is somnolence, especially in adolescents and adults. Anticholinergic toxicity and delirium may occur, characterized by dry mouth, confusion, and fixed and dilated pupils [21]. Children can become hyperexcitable or ataxic, and may even develop hallucinations or convulsions. A flushed face, fever, dilated pupils, and shortness of breath suggest atropine-like intoxication.

Buspirone

The most commonly experienced symptoms of toxicity are severe drowsiness or dizziness, pinpoint pupils, nausea, vomiting, or gastric distress.

Abuse/dependence

Benzodiazepines

Parents and children should be cautioned about this possibility, and risks should be openly discussed. A predictably vulnerable patient who has abused other drugs or alcohol should not be treated with benzodiazepines, and might be considered for antihistamines or buspirone instead. These drugs are highly abusable. This may be particularly problematic for impulse-ridden or substance-abusing adolescents, especially alprazolam in view of the potential for severe withdrawal seizures. Helpful preventive measures include short-term treatment (less than three months), and gradual tapering, especially for the shorter half-life agents, rather than abrupt discontinuation.

Antihistamines

It is rare for antihistamines to be abused as these agents have few reinforcing effects and many unpleasant side-effects [21].

Buspirone

There are no reports of abuse or dependence with buspirone. On the contrary, buspirone has been used in the treatment of anxiety in adults recently detoxified from alcohol [166]. In a comparative study of drug effects and abuse liability of lorazepam, buspirone and secobarbital in nondependent adult subjects, results indicated that dose escalation was not likely to occur in any of these medications [167].

Drug interactions

See Table 13.1.

Available preparations and cost

See Tables 13.2 and 13.3.

Initiation and maintenance of treatment

Benzodiazepines

The following recommendations are suggested as general guidelines for use; however, dosing and titration must be tailored to individual patients.

Doses are usually given in children and adolescents on a bid, tid, or qid basis, depending on the individual drug and the child (see Table 13.4). Prepubertal children tend to have more efficient hepatic metabolism and renal excretion, and thus they often need more frequent administration of these medications than adolescents or adults.

Among the benzodiazepines, an approximate dose equivalency can be described by focusing specifically on the sedative properties (see Table 13.5). These equivalencies may not apply to other properties and uses.

See Tables 13.4 and 13.5.

Table 13.1 Drug interactions with anxiolytics and sedatives

Benzodiazepines	Drugs whose activity or blood levels may increase • alcohol • neuroleptics • sedatives (narcotic, analgesic, recreational) • antidepressants • phenytoin • zidovudine Drugs that may increase the activity or blood level of benzodiazepines: • antimicrobials (erythromycin, isoniazid) • disulfuram • fluoxetine • oral contraceptives • cimetidine • alcohol • sedatives • neuroleptics • MAOIs • Isoniazid • Phenytoin • digoxin Drugs whose activity may be impaired: • carbamazepine Drugs that may decrease the activity or lower blood level of benzodiazepines: • antacids • heavy tobacco use Drugs that may produce adverse reactions: • MAOIs (central excitatory syndrome)
Buspirone	Drugs whose activity or blood levels may increase: • neuroleptics (theoretical and one report of increased haloperidol levels, Sussman, 1987) Drugs that may produce adverse reactions: • trazodone (one report of hepatic toxicity) • MAOIs (theoretical risk of central excitatory syndrome) • neuroleptics (theoretical risk of increased effects of dopamine antagonism) • digoxin (may be displaced from protein binding sites)
Antihistamines	Drugs whose activity or blood levels may increase: • alcohol • sedatives (narcotic, analgesic, recreational) • MAOIs Drugs whose activity may be decreased: • ototoxic medications • apomorphine • epinephrine (pressor effect) Drugs that may produce adverse reactions: • potentiation of anticholinergic side effects and possible toxicity with any anticholinergic agent

Table 13.2 Sample of available benzodiazepines, usual adult doses, and costs

Compound (brand name)	How available	Age range	Adult half-life (hours)	Usual adult daily dose for anxiety	Approximate daily cost*
Lorazepam (Ativan)	INJ – 2, 4 mg/ml TAB – 0.5, 1.0, 2.0 mg	≥ 12 years	12	2–6 mg/day divided	$2.58
Prazepam (Centrax)	TAB – 5, 10, 20 mg	≥ 18 years	30–200	20–60 mg/day divided	$2.81
Chlordiazepoxide (Librium)	CAP – 5, 10, 25 mg	≥ 12 years	24–48	5–10 mg b.i.d. or t.i.d.	$1.55†
	TAB – 5, 10, 25 mg				
Oxazepam (Serax)	TAB – 15	≥ 6 years	6–11	10–15 mg t.i.d. to q.i.d.	$2.08
	CAP – 10, 15, 30 mg				
Clorazepate (Tranxene)	TAB – 3.75, 7.5, 15 mg	≥ 9 years	30–200	30 mg/day divided	$4.81†
	SR – 11.25, 22.5 mg				
Diazepam (Valium)	INJ – 5 mg/ml	≥ 6 months	20–100	2–10 mg t.i.d. to q.i.d.	$1.60†
	TAB – 2, 5, 10 mg				
	SR – 15 mg				
Alprazolam (Xanax)	TAB – 0.25, 0.5, 1.0, 2.0 mg	≥ 18 years	6–27	0.25–0.5 mg/t.i.d.(for anxiety)	$4.33
	SR – 0.5, 1, 2, 3 mg			5–6 mg/day divided (for panic disorder)	
Temazepam (Restoril)	CAP – 7.5, 15, 22.5, 30 mg	≥ 18 years	9–12	15 mg q.h.s.	$0.84†
Midazolam (Versed)	INJ – 1, 5 mg/ml	≥ 18 years	1–12	No approved psychiatric indication	NA
Flurazepam (Dalmane)	CAP – 15, 30 mg	≥ 15 years	40–100	15 or 30 mg q.h.s.	$0.74†
Quazepam (Doral)	TAB – 7.5, 15 mg	≥ 18 years	40–100	7.5 or 15 mg q.h.s.	$0.88
Triazolam (Halcion)	TAB – 0.125, 0.25 mg	≥ 18 years	2–6	0.25 mg q.h.s.	$0.89

*Cost estimates based on median effective adult dose for primary psychiatric indication and average wholesale price as published in *Prescription Pricing Guide*, Medi-Span, Inc., June 1992.
†Generic available.

Abbreviations: INJ – injectable; TAB – tablet; CAP – capsule; SR – sustained release; b.i.d – twice per day; t.i.d – three times per day; q.i.d – 4 times per day; q.h.s – every night.

Table 13.3 Sample of available antihistamine agents, usual adult doses, and costs

Agent (brand name)	Available forms	Adult half-life (hours)	Dose range	Psychiatric indications	Approximate daily cost*
Diphenhydramine (Benadryl)	CAP – 25 mg INJ – 1, 5, 50 mg/ml TAB – 12.5, 25 mg LIQ – 12.5 mg/5 ml	3–14	≤ 5 mg/kg/day, div q.i.d. Max. 400 mg/day 50–100 mg as hypnotic	EPS Hypnotic	$0.37†
Hydroxyzine (Atarax, Vistaril)	TAB – 10, 25, 50 mg LIQ – 10 mg/ 5 ml INJ – 25, 50 mg/ml	3–29	50–100 mg/day, divided 0.6 mg/kg as sedative	Anxiety Sedation	$0.89†
Cyproheptadine (Periactin)	TAB – 4 mg LIQ – 2 mg/ 5 ml	< 5	0.25 mg/kg/day, divided Max. 16 mg/day	None	NA
Promethazine (Phenergan)	TAB – 12.5, 25, 50 mg SUP – 12.5, 25, 50 mg LIQ – 6.25 mg/5 ml INJ – 25, 50 mg/ml	< 5	1.1 mg/kg single dose Usual dose ≤ 50 mg	Hypnotic Sedation	$0.31†

*Cost estimates based on median effective adult dose for primary psychiatric indication and average wholesale price as published in *Prescription Pricing Guide*, Medi-Span, Inc., June 1992.

†Generic available.

Abbreviations: CAP – capsule; TAB – tablet; INJ – injectable; LIQ – liquid; SUP – suppository; div – divided; q.i.d – four times per day; EPS – extrapyramidal symptoms.

Table 13.4 Oral dosage and treatment regimen for anxiety and sleep disorders

	Usual daily dose (mg)	Starting dose (mg per day)	Rate of increase	Maximum daily dose (mg)
Adolescents				
Lorazepam	0.5–6	0.5–1	0.5–1 mg q3-4d	10
Diazepam	2–20	0.5–1	0.5–1 mg q5-7d	20–30
Alprazolam	0.75–4	0.25–0.5	0.25–5 mg q3-4d	8–10
Clonazepam	0.5–3	0.25–0.5	0.25 mg q5-7d	3
Prepubertal children				
Lorazepam	0.25–3	0.25–0.5	0.25–0.5 mg q3-4d	4
Diazepam	1–10	0.5	0.5 mg q5-7d	10–15
Alprazolam	0.25–2	0.25	0.25 mg q3-4d	1–4
Clonazepam	0.25–2	0.125–0.25	0.25–0.5 q5-7d	4

q3-4d – every 3-4 days; q5-7d – every 5-7 days.

Table 13.5 Dose equivalencies for oral administration of benzodiazepines [168]

	Dose equivalency (mg)	Brand name in United States
Clonazepam	0.25	Klonopin
Alprazolam	0.5	Xanax
Triazolam	0.5	Halcion
Lorazepam	1.0	Ativan
Diazepam	5.0	Valium
Clorazepate	7.5	Tranxene
Halazepam	20.0	Paxipam
Chlordiazepoxide	25.0	Librium
Flurazepam	30.0	Dalmane
Temazepam	30.0	Restoril

Antihistamines

Diphenhydramine

Age limit: not for neonatal or premature infants.

Dose limit: 300 mg/day (for children over 20 lbs).

Indications: allergic reactions; motion sickness; drug-induced parkinsonism; Parkinson's disease.

Hydroxyzine

Age limit: not for neonatal or premature infants.

Dose limit: 100 mg qid for over age six years; 50 mg qid for under age six years.

Indications: anxiety.

Pruritis; pre- or postoperative sedation; nausea and vomiting.

Buspirone

Dosage and titration schedules have not been established for children or adolescents, but reasonable estimates can be made. For adolescents, a usual daily dose of 20 mg daily is reasonable; a starting dose might be 5–10 mg bid, increasing by 5–10 mg/day every 3–4 days, up to a maximum dose of about 60 mg daily (the daily dosage maximum for adults).

For prepubertal children, an expected daily dose of about 10–15 mg daily is reasonable; it is usually prudent to start at 2.5–5 mg daily or bid, with dose increases of 2.5 mg every 3-4 days, up to a maximum of about 20 mg daily. These are suggested estimates derived from usage in adults. Dose and titration need to be adjusted according to tolerability and therapeutic response of each individual.

In adults, therapeutic effects may take 1–2 weeks to appear, and maximal effects may not occur until 3–4 weeks. It is unusual to see improvement before one week.

Management of specific side-effects

Benzodiazepines

Sedation and cognitive impairment

There is no specific antidote to these adverse effects, but gradual dose titration, avoidance of excessive doses, and lowering of dose when necessary can be helpful. Gradual dose elevations and careful titration can be helpful, at least to a degree. Most children will accommodate to the sedative effects within days to weeks.

Behavioral disinhibition

Potential worsening of anxiety, excitement, agitation or aggression may occur, particularly in younger children. If the symptoms do not attenuate within a few days, the medication should be tapered and discontinued. Dose reduction or discontinuation is initially recommended but switching to another medication is often necessary. Explosive outbursts usually subside as medication is withdrawn but it may take several days before disinhibition is fully eliminated.

Since concomitant treatment with other medications may result in drug-drug interactions that complicate the clinical picture, no other medications should be given in the emergency setting. A toxic screen should be obtained to rule out concurrent involvement of alcohol or other recreational drugs. Behavioral management, and at times inpatient treatment, may be necessary

Rebound insomnia and other withdrawal symptoms
With abrupt discontinuation of benzodiazepines after a steady-state level is achieved, or even following the short-term use of short-acting agents, insomnia and other withdrawal symptoms may emerge. In theory, children may be at greater risk for rebound insomnia due to their faster metabolic clearance of the medications. Gradual reduction by tapering the dose is recommended.

Benzodiazepines can induce definite physiologic and psychological dependence, and may lead to serious withdrawal symptoms on discontinuation. The risk of physical or psychological dependence increases for patients on high doses for more than two months. Most withdrawal symptoms are mild, but occasionally more severe problems can occur. Clinically significant withdrawal symptoms may include anxiety, irritability, shakiness, tremors, sweating, body aches and pains, muscle cramping, vomiting, and sleep disruption. With short-acting drugs, rebound insomnia may occur after discontinuation of even short-term usage. In more severe situations, seizures and delirium may develop.

Teratogenicity
Prevention of pregnancy is recommended as a precaution, in view of the lack of definitive data in the literature.

Antihistamines
Sedation
Usually sedation diminishes over the course of a week or two, but sometimes dose reduction is necessary.

Anticholinergic effects
Most patients accommodate to the anticholinergic effects within a couple of weeks. If waiting or dosage reductions are not effective, symptomatic management of these side-effects may include use of hard, sugar-free candy for dry mouth or stool softeners for constipation.

Gastrointestinal effects
Administration of the medication with meals may ameliorate these symptoms.

Tics and dyskinesias
Dose reduction or discontinuation is recommended.

Buspirone

Sedation
Dose reduction is usually helpful.

Dizziness and lightheadedness
These usually improve over time but temporary dose reduction may be necessary. Headache is usually transient, but sometimes requires dose reduction. Nausea can be reduced by taking the medication with food.

How to withdraw medication

Benzodiazepines
Benzodiazepines should be slowly tapered, usually over several weeks (and occasionally longer). Generally the initial reductions should be no more than 25% of the dose; reductions of about 10% per week may be reasonable. Dangers in withdrawal are greatest with short-acting drugs abruptly stopped (as long-acting drugs tend to self-taper), but significant risks may still emerge up to three weeks after discontinuation of long-acting drugs [20].

Antihistamines
Withdrawal effects of antihistamines are usually not significant, but cholinergic rebound may occasionally occur if high doses (>200 mg/day) are abruptly discontinued. Symptoms may include diarrhea or malaise. Gradual reduction of dose over several days to weeks is recommended.

Buspirone
No significant withdrawal effects have been reported in adult studies. Rebound anxiety has not been described, even when the medication is suddenly discontinued.

References

1 Stein L, Wise CD, Berger BD: Antianxiety action of benzodiazepines. Decrease in activity of serotonin neurons in the punishment system. In: Garattini S, Mussini E, Randall L (eds) *The Benzodiazepines*. New York, NY: Raven, 1973, pp. 299–326.
2 Wise CD, Berger BD, Stein L: Benzodiazepines: anxiety-reducing activity by reduction of serotonin turnover in the brain. *Science* 1972; **177**: 180–3.
3 Grant SJ, Huang YH, Redmond Jr. DE: Benzodiazepines attenuate single unit activity in the locus coeruleus. *Life Sciences* 1980; **27**: 2231–6.

4 Taylor DP, Riblet LA, Stanton HC et al.: Dopamine and antianxiety activity. *Pharmacology Biochemistry and Behavior* 1982; **17**: 25–35.

5 Sepinwall J, Cook L: Relationship of γ-aminobutyric acid (GABA) to antianxiety effects in benzodiazepines. *GABA Neurotransmission* 1980; **5**: 839–48.

6 Kanto J, Sellman R, Haataja M et al.: Plasma and urine concentrations of diazepam and its metabolites in children, adults and in diazepam-intoxicated patients. *Int J Clin Pharmacol Biopharm* 1978; **16**: 258–64.

7 Coffey B, Shader RI, Greenblatt DJ: Pharmacokinetics of benzodiazepines in children and adolescents. *J Clin Psychopharmacol* 1983; **3**: 217–25.

8 Ciraulo DA, Antal EJ, Smith RB et al.: The relationship of alprazolam dose to steady-state plasma concentrations. *J Clin Psychopharmacol.* 1990; **10**: 27–32.

9 Simons KJ, Watson WT, Martin TJ et al.: Diphenhydramine: pharmacokinetics and pharmacodynamics in elderly adults, young adults, and children. *J Clin Pharmacol* 1990; **30**: 665–71.

10 del Cuvillo A, Sastre J, Montoro J et al.: Use of antihistamines in pediatrics. *J Investig Allergol Clin Immunol* 2007; **17**: 28–40.

11 Simons ER, Simons KJ: Levocetirizine: pharmacokinetics and pharmacodynamics in children age 6 to 11 years. *J Allergy Clin Immunol* 2005; **116**: 355–61.

12 Ortiz A, Pohl R, Gershon S: Azaspirodecandiones in generalized anxiety disorder: buspirone. *J Affect Disord* 1987; **13**: 131–43.

13 Gammans RE, Mayol RF, LaBudde JA: Metabolism and disposition of buspirone. *Am J Med* 1986; **80**: 41–51.

14 Salazar DE, Frackiewicz EJ, Dockens R et al.: Pharmacokinetics and tolerability of buspirone during oral administration to children and adolescents with anxiety disorder and noraml healthy adults. *J Clin Pharmacol* 2001; **41**: 1351–8.

15 Costello EJ, Egger HL, Angold A: The developmental epidemiology of anxiety disorders: phenomenology, prevalence, and comorbidity. *Child Adolesc Psychiatr Clin N Am* 2005; **14**: 631–48.

16 Rynn M, Puliafico A, Heleniak C et al.: Advances in pharmacotherapy for pediatric anxiety disorders. *Depression and Anxiety* 2011; **28**: 76–87.

17 Witek MW, Rojas V, Alonso C et al.: Review on benziodiazepine use in children and adolescents. *Psychiatr Q* 2005; **76**: 283–96.

18 Birmaher B, Yelovich AK, Renaud J: Pharmacologic treatment for children and adolescents with anxiety disorders. *Pediatr Clin North Am* 1998; **45**: 1187–204.

19 Zito JM, Safer DJ, dosReis S et al.: Psychotropic practice patterns for youth: a 10-year perspective. *Arch Pediatr Adolesc Med* 2003; **157**: 17–25.

20 Coffey BJ: Anxiolytics for children and adolescents: traditional and new drugs. *J Clin Adolesc Psychopharmacol* 1990; **1**: 57–83.

21 Rosenberg DR, Holttum J, Gershon S: *Textbook of Pharmacotherapy for Child and Adolescent Psychiatric Disorders.* New York, NY: Brunner/Mazel, 1994.

22 Whitaker A, Johnson J, Shaffer D et al.: Uncommon troubles in young people: prevalence estimates of selected psychiatrists disorders in a nonreferred adolescent population. *Arch Gen Psychiatry* 1990; **47**: 487–96.

23 Bowen RC, Offord DR, Boyle MH: The prevalence of overanxious disorder and separation anxiety disorder: results from the Ontario Child Health Study. *J Am Acam Child AdolescPsychiatry* 1990; **29**: 753–8.

24 Anderson JC, Williams S, McGee R et al.: DSM-III disorders in preadolescent children: prevalence in a large sample from the general population. *Arch Gen Psychiatry* 1987; **44**: 69–76.

25 Keller MB, Lavori PW, Wunder J et al.: Chronic course of anxiety disorders in children and adolescents. *J Am Acad Child Adolesc Psychiatry* 1992; **31**: 595–9.

26 Benjamin RS, Costello EJ, Warren M: Anxiety disorders in a pediatric sample. *J Anxiety Disord* 1990; **4**: 293–316.

27 Simeon JG, Ferguson HB: Alprazolam effects in children with anxiety disorders. *Can J Psychiatry* 1987; **32**: 570–4.

28 Simeon JG, Ferguson HB, Knott V et al.: Clinical, cognitive, and neurophysiological effects of alprazolam in children and adolescents with overanxious and avoidant disorders. *J Am Acad Child Adolesc Psychiatry* 1992; **31**: 29–33.

29 Ansseau M, Papart P, Gerard MA et al.: Controlled comparison of buspirone and oxazepam in generalized anxiety. *Neuropsychobiology* 1990; **24**: 74–8.

30 Cohn JB, Wilcox CS: Low-sedation potential of buspirone compared with alprazolam and lorazepam in the treatment of anxious patients: a double blind study. *J Clin Psychiatry* 1986; **47**: 409–12.

31 Enkelmann R: Alprazolam versus buspirone in the treatment of outpatients with generalized anxiety disorder. *Psychopharmacology* 1991; **105**: 428–32.

32 Feighner JP, Merideth C, Hendrickson G: A double blind comparison of buspirone and diazepam in outpatients with generalized anxiety disorder. *J Clin Psychiatry* 1982; **43**: 103–7.

33 Newton RE, Casten GP, Alms DR et al.: The side effect profile of buspirone in comparison to active controls and placebo. *J Clin Psychiatry* 1982; **43**: 100–2.

34 Cutler NR, Hesselink JM, Sramek JJ: A phase II multicenter dose-finding, efficacy and safety trial of ipsaprione in outpatients with generalized anxiety disorder. *Prog Neuropsychopharmacol Biol Psychiatry* 1994; **18**: 447–63.

35 Coffey B: Review and update: benzodiazepines in childhood and adolescence. *Psychiatr Ann* 1993; **23**: 332–9.

36 Kutcher SP, Reiter S, Gardner DM et al.: The pharmacotherapy of anxiety disorders in children and adolescents. *Psychiatr Clin North Am* 1992; **15**: 41–67.

37 Maletic V, March J, Johnston H: Child and adolescent psychopharmacology. In: Jefferson J, Greist J (eds) *Psychiatric Clinics of North America: Annual Drug Therapy.* Philadelphia, PA: Saunders, 1994, pp. 101–4.

38 Popper CW: Psychopharmacologic treatment of anxiety disorders in adolescents and children. *J Clin Psychiatry* 1993; **54**: 52–63.

39 Kranzler HR: Use of Buspirone in an adolescent with overanxious disorder. *J Am Acad of Child Adolesc Psychiatry* 1988; **27**: 789–90.

40 Simeon JG, Knott VJ, Dubois C et al.: Buspirone therapy of mixed anxiety disorders in childhood and adolescence: a pilot study. *J Child Adolesc Psychopharmacol.* 1994; **4**: 159–70.

41 Malhotra S, Santosh PJ: An open clinical trial of buspirone in children with attention-deficit/hyperactivity disorder. *J Am Acad Child Adolesc Psychiatry* 1998; **37**: 360–3.

42 Pishkin V, Shurley JT, Wolfgang A: Psychophysiological and cognitive indices in an acute double-blind study with hydroxyzine in psychiatric patients. *Arch Gen Psychiatry* 1967; **16**: 471–8.

43 Rickels K, Weisman K, Norstad N et al.: Buspirone and diazepam in anxiety: a controlled study. *J Clin Psychiatry* 1982; **43**: 81–6.

44 Goldberg HL, Finnerty R: Comparison of buspirone in two separate studies. *J Clin Psychiatry* 1982; **43**: 87–91.

45 Uhlenhuth EH: Buspirone: a clinical review of a new, non-benzodiazepine anxiolytic. *J Clin Psychiatry* 1982; **43**: 109–16.

46 Wheatley D: Buspirone: multicenter efficacy study. *J Clin Psychiatry* 1982; **43**: 92–4.

47 King NJ, Gullone E, Tonge BJ, Ollendick TH: Self-reports of panic attacks and manifest anxiety in adolescents. *Behav Res Ther* 1993; **31**: 111–16.

48 Black B, Robbins DR: Case study: panic disorder in children and adolescents. *J Am Acad Child Adolesc Psychiatry* 1990; **29**: 36–44.

49 Klein DF, Mannuzza S, Chapman T et al.: Child panic revisited. *J Am Acad Child Adolesc Psychiatry* 1992; **31**: 112–14.

50 Moreau D, Follet C: Panic disorder in children and adolescents. *Child Adolesc Psychiatr Clin N Amer* 1993; **2**: 581–602.

51 Von Korff MR, Eaton WM, Keyl PM: The epidemiology of panic attacks and panic disorder results of three community surveys. *Am J Epidemiol* 1985; **122**: 970–81.

52 Hayward C, Killen JD, Hammer LD et al.: Pubertal stage and panic attack history in sixth- and seventh-grade girls. *Am J Psychiatry* 1992; **149**: 1239–43.

53 Bernstein GA, Borchardt CM, Perwien AR: Anxiety disorders in children and adolescents: a review of the past 10 years. *J Am Acad Child Adolesc Psychiatry* 1996; **35**: 1110–19.

54 Payne K, Mattheyse FJ, Libenberg D et al.: The pharmacokinetics of midazolam in paetiatric patients. *Eur J Clin Pharmacol* 1989; **37**: 267–72.

55 Pollack MH, Otto MW, Sabatino S et al.: Relationship of childhood anxiety to adult panic disorder: correlates and influence on course. *Am J Psychiatry* 1996; **153**: 376–81.

56 Aden K, Thein SG: Alprazolam compared to diazepam and placebo in the treatment of anxiety. *J Clin Psychiatry* 1980; **41**: 245–8.

57 Andersch S, Rosenberg NK, Kullingsjo H et al.: Efficacy and safety of alprazolam, imipramine and placebo in treating panic disorder: A Scandinavian multicenter study. *Acta Psychiatr Scand Suppl* 1991; **365**: 18–27.

58 Maletzky B: Anxiolytic efficacy of alprazolam compared to diazepam and placebo. *J Int Med Res* 1980; **8**: 139–43.

59 Schatzberg AF: Overview of anxiety disorders: prevalence, biology, course, and treatment. *J Clin Psychiatry* 1991; **52**: 5–9.

60 Spier SA, Tesar GE, Rosenbaum JF et al.: Treatment of panic disorder and agoraphobia with clonazepam. *J Clin Psychiatry* 1986; **47**: 238–42.

61 Biederman J: Clonazepam in the treatment of prepubertal children with panic-like symptoms. *J Clin Psychiatry* 1987; **48**: 38–42.

62 Kutcher S, Mackenzie S: Successful clonazepam treatment of adolescents with panic disorder. *J Clin Psychopharmacol* 1988; **8**: 229–301.

63 Ballenger JC, Carek DJ, Steele JJ et al.: Three cases of panic disorder with agoraphobia in children. *Am J Psychiatry* 1989; **146**: 922–4.

64 Woods SW, Nagy LM, Koleszar AS et al.: Controlled trial of alprazolam supplementation during imipramine treatment of panic disorder. *J Clin Psychopharmacol* 1992; **12**: 32–8.

65 Sheehan DV, Raj AB, Sheehan KH et al.: Is buspirone effective for panic disorder? *J Clin Psychopharmacol* 1990; **10**: 3–11.

66 Pohl R, Balon R, Yeragain VK et al.: Serotonergic anxiolytics in the treatment of panic disorder: a controlled study with buspirone. *Psychopathology* 1989; **22**: 60–7.

67 Gastfriend DR, Rosenbaum JF: Adjunctive buspirone in benzodiazepine treatment of four patients with panic disorder. *Am J Psychiatry* 1989; **146**: 914–16.

68 Last CG, Perrin S, Hersen M et al.: DSM-III-R anxiety disorders in children: sociodemographic and clinical characteristics. *J Am Acad Child Adolesc Psychiatry* 1992; **31**: 1070–6.

69 Bernstein GA, Borchardt CM: Anxiety disorders of childhood and adolescence: a critical review. *J Am Acad Child Adolesc Psychiatry* 1991; **30**: 519–32.

70 D'Amato G: Chlordiazepoxide in management of school phobia. *Dis Nerv Sys* 1962; **23**: 295.

71 Kraft IA, Ardali C, Duffy JH et al.: A clinical study of chloridazepoxide used in psychiatric disorders of children. *Int J Neuropsychiatry* 1965; **1**: 433–7.

72 Klein RG, Last CG: *Developmental Clinical Psychology and Psychiatry: Anxiety disorders in children.* Thousand Oaks, CA: Sage Publications, 1989.

73 Bernstein GA, Garfinkel BD, Borchardt CM: Comparative studies of pharmacotherapy for school refusal. *J Am Acad Child Adolesc Psychiatry* 1990; **29**: 773–81.

74 Graee F, Milner J, Rizzotto L et al.: Clonazepam in childhood anxiety disorders. *J Am Acad Child Adolesc Psychiatry* 1994; **33**: 372–6.

75 Balon R: Chlordiazepoxide in management of school phobia. *Can J Psychiatry* 1994; **39**: 581–2.

76 Golbin AZ, Sheldon SH: Parasomnias in Pediatric Sleep Medicine. Philadelphia, PA: W.B. Saunders, 1992.

77 McLeer SV, Deblinger E, Atkins MS et al.: Post-traumatic stress disorder in sexually abused children. *J Am Acad Child Adolesc Psychiatry* 1988; **27**: 650–4.

78 Terr LC: Chowchilla revisited: the effects of psychic trauma four years after a school-bus kidnapping. *Am J Psychiatry* 1983; **140**: 1543–50.

79 Terr LC: Acute responses to external events and posttraumatic stress disorder. In: Lewis M (ed.) *Child and Adolescent Psychiatry: A Comprehensive Textbook,* 2nd edn. Baltimore, MD: Williams & Wilkins, Baltimore, 753–63.

80 Donnelly CL, Amaya-Jackson L: Post-traumatic stress disorder in children and adolescents—epidemiology, diagnois and treatment options. *Pediatr Drugs* 2002; **4**: 159–70.

81 Braun P, Greenberg D, Dasberg H et al.: Core symptoms of posttraumatic stress disorder unimproved by alprazolam treament. *J Clin Psychiatry* 1990; **51**: 236–8.

82 Risse SC, Whitters A, Burke J et al.: Severe withdrawal symptoms after discontinuation of alprazolam in eight patients with combat-induced posttraumatic stress disorder. *J Clin Psychiatry* 1990; **51**: 206–9.

83 Feldman TB: Alprazolam in the treatment of posttraumatic stress disorder. *J Clin Psychiatry* 1987; **48**: 216–17.

84 Wells BG, Chu CC, Johnson R et al.: Buspirone in the treatment of posttraumatic stress disorder. *Pharmacotherapy* 1991; **11**: 340–3.

85 Griest JH: Treatment of obsessive compulsive disorder: psychotherapies, drugs, and other somatic treatment. *J Clin Psychiatry* 1990; **51**: 44–50.

86 Hewlett WA, Vinogradov S, Agras WS: Clonazepam treatment of obsessions and compulsions. *J Clin Psychiatry* 1990; **51**: 158–61.

87 Dominguez RA, Mestre SM: Management of treatment-refractory obsessive compulsive disorder patients. *J Clin Psychiatry* 1998; **55**: 86–92.

88 Jenike MA, Baer L: An open trial of buspirone in obsessive-compulsive disorder. *Am J Psychiatry* 1988; **145**: 1285–6.

89 Pato MT, Pigott TA, Hill JL: Controlled comparison of buspirone and clomipramine in obsessive-compulsive disorder. *Am J Psychiatry* 1991; **148**: 127–9.

90 Alessi N, Bos T: Buspirone augmentation of fluoxetine in a depressed child with obsessive-compulsive disorder. *Am J Psychiatry* 1991; **148**: 1605–6.

91 Markovitz PJ, Stagno SJ, Calabrese JR: Buspirone augmentation of fluoxetine in obsessive-compulsive disorder. *Am J Psychiatry* 1990; **147**: 798–800.

92 Grady TA, Pigott TA, L'Heureux F et al.: Double-blind study of adjuvant buspirone for fluoxetine-treated patients with obsessive compulsive disorder. *Am J Psychiatry* 1993; **150:** 819–21.

93 Pigott TA, L'Heureux F, Hill JL et al.: A double-blind study of adjuvant buspirone hydrochloride in clomiprane-treated patients with obsessive-compulsive disorder. *J Clin Psychopharmacol* 1992; **12:** 11–18.

94 Zwier KJ, Rao U: Buspirone use in an adolescent with social phobia and mixed personality disorder (cluster A type). *J Am Acad Child Adolesc Psychiatry* 1994; **33:** 1007–11.

95 Gittelman-Klein R, Spitzer R, Cantwell D: Diagnostic classifications and psychopharmacologic indications. In: Werry JS (ed.) *Pediatric Psychopharmacology: The Use of Behavior Modifying Drugs in Children.* New York, NY: Brunner/Mazel, 1978.

96 Gittelman-Klein R, Klein DF: Separation anxiety in school refusal and its treatment with drugs. In: Hersov L & Berg I (eds) Out of School. John Wiley & Sons, New York, 1980, pp. 321–41.

97 Gittelman R: Anxiety Disorders of Childhood. New York, NY: Guilford, 1986.

98 Pfefferbaum B, Overall JE, Boren HA et al.: Alprazolam in the treatment of anticipatory and acute situational anxiety in children with cancer. *J Am Acad Child Adolesc Psychiatry* 1987; **26:** 532–5.

99 Hennes HM, Wagner V, Bonadio WA et al.: The effect of oral midazolam on anxiety of preschool children during laceration repair. *Ann Emerg Med* 1990; **20:** 713–16.

100 Shapira J, Kupietzky A, Kadari A et al.: Comparison of oral midazolam with and without hydroxyzine in the sedation of pediatric dental patients. *Pediatr Dent* 2004; **26:** 492–6.

101 Samarkandi A, Naguib M, Riad W et al.: Melatonin vs. midazolam premedication in children: a double-blind placebo-controlled study. *Eur J Anaesthesiology* 2005; **22:** 189–96.

102 Karl HW, Milgrom P, Domoto P et al.: Pharmacokinetics of oral triazolam in children. *J Clin Psychopharmacol* 1997; **17:** 169–72.

103 Tweedy CM, Milgrom P, Kharasch ED et al.: Pharmacokinetics and clinical effects of sublingual triazolam in pediatric dental patients. *J Clin Psychopharmacol* 2001; **21:** 268–72.

104 Aman MG, Werry JS: Methylphenidate and diazepam in severe reading retardation. *J Am Acad Child Adolesc Psychiatry* 1982; **21:** 31–7.

105 Petti TA, Fish B, Shapiro T et al.: Effects of chlordiazepoxide in disturbed children: a pilot study. *J Clin Psychopharmacol* 1982; **2:** 270–3.

106 Quiason N, Ward D: Buspirone for aggression. *J Am Acad Child Adolesc Psychiatry* 1991; **30:** 1026.

107 Ratey J, Sovner R, Parks A et al.: Buspirone treatment of aggression and anxiety in mentally retarded patients: a multiple-baseline, placebo lead-in study. *J Clin Psychiatry* 1991; **52:** 159–62.

108 Ratey JJ, Sovner R, Mikkelsen E et al.: Buspirone therapy for maladaptive behavior and anxiety in developmentally disabled persons. *J Clin Psychiatry* 1989; **50:** 382–4.

109 Pfeffer CR, Jiang H, Domeshek LJ: Buspirone treatment of psychiatrically hospitalized prepubertal children with symptoms of anxiety and moderately severe aggression. *J Child Adolesc Psychopharmacol* 1997; **7:** 145–55.

110 Gonce M, Barbeau A: Seven case of Gilles de la Tourette's syndrome: partial relief with clonazepam: a pilot study. *Can J Neurol Sci* 1977; **4:** 279–83.

111 Steingard RJ, Goldberg M, Lee D et al.: Adjunctive clonazepam treatment of tic symptoms in children with comorbid tic disorders and ADHD. *J Am Acad Child Adolesc Psychiatry* 1994; **33:** 394–9.

112 Owens JA, Rosen CL, Mindell JA: Medication use in the treatment of pediatric insomnia: results of a survey of community-based pediatricians. *Pediatrics* 2003; **111:** 628–35.

113 Schnoes CJ, Kuhn BR, Workman EF et al.: Pediatric prescribing practices for clonidine and other pharmacological agents for children with sleep disturbances. *Clinical Pediatrics* 2006; **45:** 229–38.

114 Hishikawa Y. Appropriate use of benzodiazepines in insomnia: Clinical update. *J Clin Psychiatry* 1991; **52:** 10–13.

115 Coleman RM, Roffwarg HP, Kennedy SJ et al.: Sleep-wake disorders based on a polysomnographic diagnosis: a national cooperative study. *JAMA* 1982; **247:** 997–1003.

116 Dahl RE: The pharmacologic treatment of sleep disorders. *Pediatr Psychopharmacol* 1992; **15:** 161–78.

117 Bootzin RR, Perlis ML: Nonpharmacological treatments of insomnia. *J Clin Psychiatry* 1992; **53:** 37–41.

118 Gillin JC: Relief from situational insomnia: pharmacologic and other options. *Postgrad Med J* 1992; **92:** 157–70.

119 Glick BS, Schulman D, Turecki S: Diazepam (Valium) treatment in childhood sleep disorders. A preliminary investigation. *Dis Nerv Sys* 1971; **32:** 565–66.

120 Rapoport J, Mikkelsen E, Werry J: Antimanic, antianxiety, hallucinogenic and miscellaneous drugs. In: Werry JS (ed.) *Pediatric Psychopharmacology: The Use of Behavioral Modifying Drugs in Children*. New York, NY: Brunner/Mazel, 1978.

121 Bonnet MH, Kramer M, Roth T: A dose response study of the hypnotic effectiveness of alprazolam and diazepam in normal subjects. *Psychopharmacology* 1981; **75:** 258–61.

122 Tietz EI, Roth T, Zorick FJ et al.: The acute effect of quazepam on the sleep of chronic insomniacs. A dose-response study. *Arzneimittelforschung* 1981; **31:** 1963–6.

123 Uhthoff HK, Brunet JA, Aggerwal A et al.: A clinical study of quazepam in hospitalized patients with insomnia. *J Int Med Res* 1981; **9:** 288–91.

124 Rickels K, Gingrich Jr. RL, Morris RJ et al.: Triazolam in insomniac family practice patients. *Clin Pharmacol Ther* 1975; **18:** 316–24.

125 Roth T, Kramer M, Schwartz JL: Triazolam: a sleep laboratory study of a new benzodiazepine hypnotic. *Curr Ther Res Clin Exp* 1974; **16:** 117–23.

126 Roehrs T, Vogel G, Sterling W et al.: Dose effects of temazepam in transient insomnia. *Arzneimittel-Forschung* 1990; **40:** 859–62.

127 Kales A, Manfredi RL, Vgontzas AN et al.: Rebound insomnia after only brief and intermittent use of rapidly eliminated benzodiazepines. *Clin Pharmacol Ther* 1991; **49:** 468–76

128 Roehrs T, Merlotti L, Zorick F et al.: Rebound insomnia in normals and patients with insomnia after abrupt and tapered discontinuation. *Psychopharmacology* 1992; **108:** 67–71.

129 Roehrs T, Merlotti L, Zorick F et al.: Rebound insmonia and hypnotic self administration. *Psychopharmacology* 1992; **107:** 480–4.

130 Salzman C: The APA Task Force report on benzodiazepine dependence, toxicity, and abuse. *Am J Psychiatry* 1991; **148:** 151–2.

131 Quinn DM: Prevalence of psychoactive medication in children and adolescents. *Can J Psychiatry* 1986; **31:** 575–80.

132 Lahmeyer H, Wilcox CS, Kann J et al.: Subjective efficacy of zolpidem in outpatients with chronic insomnia: a double-blind comparison with placebo. *Clinical Drug Investigation* 1997; **13**: 134–44.

133 Roth T, Roehrs T, Vogel G: Zolpidem in the treatment of transient insomnia: a double-blind, randomized comaprison with placebo. *Sleep* 1995; **18**: 246–51.

134 Elie R, Ruther E, Farr I et al.: Sleep latency is shortened during 4 weeks of treatment with zalepon, a novel nonbenzodiazepine hypnotic. Zaleplon Clinical Study Group. *J Clin Psychiatry* 1999; **60**: 536–44.

135 Manfredi RL, Kales A, Vgontzas AN et al.: Buspirone: desative or stimulant effect? *Am J Psychiatry* 1991; **148**: 1213–17.

136 De Roeck J, Cluydts R, Schotte C et al.: Explorative single-blind study on the sedative and hypnotic effects of buspirone in anxiety patients. *Acta Psychiatr Scand Suppl* 1989; **79**: 129–35.

137 Carruthers SG, Shoeman DW, Hignite CE et al.: Correlation between plasma diphenhydramine level and sedative and antihistamine effects. *Clin Pharmacol Ther* 1978; **23**: 375–82.

138 Teutsch G, Mahler DL, Brown CR et al.: Hypnotic efficacy of diphenhydramine, methyapyrilene, and pentobarbital. *Clin Pharmacol Ther* 1975; **17**: 195–201.

139 Kudo Y, Kurihara M: Clinical evaluation of diphendramine hydrochloride for the treatment of insomnia in psychiatric patients: a double-blind study. *J Clin Pharmacol* 1990; **30**: 1041–8.

140 Rickels K, Morris RJ, Newman H et al.: Diphenhydramine in insomniac family practice patients: a double-blind study. *J Clin Pharmacol* 1983; **23**: 234–42.

141 Sunshine A, Zighelboim I, Laska E: Hypnotic activity of diphenhydramine, methapyrilene, and placebo. *J Clin Pharmacol* 1978; **18**: 425–31.

142 Borbely AA, Youmbi-Balderer G: Effect of diphenhydramine on subjective sleep parameters and on motor activity during bedtime. *In J Clin Pharmacol Ther Toxicol* 1988; **26**: 392–6.

143 Meulman JR, Nelson RC, Clark Jr. RL: Evaluation of temazepam and diphenhydramine as hypnotics in a nursing-home population. *Drug Intell Clin Pharmacy* 1987; **21**: 716–20.

144 Adam K, Oswald I: The hypnotic effects of an antihistamine: promethazine. *Br J Clin Pharmacol* 1986; **22**: 715–17.

145 Schubert DS: Hydroxyzine for acute treatment of agitation and insomnia in organic mental disorder. *Psychiatr Univ Ott.* 1984; **9**: 59–60.

146 Russo RM, Gururaj VJ, Allen JE: The effectiveness of diphenhydramine HCI in pediatric sleep disorders. *J Clin Pharmacol* 1976; **16**: 284–8.

147 Pelayo R, Chen W, Monzon S et al.: Pediatric sleep pharmacology: you want to give my kid sleeping pills? *Pediatr Clin North Am* 2004; **51**: 117–34.

148 Glassman JN, Darko D, Gillin, JC: Medication-induced somnambulism in a patient with schizoaffective disorder. *J Clin Psychiatry* 1986; **47**: 523–4.

149 Lauerma H: Nocturnal wandering caused by restless legs and short-acting benzodiazepines. *Acta Psychiatr Scand* 1991; **83**: 492–3.

150 Reid WH, Haffke EA, Chu CC: Diazepam in intractable sleepwalking: a pilot study. *Hillside J Clin Psychiatry* 1984; **6**: 49–55.

151 Cooper AJ: Treatment of coexistant night terrors and somnambulism in adults with imipramine and diazepam. *J Clin Psychiatry* 1987; **48**: 209–10.

152 Linscheid TR, Rasnake LK: Sleep disorders in children and adolescents. In: Garfinkel BD, Carlson GA, Weller EB (eds) *Psychiatric Disorders in Children and Adolescents.* Philadelphia, PA: WB Saunders, 1990.

153 Fisher C, Kahn E, Edwards A et al.: A psychophysiological study of nightmares and night terrors. The suppression of stage 4 night terrors with diazepam. *Arch Gen Psychiatry* 1973; **28**: 252–9.

154 Popovicu L, Corfariu O: Efficacy and safety of midazolam in the treatment of night terrors in children. *Br J Clin Pharmacol* 1983; **16**: 97S–102S.

155 Schenck CH, Bundle SR, Patterson AL et al.: Rapid eye movement sleep behavior disorder. A treatable parasomnia affecting older adults. *J Amer Med Assoc* 1987; **257**: 1786–9.

156 Schenck CH, Bundle SR, Smith SA et al.: REM behavior disorder in a 10-year old girl and aperiodic TEM and NREM sleep movements in an 8-year old brother. *Sleep Res* 1986; **15**: 162.

157 Schenck CH, Milner DM, Hurwitz TD et al.: A polysomnographic and clinical report on sleep-related injury in 100 adult patients. *Am J Psychiatry* 1989; **146**: 1166–73.

158 Schneck CH, Mahowald MW, Kim SW et al.: Prominent eye movements during NREM and REM sleep behavior disorder associated with Fluoxetine treatment of depression and obsessive compulsive disorder. *Sleep* 1992; **15**: 226–35.

159 *Physicians Desk Reference*, 64th edn. PDR Network, LLC: Montvale, NJ.

160 Green WH: *Child and Adolescent Psychopharmacology*, 3rd edn. Philadelphia, PA: Lippincot Williams & Wilkins, 2010.

161 Ornoy A, Arnon J, Shechtman S et al.: Is benzodiazepine use during pregnancy really teratogenic? *Reproductive Toxicology* 1998; **12**: 511–15.

162 Iqbal MM, Sobhan T, Ryals T: Effects of commonly used benzodiazepines on the fetus, the neonate, and the nursing infant. *Psychiatric Services* 2002; **53**: 39–49.

163 Wikner BN, Stiller CO, Bergman U et al.: Use of bendoziazepines and benzodiazepine receptor agonists during pregnancy: neonatal outcome and congenital malformations. *Pharmacoepidemiol Drug Saf* 2007; **16**: 1203–10.

164 Mattila MJ, Aranko K, Seppala T: Acute effects of buspirone and alcohol on psychomotor skills. *J Clin Psychiatry* 1982; **42**: 56–61.

165 Rall TW: Hypnotics and sedatives: ethanol. In: Gilman AF, Rall TW, Nies AS, Taylor P (eds) *Goodman and Gilman's The Pharmacological Basis of Therapeutics*, 8th edn. New York, NY: Pergamon, 1990.

166 Tollefson GD, Montague-Clouse J, Tollefson SL: Treatment of comorbid generalized anxiety in a recently detoxified alcoholic population with a selective serotonergic drug (buspirone). *J Clin Psychopharmacol* 1992; **12**: 19–26.

167 Sellers EM, Schneiderman JF, Romach MK et al.: Comparative drug effects and abuse liability of lorazepam, buspirone, and secobarbital in nondependent subjects. *J Clin Psychopharmacol* 1992; **12**: 79–85.

168 Hyman S, Arana G: *Handbook of Psychiatric Drug Therapy*. Boston, MA: Little, Brown & Co, 1987.

CHAPTER 14

Adrenergic Agents in Child and Adolescent Psychiatry*

*Lawrence David Scahill***

Yale Child Study Center, New Haven, USA

Clonidine and guanfacine

Clonidine, an alpha-2 adrenergic agonist with known antihypertensive efficacy, has been used in the treatment of Tourette syndrome, Attention-deficit hyperactivity disorder (ADHD), pervasive developmental disorders and substance abuse since the late 1970s [1, 2]. Interest in guanfacine has emerged since the early 1990s for the treatment of ADHD and Tourette syndrome (TS) [3]. Although commonly used in practice, clonidine was not approved by the U.S. Food and Drug Administration for any indication in children until late 2010. At that time, a new extended release formulation of clonidine was approved for the treatment of children with ADHD. An extended release formulation of guanfacine was approved for the treatment of children with ADHD in 2009.

Clonidine activates presynaptic alpha-2 receptors on norepinephrine neurons in the locus coeruleus. These neurons are known to play a role in arousal, heart rate and blood pressure. Stimulation of these receptors results in reduced firing of these neurons and inhibition of central noradrenergic system through negative feedback. This mechanism of action fits with the longstanding belief that the hyperactivity, impulsiveness and distractibility in children with ADHD are due to overarousal. Based on accumulated preclinical evidence since the late 1980s, guanfacine has been shown to stimulate alpha-2 receptors in the prefrontal cortex (PFC). This action may improve attention and decrease impulsive behavior with less

*This work was partially supported by Yale, RUPP grant U10MH66764; Yale CTSA grant, UL1 RR024139, Yale STAART grant, U54-MH066494.

**Dr. Scahill's disclosures: Boehringer-Ingelheim, consultant; NeuroSearch, consultant; Pfizer, consultant; Shire, research support; Seaside, research support.

sedation [3]. The differences between guanfacine and clonidine are described in greater detail below.

Chemical properties
See Table 14.1 and Figure 14.1.

Clonidine
Oral clonidine is rapidly and almost completely absorbed from the GI tract. The half-life is eight to 16 hours and peak plasma concentrations occur within one to three hours. It is lipophilic and crosses the blood-brain barrier easily. Clonidine has no active metabolites; 35% metabolized in the liver and 65% excreted unchanged in the urine [4]. In keeping with peak plasma levels, sedation effects are most prominent 30 to 90 minutes after oral dose. The effects on target behaviors such as hyperactivity, impulsiveness or tics last from two to six hours—resulting in the need for multiple doses during the day. This is in contrast to its antihypertensive and cardiac effects, which begin within a half hour to one hour of ingestion and last for six to eight hours [4].

Skin patch
Clonidine is also available as a weekly transdermal patch. The clonidine skin patch is available in proprietary form: Catapres-TTS 1, 2, and 3, which correspond to oral clonidine doses of 0.1, 0.2, and 0.3 mg per day. Recently a generic transdermal product has become available. This product is less expensive but initial experience suggests that it may not adhere as well as the branded product. The chief advantage of the patch is more even dosing throughout the day. Plasma concentration of clonidine depends on the dose of the patch and creatinine clearance. In healthy children, renal function is normal and an unlikely source of variability in response.

One common question raised by parents is whether the child can engage in swimming. The clonidine skin patch appears to be resilient to brief water exposure such as the shower or bath. But the patch may fall off after extended exposure, such as swimming for several hours. Some parents develop ingenious solutions such as placing a large band-aid over the patch. Whether such solutions affect the drug delivery is not known. Thus, parents should be advised to check on the adherence of the patch and evidence of continued benefits after long exposure to water.

In late 2010, the U.S. Food and Drug Administration approved an extended-release formulation of clonidine to be sold under the trade name, Kapvay. When available, the product will come in a 0.1 mg and 0.2 mg tablet. As with many other extended release compounds, this product cannot be crushed or cut in half. The package insert [5] (available at

Table 14.1 Pharmacokinetic properties of adrenergic agents

Generic name	Selectivity	Peak plasma concentration (hours)	Plasma half-life (hours)	Metabolism and excretion	Comments
Clonidine*	Alpha-2	1–3	8–12	35% hepatic and 65% renal	Highly lipophilic; easily penetrates blood-brain barrier
Guanfacine*	Alpha-2	1–4	12–24	Renal	May be better tolerated by children and adolescents than clonidine with fewer adverse effects
Propranolol	Beta-1 and Beta-2	1–2	4–6	Hepatic	Highly lipophilic; potent central and peripheral effects
Nadolol	Beta-1 and Beta-2	2–4	20	Renal	Hydrophilic, low bioavailability, does not easily cross blood-brain barrier
Pindolol	Beta-1 and Beta-2	1–2	3–4	50% Hepatic	5HT 1A receptor antagonist

5HT-1A = 5-Hydroxy-tryptamine-1A.

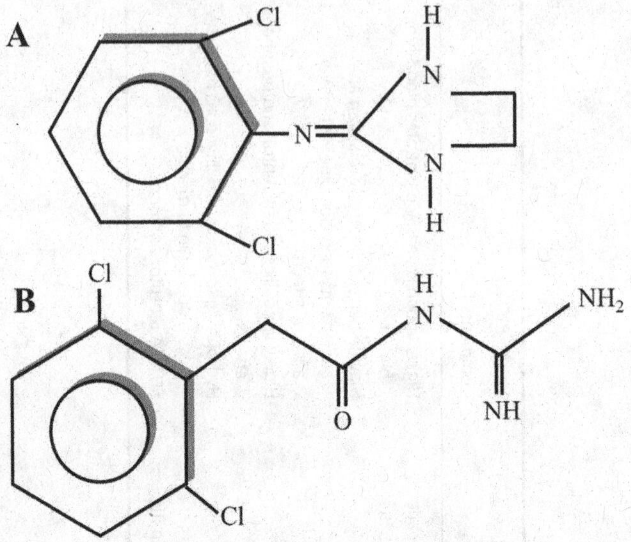

Figure 14.1 (A) Molecular structure of clonidine. (B) Molecular structure of guanfacine.

www.accessdata.fda.gov/drugsatfda_docs/label/2010/022331s001s002lbl. pdf) indicates this formulation should be administered twice a day (morning and bedtime). This extended release clonidine is approved as monotherapy for ADHD or as adjunctive treatment with a stimulant. Results of two clinical trials are summarized on the FDA website. In the monotherapy trial, doses tested were 0.2 mg and 0.4 mg per day versus placebo. The same dosing strategy was used in the combined treatment trial with methylphenidate. Common adverse effects included sedation, fatigue, sleep disturbance and irritability. Hypotension and bradycardia appeared to be dose dependent—both occurring more often in the 0.4 mg/day dose level. Neither complaint was reported as the reason for treatment discontinuation. It is not clear at present whether the total daily dose of the new formulation should be considered "equivalent" to the existing immediate release compound.

Another extended release compound, sold under the trade name Nexiclon, was also approved for the treatment of adults with hypertension [6]. This product is administered once daily. There is not yet any information on the use of this extended release formulation of clonidine in pediatric patients for any purpose.

Case history

M.—a 9-year-old boy with ADHD, who had been started on methylphenidate nine months previously by his pediatrician, developed a dramatic increase in multiple motor and phonic tics. At the evaluation session, the child psychiatrist learned that M. had a history of mild tics that went unnoticed except by those who knew him well. Over the prior 4 to 6 weeks, multiple tics emerged that were noticed by others and evident during the examination. According to his mother, his tics occurred in all settings and often disrupted the classroom. For the first six months of stimulant treatment, M. had been on methylphenidate 10 mg (morning and noon) and 5 mg at 4 p.m. About two months prior to the consultation, the dose was raised to 15 mg (morning and noon) and 10 mg at 4 pm.

On examination, M. was healthy. He had received regular primary care from his pediatrician. His last physical examination was six months before the consultation and was normal. The family history was remarkable for positive history of tics in a maternal uncle and the maternal grandfather. There was no history of seizure disorder. Neurologic examination of the patient was unremarkable except for tics and vocalizations.

Immediately prior to the consultation, the pediatrician lowered the methylphenidate to the prior dose. Because the tics remained unchanged at the time of the consultation, the child psychiatrist recommended a two-step taper in order to discontinue the stimulant. Before starting the taper, the child psychiatrist obtained standard ADHD ratings from the parents and the classroom (e.g., the ADHD Rating Scale) [7]. Although it could not be completely attributed to the discontinuation of the stimulant, a month later his tics were rated as much better. Off medication, ADHD ratings by both parent and teacher showed return of ADHD target symptoms.

Clonidine, 0.05 mg (half of a 0.1 mg tablet), was initiated at bedtime. Four days later, a dose of 0.05 mg was added in the morning. Subsequently, the dose was increased by a 0.05 mg increment every four days to an ultimate dose of 0.05 mg at 8 a.m., 12 noon, 4 p.m. and 8 p.m. His mother reported a modest decrease in tics and some improvement in ADHD (corroborated by teacher ADHD rating). Given the stability of his tics and incomplete response to clonidine for ADHD, methylphenidate was reintroduced at 5 mg (morning and noon) and 2.5 at 4 p.m.; then increased to 10, 10 and 5 mg doses on the same schedule. Tics remained stable and ADHD symptoms improved at school and at home. This treatment plan is consistent with a study by the TS Study Group [8] (see below).

Clinical applications of clonidine
See Box 14.1.

Treatment of ADHD
Stimulants are the first-line treatments for ADHD (see Chapter 6). However, some families may be opposed to using stimulant medication and some children do not show positive response to stimulants. Thus, there is a place for nonstimulants such as clonidine and guanfacine in the treatment of ADHD.

Box 14.1   Clinical applications for clonidine and guanfacine in children and adolescents

FDA-approved indications:
- Extended-release guanfacine approved for ADHD in children 5 to 17 years
- Extended release clonidine approved for ADHD in children 6 to 17 years

Uses with empirical evidence:
- TS
- ADHD
- ADHD in combination with psychostimulant*
- Sleep latency problems (spontaneous or stimulant-induced in ADHD) (clonidine > guanfacine)

Possible uses:
- Hyperactivity in developmental disorders (e.g., autism, fragile-X syndrome)
- PTSD

ADHD = attention deficit hyperactivity disorder; FDA = Food and Drug Administration; TS = Tourettes syndrome; PTSD = post traumatic stress disorder.
*Two recently extended release clonidine products have been approved (Nexiclon and Kapvay). Kapvay is approved for the treatment of children with ADHD as monotherapy or in combination with a psychostimulant. Nexiclon is approved for the treatment of adults with hypertension.

Early trials with clonidine targeting ADHD have been extensively reviewed by Connor [9]. The review noted that many of these early studies involved small sample sizes and provided somewhat mixed results. Overall, however, clonidine was judged to be superior to placebo. Since then, a federally funded trial was completed and provides useful information on the use of clonidine in children with ADHD with TS [8]. As in the above case example, children with TS often have ADHD. For example, up to two-thirds of clinically ascertained children with TS have ADHD [10]. Traditionally, stimulant medications have been avoided in children with tic disorders due to concern about tic exacerbation. Although stimulant medication may increase tics in some cases, accumulated data from several studies over the past two decades challenge this absolute contraindication (see [11] for a review).

In a four-group, 16-week trial, 136 children (age seven to 14 years) were randomly assigned to clonidine, methylphenidate (MPH), the combination of clonidine + MPH or placebo [8]. In the MPH only group, the mean dose was approximately 26 mg/day given in two divided doses; the mean dose of clonidine was 0.25 mg/day given in two or three doses. Doses of each active drug were similar when administered in the combined treatment group. All three active treatments were superior to placebo, but the magnitude of the effect was modest for the monotherapies. After adjusting for placebo, there was a 21% decrease on the Conners' Teacher Questionnaire in the clonidine group, 16% for the methylphenidate group and 37% for combined treatment group. Results were similar on parent ratings. There was a modest improvement in tics for all active treatment groups and no difference between groups. In all treatment groups, including placebo, approximately 20% of subjects reported an increase in tics. Sedation was more common in the clonidine only group and insomnia was more common in the methylphenidate group. Combined treatment appeared to attenuate both of these adverse effects [8].

Palumbo et al. [12] conducted a trial with the same four-group design in 122 children (age seven to 12 years of age) with ADHD uncomplicated by TS. The average dose of clonidine alone, methylphenidate alone and combined treatments were similar to the prior study conducted by the TS Study Group. In the Palumbo et al. [12] study, neither clonidine alone nor methylphenidate alone was superior to placebo on the Conners' Teacher Questionnaire. As in the TS Study Group trial, however, the combination of clonidine and methylphenidate showed a significant improvement of the Conners' Teacher Questionnaire. On the Conners' Parent Questionnaire, clonidine showed a significant decrease compared to placebo; methylphenidate alone did not. Combined treatment demonstrated superiority to placebo on parent ratings [12].

This trial included a careful comparison of adverse effects across the four groups. In the clonidine-only group, drowsiness, bradycardia and hypotension were more common than the other treatment groups, but clonidine was not associated with alterations in the electrocardiogram [13]. Although the rate of study withdrawal due to adverse effects was no different across the four groups, the overall frequency of adverse events was greatest in the clonidine only treatment group.

Treatment of tics in Tourette syndrome

Although haloperidol and pimozide are approved for the treatment of tics for patients with TS, these medications are not considered first line due to concern about short- and long-term adverse effects. The potentially more favorable adverse effect profile of the atypical antipsychotics has also resulted in increased use of these compounds in TS [14] (see Chapter 10, antipsychotics). However, weight gain is an emerging concern with the atypical antipsychotics. Thus, although it is often not as effective as the antipsychotic medications for tics, clonidine is among the most frequently prescribed agent for this condition [14]. As noted above, clonidine is also used in children with TS for the treatment of co-existing ADHD, which contributes to its frequent use in this population.

Despite the common use of clonidine for tics in children with TS, it has been poorly studied for this purpose. Leckman et al. [15] conducted a 12-week, double-blind trial of clonidine versus placebo in 40 pediatric subjects with TS. In doses ranging from 0.3 to 0.5 mg per day in three or four divided doses, clonidine was superior to placebo [15]. This finding has not been replicated in other smaller trials of clonidine in TS [14].

Treatment of pervasive developmental disorders (PDDs) (also called autism spectrum disorders)

The PDDs, which commonly include autism, Asperger's disorder, and pervasive developmental disorder—not otherwise specified, are characterized by extreme deficits in social interaction and communication as well as unusual preoccupations and restrictive interests. The differential diagnosis is based on the presence of symptoms from some or all of these domains. In addition to the essential features, some children with PDD exhibit disruptive and explosive behavior; others are hyperactive and impulsive [16, 17]. Currently, risperidone and aripiprazole are approved for the treatment of tantrums, aggression and self-injury in children with autistic disorder. Medications from several different classes (including alpha 2 agonists) are used to treat target problems in children with PDD [18].

Clonidine is also used to treat hyperactivity and impulsiveness in children with pervasive developmental disorders (PDD) [18]. Evidence supporting the use of clonidine in this population is meager [19]. Although safety is not a major concern, adverse effects, such as sedation and irritability, often occur in children with PDD and often prompt discontinuation [19, 20].

Treatment of sleep problems

Sleep problems (trouble falling asleep, staying asleep or waking too early) are common complaints in pediatric primary care and child mental health settings [21]. Sleep problems also accompany many psychiatric conditions and become a target for pharmacological intervention. Because of its perceived safety and predictable sedative effects, clonidine is often used as a sleep aid in children and adolescents.

Sleep experts recommend behavioral approaches before resorting to medications such as clonidine. However, in cases for whom behavioral interventions have not succeeded following an adequate trial, clonidine may be a useful intervention [22]. The drug may be given 30 to 40 minutes before bedtime and should be accompanied by decreased stimulation from television, video games and loud music to make full use of the peak sedative effects. The typical bedtime dose ranges from 0.05 to 0.20 mg (in older children); doses above 0.3 mg are not recommended. Because tolerance to the sedative effects often occurs with clonidine, the dose often has to be increased to aid sleep onset. Thus, the starting dose should be the smallest needed to promote sleep onset. In addition to monitoring sleep onset, checking for midsleep awakening is also warranted.

Taken together, available evidence suggests than clonidine is safe and effective for the treatment of ADHD, though the magnitude of benefit appears lower than stimulants [12]. The combination of clonidine and methylphenidate appears safe and more effective than either drug alone, at least in some cases. The combination may in fact offset some of the adverse effects associated with monotherapy with either drug. Two extended release products have been approved for the treatment (see below). Clonidine can also improve tics—but the magnitude of benefit may be modest. The use of clonidine as a sleep aid is common. Behavioral techniques ought to be the first line and should be continued—even after the use of clonidine has been initiated.

Guanfacine

The half-life of immediate release guanfacine is approximately 17 hours. Peak plasma levels occur within two to three hours of oral administration and steady state blood levels are typically achieved within four to five days (see Table 14.1). Compared to clonidine, guanfacine is less sedating and is less effective for hypertension [23]. Clonidine binds at imidazoline receptors in the medulla, which likely accounts for its larger effects on blood pressure. The greater sedative effect of clonidine appears to be due to its higher affinity for alpha-2C receptors, located on dendrites of the locus coeruleus. Clonidine also binds to alpha-2B receptors in the thalamus, which presumably contributes to the sedative effects. By contrast, guanfacine is less potent at presynaptic alpha-2 receptors and does not bind to alpha 2B, 2C or imidazoline receptors. The newer, extended-release formulation of guanfacine has a similar half-life to the immediate-release compound (approximately 17 hours). However, it has a more gradual rise in plasma concentration (peak level occurs at about five hours) and longer duration of action allowing it to be given once daily [24].

Treatment of ADHD

Several open-label trials provided initial evidence of efficacy and tolerability of immediate release guanfacine for the treatment of ADHD (reviewed in [3]). Scahill et al. [25] conducted an eight-week randomized, double-blind, placebo-controlled study of guanfacine in 34 medication-free subjects 7–14 years of age with ADHD and a tic disorder [25]. Of these, 23 subjects reported prior failed treatment with a stimulant. The modal dose of guanfacine in the study was 1 mg in the morning, 0.5 mg in the afternoon, and 1 mg at bedtime (range 1.5 to 3.0 mg per day). On the teacher-rated ADHD Rating Scale (ADHD-RS) [7] the guanfacine group showed a 37% decrease compared to 8% for placebo ($p \leq 0.006$)

[25]. Significant benefit was observed on the teacher-rated Inattention and Hyperactivity subscales of the ADHD-RS. Parent ratings also showed improvement—but the difference was not significant. The subjects in this trial had relatively mild tics, but tics also showed significant improvement in the guanfacine group compared to placebo. Guanfacine was well tolerated with no significant decreases in heart rate or blood pressure. One subject in the guanfacine group withdrew from the study because of moderate to severe sedation.

The extended-release formulation was introduced in the fall of 2009. Two large-scale pivotal trials have been completed showing clear bene-fit over placebo [26, 27]. These two trials used a similar design involving multiple fixed doses of extended-release guanfacine versus placebo. For example, in a five-week trial by Biederman et al. [26] 345 subjects (age six to 17 years) were randomly assigned to 2, 3, 4 mg doses of extended release guanfacine or placebo. All subjects assigned to active medication were started on 1 mg dose with weekly increases in 1 mg increments un-til the assigned dose was achieved. Thus, children assigned to the 4 mg dose were on that dose for only 2 weeks. All active doses were superior to placebo. However, the brief duration of the trial and the fact that sub-jects on the 3 and 4 mg dose were observed on the assigned dose for 2 to 3 weeks makes it difficult to interpret the results. The placebo-controlled trial reported by Sallee et al. [27] used a similar design and also provides ambiguous results about the optimal dose.

In a separate study, Sallee et al. [28] enrolled 259 subjects in a two-year open-label trial. Of these, 53 subjects were also on a stimulant [28]. Overall, only 60 (23.2%) subjects completed the two-year study. The figure presented in the report suggests that about half of the subjects re-mained on study for about one year. Reasons for study exit varied and were not always clear. For example, reasons for drop out of 155 sub-jects were described as either: "withdrew consent" or "lost to follow up" or "other." Only 31 (12%) reportedly exited due to adverse events. Whether subjects in the "withdrew consent" or "lost to follow up" or "other" categories were motivated by lack of efficacy or adverse effects is not completely clear. Sedation or fatigue was reported in 59% of sub-jects on monotherapy compared to 11% of those on combined treatment with a stimulant. Not surprisingly, these complaints were more com-mon early in treatment. Bradycardia (heart rate 50 or lower) occurred in 15 subjects; 21 subjects showed a 30 to 60 ms increase in QTc. How-ever, no subject exceeded the QTc threshold of 480 ms. Approximately a fourth of the sample showed a drop in blood pressure (for example, diastolic reading 50 mmHg or lower for children 6 to 12 years). Despite these measured changes in blood pressure, syncope was reported in 2% of subjects [28].

Although the report offers information on dosing, the optimal dose remains somewhat uncertain. On the ADHD-Rating Scale, there was an overall reduction of over 50% in the group treated with extended release guanfacine only. This percent decline in symptom severity was the same across the 1 mg, 2 mg, 3 mg and 4 mg per day dose. Examination of the weight-adjusted dose suggests that 0.05 to 0.08 mg/kg/day can be used as a target dose [28].

Spencer et al. [29] enrolled 75 subjects (age six to 17 years) in a six-week open-label trial of extended release guanfacine added to ongoing stable treatment with methylphenidate (n = 42) or amphetamine (n = 33). To be eligible, subjects had to be rated as achieving a suboptimal response to stimulant treatment. As in the prior trials, the dose was started at 1 mg/day with planned weekly increases. In this trial, however, clinicians were allowed to delay an increase or reduce the dose to manage adverse effects. The mean dose of extended release guanfacine was 3 mg (weight-adjusted 0.07 mg/kg/day) at the end of the six-week trial. Added extended guanfacine resulted in a 50% decline in the ADHD Rating Scale overall. The group on methylphenidate appeared to show greater benefit than the group on amphetamine. Although adverse events were common, there were no serious adverse effects. Five subjects withdrew due to adverse effects (one due to marked fatigue, the other four events leading to discontinuation were not specified). The most common adverse events were sedation and fatigue, which were reported in over 50% of subjects. Twenty subjects showed measureable decreases in blood pressure (of these, 15 events occurred on the 4 mg/day dose). Lightheadedness or syncope was not reported. There were no clinically meaningful changes on the cardiograms for any subject [29].

Treatment of tics

The sample that participated in the Scahill et al. [25] trial also had chronic tic disorder, although the tics were mild. Nonetheless, there was a 30% decrease in the total tic score of a clinician-rated tic severity scale, compared to no change on placebo. In a trial of 24 children with TS, Cummings et al. [30] saw no difference in tic severity between guanfacine and placebo-treated. However, the decrease in tics in this trial was similar in magnitude to that observed in the study by Scahill et al. [25]—suggesting that the small sample size limited the detection of difference between drug and placebo.

Treatment of PDD

The RUPP Autism Network conducted an open-label trial of immediate release guanfacine in 25 children with PDD and hyperactivity [31]. This pilot trial included 23 boys and two girls with a mean age of nine

($\pm$ 3.14) years with a documented history of failed treatment with methylphenidate. After eight weeks of treatment, the parent-rated measure of hyperactivity subscale improved by 40% and the teacher-rated scale decreased by 25%. Twelve of the 25 subjects (48%) were rated as Much Improved or Very Much Improved on the Clinical Global Impression for Improvement. The doses ranged from 1.0 to 3.0 mg/day given in two or three divided doses. Irritability led to discontinuation in four subjects. Other common adverse effects included sedation, sleep disturbance (insomnia or mid-sleep awakening), and constipation. There were no significant changes in pulse, blood pressure or electrocardiogram [31].

Handen et al. [32] evaluated immediate release guanfacine in 11 children (ten boys and one girl, age range 5 to 9 years) with developmental disabilities accompanied by prominent symptoms of ADHD. Approximately half of the participants were randomly assigned to receive guanfacine for four weeks followed by a one-week washout and another week of placebo. The other half of the sample received a week of placebo followed by four weeks of guanfacine and then the one-week washout. The target dose was 3 mg/d (range 1–3 mg) given in three divided doses (morning, noon, and late afternoon). The mean change on the ABC hyperactivity subscale was significant showing 35% placebo-adjusted change; five of 11 subjects (45%) achieved 50% or greater improvement. Drowsiness occurred in five subjects and limited planned dose increases in three subjects. The rationale for this target dose and relatively rapidly increasing dose schedule is not clear.

Taken together, these two pilot trials provide encouraging preliminary results for the use of guanfacine in children with pervasive developmental disabilities accompanied by hyperactivity and impulsiveness. It appears to be better tolerated than clonidine in the treatment of children with developmental disabilities. Compared to typically developing children ADHD or TS, children with PDD appear to be more vulnerable to adverse effects.

Box 14.2   Contraindications to clonidine and guanfacine use

Absolute:
None

Relative:
Co-existing depression (clonidine > guanfacine)
Personal or family history of syncope (clonidine > guanfacine)
Cardiovascular disorders (clonidine > guanfacine)
Renal disease (guanfacine > clonidine)
Liver disease (clonidine > guanfacine)
Raynaud's phenomenon
Diabetes (drug may cause increase in growth hormone secretion followed by rise
   in glucose)

Box 14.3   Adverse effects of clonidine and guanfacine*

Common
- Sedation
- Hypotension
- Dizziness
- Constipation
- Irritability
- Mid-sleep awakening
- Dry mouth
- Sexual dysfunction (delayed ejaculation)

Uncommon
- Depression
- Urticaria
- Skin irritation with clonidine skin patch
- Vivid dreams/nightmares
- Appetite increase or decrease
- Weight gain

---

*Guanfacine associated with lower frequency of adverse effects than clonidine.

The introduction of the extended release product of guanfacine offers new options for treating this clinical population. Guidance on the use of extended release guanfacine for the treatment of children with PDD awaits further study.

Adverse effects

The common adverse effects of sedation and fatigue of clonidine and guanfacine (see Box 14.3) can often be managed by lowering the dose and slowing the pace of dose escalation. Blood pressure and pulse should be measured at baseline and monitored during the dose adjustment phase. Careful attention to sleep patterns before initiating treatment and monitoring change after starting treatment is warranted. Although presumably rare, there have been case reports of mania after starting guanfacine [33].

Clinical considerations when prescribing clonidine or guanfacine

Rebound hypertension

For children treated chronically with clonidine or guanfacine, abrupt withdrawal should be avoided. Rebound hypertension, increased heart rate, anxiety and distress have been documented following abrupt discontinuation of clonidine [34]. The risk of rebound hypertension is lower with guanfacine [35] but gradual taper is also recommended. Considering the immediate release compounds, the rate of decrease can be a 25% drop every three to four days. The risk of rebound effects may be lower with the extended release formulations of clonidine or guanfacine but abrupt discontinuation should still be avoided.

Overdose

Overdose with clonidine or guanfacine can be a life-threatening medical emergency. Characteristic symptoms of overdose include decreased or absent reflexes, lethargy or somnolence, dilated pupils, hypotension and bradycardia, hypoventilation, and irritability. Large overdoses may be accompanied by seizures, apnea and cardiac arrhythmias. The treatment of clonidine or guanfacine overdose includes stopping the drug, monitoring respiratory status and symptomatic treatment of blood pressure, bradycardia, and seizures.

Dose schedule for clonidine and guanfacine

As shown in Box 14.4 and Table 14.2, clonidine and guanfacine doses differ by a factor of 10. Bearing this difference in mind, the dosing strategy is similar. To reduce daytime sleepiness and fatigue, immediate-release clonidine or guanfacine is usually started at bedtime [15, 25]. In school-age children and adolescents, the recommended starting dose of clonidine is 0.05 mg at bedtime (half of the smallest available tablet of 0.1 mg) and 0.5 mg for guanfacine (half the 1.0 mg tablet). The dose may be increased to a half tablet morning and night after four or five days, then a half tablet three times a day (for example, 8 a.m., 3 p.m. and 8 p.m.). Because of the differences in pharmacokinetics, immediate release clonidine is often administered four times a day and three times a day with guanfacine. Thus, a

---

Box 14.4   Guide to use of immediate release clonidine for children and adolescents with Tourette Syndrome (TS) and attention deficit hyperactivity disorder (ADHD)

- Start with 0.05 mg at bed time, add 0.05 mg dose in the morning after three to five days, add mid-day or early afternoon dose after three to five days*
- Common dose 0.2–0.3 mg/day in three or four divided doses
- After stable oral dose is achieved, may switch to skin patch of same dose (adjustment up or down may be necessary)
- Food and Drug Administration (FDA) approved*

---

* In young children the dose may begin at 0.025 mg and proceed with 0.025 mg increments on the schedule described above. A new extended-release product was approved for the treatment of ADHD in 2010. Clinical information is limited at present.

Table 14.2 Guide to use of guanfacine in children and adolescents with Tourette syndromee (TS), attention deficit hyperactivity disorder (ADHD) and pervasive developmental disorder (PDD)

Immediate release	Extended release
Start with 0.5 mg at bedtime, add 0.5 mg dose in the morning after three to five days, add dose at 3–4 p.m. after three-to-five days*	Start with 1.0 mg, increase weekly in 1 mg increments to 3 or 4 mg per day as tolerated**
Common dose 2.5 to 3 mg per day given in three divided doses	Common dose 3 mg per day
Not FDA approved	FDA approved for ADHD

*In young children, may begin with 0.25 mg and proceed with 0.25 mg increments on schedule described above.
*Tablets cannot be broken in half or crushed.

usual maintenance dose of clonidine would be 0.05 mg at 8 a.m., 12 noon, 4 p.m. and 0.1 at 8 p.m., bedtime. The usual maintenance dose of guanfacine is 1.0 mg at 8 a.m., 0.5 mg at 3:30 p.m. and 1.0 mg at bedtime. The dosing strategies with the extended release are presented in Table 14.2.

Beta-blockers

Beta-adrenergic blocking agents are competitive antagonists of epinephrine and norepinephrine at the beta-adrenergic receptors, which are located in the central nervous system and in the periphery. Two broad types of beta receptors have been identified: beta-1 and beta-2 subtypes. Beta blocking drugs differ in their affinity for beta receptor subtypes. For example, propranolol (see Figure 14.2) and nadolol have affinity for both beta receptor subtypes. Atenolol more selectively blocks beta-1 receptors, but has limited use in psychiatry. In addition to antagonist properties for both beta receptor subtypes, pindolol is a beta-adrenergic partial agonist, which may attenuate the heart rate reducing effects of propranolol. Pindolol is also a

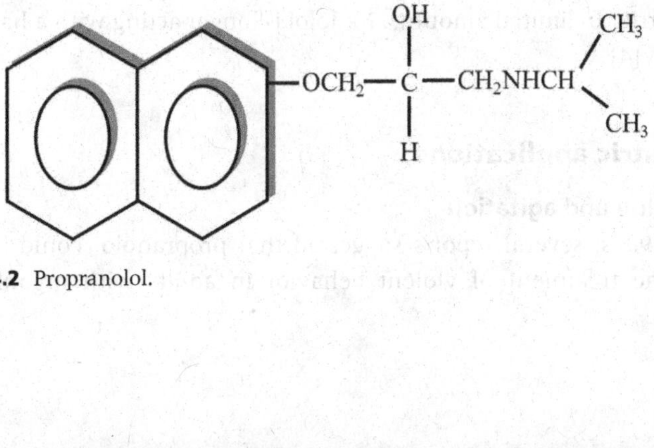

Figure 14.2 Propranolol.

5 HT1A receptor antagonist in the brain, which may have additive effects to antidepressants [36].

The primary effect of the beta-blockers is to turn down noradrenergic activity resulting in decreased heart rate and peripheral vascular resistance (especially in individuals with hypertension) [4]. Beta-1 receptors appear to play the central role in reducing heart rate and strengthening cardiac contraction. Beta-2 receptors are found in glial cells in brain. However, beta-2 receptors are also present in the lungs and blood vessels, where they produce bronchodilation and vasodilation. This effect on blood vessels likely plays a role in reducing hypertension. The relative importance of the central versus peripheral effects of beta-blockers in psychiatric applications remains unresolved and varies by agent. For example, nadolol has prominent peripheral, but little or no central effects [4]. There are over 20 beta-blockers on the market for the treatment of cardiovascular disorders and migraine. Although no beta-blocker is approved for any psychiatric indication, propranolol, pindolol and nadolol are used for various target problems such as aggression, anxiety, ADHD, akathisia and augmentation for the treatment of depression. Support from carefully conducted studies is meager in adults and all but non-existent in children.

Chemical properties

Pharmacokinetic data for propranolol, pindolol and naldolol in children and adolescents are not available. Studies in adults show that propranolol is well absorbed in the gastrointestinal system and is substantially metabolized in the first pass through the liver. Variation in first-pass metabolism contributes to wide differences in plasma levels across individuals [4]. Propranolol has peak effects of one to two hours and has about a four-hour half life. Pindolol is also well absorbed following oral administration and has a half-life of four hours. Compared to propranolol, pindolol is less lipophilic—although it does cross the blood brain barrier. Because propranolol and pindolol are relatively short acting, they are usually administered twice a day. In contrast, nadolol is less well absorbed in the gastrointestinal tract, is far less lipophilic, and crosses the blood brain barrier in limited amounts. Nadolol is longer acting with a half-life of 20 hours [4].

Psychiatric applications

Aggression and agitation

In the 1980s, several reports suggested that propranolol could be helpful in the treatment of violent behavior in adults with organic brain disease [37–41]. Williams et al. [42] treated 30 patients (age range seven to 35 years) openly with propranolol for at least six months. All subjects had exhibited uncontrolled rage and aggressive outbursts and most were already on medication with only partial response. Eighty percent of the children showed improvement on a median dose of 160 mg of propranolol per day (range 50–1600 mg/day) without hypotension. Depression emerged in one child treated with propranolol. A review of available studies in adults indicates that both propranolol and pindolol have evidence supporting their use for the treatment of aggression and agitation. However, for both compounds the evidence is not uniform, with some trials showing significant benefit over placebo and others showing no difference between drug and placebo [43]. Thus, solid empirical support awaits further study.

Post-traumatic stress disorder

Famularo et al. [44] evaluated propranolol in 11 children with PTSD in an open, multiphase study. The dosage began with 0.8 mg/kg/day and was gradually increased to 2.5 mg/kg/day. After two weeks at the maximum dose, propranolol was gradually discontinued over the next three weeks. Scores on a PTSD rating scale were lower while subjects were on propranolol and returned to baseline when it was discontinued. More recently, 29 children (mean age 15 years) identified at high risk for PTSD upon admission to an emergency department of a large North American medical center were treated with propranolol (maximum dose 40 mg twice a day) or placebo for 10 days. The most common type of trauma was motor vehicle accident. Outcome was assessed six weeks after discontinuation of the study treatment. There was no difference between active drug and placebo as measured by the frequency of developing PTSD six weeks post-treatment. Only one subject developed PTSD during the study period [45].

Performance anxiety

Propranolol, in doses of 10–40 mg taken 30–60 minutes prior to performance, has been reported to reduce performance anxiety in adults. Performance anxiety, also known as stage fright, is characterized by physical symptoms including increased heart rate, tremor, dry mouth, hoarseness, and shortness of breath. Propranolol, which at low doses has minimal central adverse effects, could conceivably reduce some of these physical symptoms without interfering with cognition or coordination. However, propranolol has not been adequately evaluated in adults or children to support this claim [46].

Anxiety disorders

Early studies in adults with generalized anxiety disorders have shown that propranolol was less effective than benzodiazepines and antidepressants [39, 47]. The notion that a beta blocker could mitigate the intensity of somatic symptoms of anxiety (tachycardia, tremor, shortness of breath) is plausible. There is less evidence, however, that the cognitive components of anxiety (apprehension and need for reassurance) are improved by beta-blockers. Moreover, given the high frequency of depression in patients with anxiety and the potential depressive effects of propranolol, the use of propranolol in generalized anxiety should be approached with caution.

Antipsychotic-induced akathisia

Propranolol, 30–120 mg/day, given in two divided doses, has been commonly used to treat restlessness and the subjective need to move in adults treated with antipsychotic medications [48]. There is the general agreement, however, that beta-blockers are not effective for the other antipsychotic-induced adverse motor effects such as dystonia or dyskinesia [49].

The Clinical Antipsychotic Trials of Intervention Effectiveness (CATIE) study compared a traditional antipsychotic (perphenazine) to several newer antipsychotic agents (olanzapine, quetiapine, risperidone and ziprasidone) in adults with schizophrenia [50]. Akathisia occurred in all treatment groups. In addition, the partial dopamine agonist, aripiprazole, can also induce akathisia [51]. Taken together, these observations suggest that dopamine D2 receptor blockade may not completely explain akathisia. Recent evidence suggests that 5 HT 2A receptor antagonists such as mianserin and low dose mirtazapine may be better tolerated and equally effective for improving antipsychotic-induced akathisia in adults with schizophrenia [51].

Alpert et al. [52, 53] conducted a pair of trials designed to evaluate the efficacy and safety of adding nadolol to antipsychotic treatment of acutely ill subjects with schizophrenia accompanied by aggression [52, 53]. Both studies were short-term; doses ranged from 80 to 120 mg per day. In both trials, subjects receiving nadolol showed a more rapid time to beneficial effects on psychotic symptoms and aggression. Given that nadolol does not readily cross the blood-brain barrier, these results support the notion that peripheral mechanisms may play a role in improvement of psychotic symptoms, aggression, and akathisia. There are currently no data in children and adolescents. In children, where it is often difficult to differentiate akathisia from hyperactivity, beta-blockers are generally not recommended—unless it can be determined that the motor restlessness is new or significantly worsened following introduction of the antipsychotic. Even in such cases, it may be necessary to reduce the dose of the antipsychotic in order to confirm the role of the medication in the purported akathisia. If lowering the dose improves akathisia, the question is whether the child can remain on the lower dose.

Lithium-induced tremor

Tremor is a frequent adverse event in patients treated with lithium (see Chapter, 11 on lithium). The tremor associated with lithium is often bothersome to patients and noticeable to others. Tremor can occur at therapeutic blood levels and will likely be more pronounced in lithium toxicity. Thus, before starting propranolol, evaluation of the lithium level is warranted. In some cases, decreasing the dose may reduce the tremor to a tolerable level. In pediatric samples, there is insufficient guidance on dosing propranolol for treating lithium-induced tremor, thus, it should be undertaken only after lithium dose adjustment has failed and the tremor is interfering in everyday living.

Attention-deficit hyperactivity disorder

Buitelaar et al. [54] compared pindolol, methylphenidate or placebo in 52 children with ADHD, 7–13 years of age. Under double-blind conditions, pindolol 20 mg twice a day or methylphenidate 10 mg twice a day were prescribed for four weeks [54]. Although pindolol showed comparable benefit to methylphenidate on hyperactivity at home and in school, it was less beneficial than methylphenidate. Moreover, pindolol treatment was associated with parasthesias, nightmares and hallucinations in a few cases. Because of these adverse effects, the pindolol arm of the trial was stopped after 32 patients completed the study. Based on currently available information, the dose of pindolol in this trial was probably too high. Nonetheless, in the absence of data supporting the use of pindolol in the treatment of children with ADHD, it should be used with caution in this population.

Contraindications

Based on experience with adults, propranolol is contraindicated for children and adolescents with asthma, cardiac problems or diabetes [4]. Pindolol and naldolol are also non-selective beta-1 and beta-2 blockers, so these concerns would also extend to these compounds [4]. Clinical assessment would necessarily include review of medical history and measurement of vital signs. In children with a strong rationale for a trial with a beta blocker and a positive history of cardiac problems, an electrocardiogram and cardiology consult is warranted.

Box 14.5   Adverse effects of propranolol, pindolol and nadolol

Common
- Decreased heart rate
- Raynaud's phenomenon
- Lethargy
- Impotence
- Hypotension
- Dizziness on standing
- Insomnia

Uncommon
- Bronchoconstriction
- Congestive heart failure
- Depression
- Hallucinations
- Nightmares
- Nausea

Adverse effects

See Box 14.5.

Clinical considerations when prescribing propranolol, pindolol or nadolol

Before starting a beta-blocker, a careful history of cardiovascular function is warranted and the date of the last physical examination should be documented. To varying degrees, beta-blockers can reduce heart rate and blood pressure. Therefore, vital signs should be measured at baseline, monitored during the dose adjustment phase and during the maintenance phase. If the blood pressure decreases to below 90/60 mmHg or if the pulse falls below 60, the upward adjustment should be delayed and dose reduction considered. As with the alpha 2 agonists, the beta-blockers should not be stopped abruptly to avoid problematic rebound hypertension. Overdose with a beta-blocker is a medical emergency. Bradycardia, hypotension, cardiac arrest, respiratory distress, peripheral cyanosis, psychosis, and seizures may occur after overdose. Treatment of overdose is symptomatic. For example, atropine for bradycardia, digitalization and diuretics for cardiac failure, vasopressors such as epinephrine for hypotension, and isoproterenol for bronchospasm may be needed.

The beta blockers have the potential to interact with several other drugs. For example, propranolol and pindolol rely on the 2D6 pathway in the liver. In addition, they are mild 2D6 inhibitors. Thus, potent 2D6 inhibitors such as fluoxetine or paroxetine, would likely raise the dose of the beta-blocker perhaps resulting in bradycardia [55]. If propranolol or pindolol is to be added to ongoing treatment with fluoxetine, it should start at low doses with gradual increase. Nadolol, which does not depend on hepatic metabolism, might be considered. If an antidepressant is added to ongoing treatment with the beta blocker, sertraline with minimal 2D6 inhibition should be considered [55]. Although MAO inhibitors are rarely used in children and adolescents, beta blockers should be avoided in patients treated with MAOIs due to concern about hypertensive crisis.

Dose schedule for beta blockers

Clear guidelines for the use of propranolol and the other beta-blockers in children and adolescents have not been established. As noted above, doses of propranolol range widely due in part to individual differences in first pass metabolism. The study conducted by Nugent et al. [45] used a maximum propranolol dose of 40 mg twice a day in their study of children exposed to trauma. Doses used in the treatment of aggression are likely to be in the range of 80 mg twice a day [45]. The report by Buitelaar et al. [54] indicates that 40 mg twice a day may not be tolerated by children and adolescents. Pindolol may be started at 2.5 mg twice a day with gradual increases to a maximum of 10 mg twice a day is a plausible and safe dosing scheme for children and adolescents. Nadolol is given once daily. The starting dose might be 20 mg with gradual increases to a maximum of 120 mg per day.

Acknowledgements

Thanks to Michelle Hartman for assistance with manuscript preparation.

References

1 Cohen DJ, Young JG, Nathanson JA et al.: Clonidine in Tourette's syndrome. *Lancet* 1979; **2**: 551–3.

2 Gold MS, Redmond DE, and Kleber HD: Clonidine blocks acute opiate-withdrawal symptoms. *Lancet* 1978; **2**: 599–602.

3 Arnsten, AF, Scahill L, Findling RL: Alpha2-Adrenergic receptor agonists for the treatment of attention-deficit/hyperactivity disorder: emerging concepts from new data. *J Child Adolesc Psychopharmacol* 2007; **17**: 393–406.

4 Hoffman BB: Catecholamines, sympathomimetic drugs, and adrenergic receptor antagonists. In: Hardman JG, Limbird LE, Gilman AG (eds) *Goodman and Gilman's The Pharmacological Basis of Therapeutics*, 10th edn. York, NY: McGraw-Hill, 2001, pp. 215–68.

5 US Food and Drug Administration (Kapvay). www.accessdata.fda.gov/drugsatfda_docs/label/2010/022331s001s002lbl.pdf, accessed February 10, 2011.

6 US Food and Drug Administration (Nexiclon). www.accessdata.fda.gov/drugsatfda_docs/label/2010/022499s001,022500s001bl.pdf, accessed March 20, 2011.

7 DuPaul GJ, Ervin RA, Hook CL et al.: Peer tutoring for children with attention deficit hyperactivity disorder: effects on classroom behavior and academic performance. *J Appl Behav Anal* 1998; **31**: 579–92.

8 Tourette's Syndrome Study Group: Treatment of ADHD in children with Tourette's syndrome: a randomized controlled trial. *Neurology* 2002; **58**: 527–36.

9 Connor DF, Fletcher KE, Swanson JM: A meta-analysis of clonidine for symptoms of attention-deficit hyperactivity disorder. *J Am Acad Child Adolesc Psychiatry* 1999; **38**: 1551–9.

10 Centers for Disease Control and Prevention (CDC): Prevalence of diagnosed Tourette syndrome in persons aged 6–17 years—United States, 2007. *Morb Mortal Wkly Rep* 2009; **58**: 581–5.

11 Bloch MH, Panza KE, Landeros-Weisenberger A et al.: Meta-analysis: treatment of attention-deficit/hyperactivity disorder in children with comorbid tic disorders. *J Amer Acad Child Adolesc Psychiatry* 2009; **48**: 884–93.

12 Palumbo, DR, Sallee FR, Pelham WE Jr et al.: Clonodine for attention deficit/hyperactivity disorder. *J Am Acad Child Adolesc Psychiatry* 2008; **47**: 180–8.

13 Daviss WB, Patel NC, Robb AS et al.: Clonidine for attention-deficit/hyperactivity disorder: II. ECG changes and adverse events analysis. *J Am Acad Child Adolesc Psychiatry* 2008; **47**: 189–98.

14 Scahill, L, Erenberg, G, Berlin et al.: Contemporary assessment and pharmacotherapy of Tourette syndrome. *NeuroRx* 2006; **3**: 192–206.

15 Leckman JF, Hardin MT, Riddle MA et al.: Clonidine treatment of Gilles de la Tourette's syndrome. *Arch Gen Psychiatry* 1991; **48**: 324–8.

16 Research Units on Pediatric Psychopharmacology Autism Network: Risperidone in children with autism for serious behavioral problems. *NEJM* 2002; **347**: 314–21.

17 Research Units on Pediatric Psychopharmacology Autism Network: Randomized, controlled, crossover trial of methylphenidate in pervasive developmental disorders with hyperactivity. *Arch Gen Psychiatry* 2005; **62**: 1266–74.

18 Oswald, DP and Sonenklar, NA: Medication usage among children with autism spectrum disorders. *J Child Adolesc Psychopharmacol* 2007; **17**: 348–55.

19 Ristow A, Westphal A, and Scahill L: Activity in children with pervasive developmental disorders. In: Hollander E, Kolevzon A, Coyle JY (eds) *Textbook of Autism Spectrum Disorders*. Arlington, VA: American Psychiatric Publishing, 2011, pp. 479–92.

20 Jaselskis CA, Cook EH, Fletcher KE et al.: Clonidine treatment of hyperactive and impulsive children with autistic disorder. *J Clin Psychopharmacol* 1992; **12**: 322–7.

21 Owens, JA, Rosen, CL, Mindell, JA: Medication use in the treatment of pediatric insomnia: results of a survey of community-based pediatricians. *Pediatrics* 2003; **111**: e628–35.

22 Ingrassia,A, Turk, J: The use of clonidine for severe and intractable sleep problems in children with neurodevelopmental disorders–a case series. *Eur Child Adolesc Psychiatry* 2005; **14**: 34–40.

23 Ballidin J, Bergren U, Eriksson E et al.: Guanfacine as an alpha-2-agonist inducer of growth hormone secretion—a comparison with clonidine. *Psychoneuroendicrinology* 1993; **18**: 45–55.

24 Boellner SW, Pennick M, Fiske K et al.: Pharmacokinetics of a guanfacine extended-release formulation in children and adolescents with attention-deficit hyperactivity disorder. *Pharmacotherapy* 2007; **27**: 1253–62.

25 Scahill L, Chappell PB, Kim YS et al.: Guanfacine in the treatment of children with tic disorders and ADHD: a placebo-controlled study. *Am J Psychiatry* 2001; **158**: 1067–74.

26 Biederman, J., Melmed, R.D., Patel, A. et al.: A randomized, double-blind, placebo-controlled study of guanfacine extended release in children and adolescents with attention-deficit/hyperactivity disorder. *Pediatrics* 2008; **121**: E73–E84.

27 Sallee, FR, McGough, J, Wigal, T et al.: Guanfacine extended release in children and adolescents with Attention Deficit-Hyperactivity Disorder: a placebo controlled trial. *J Am Acad Child Adolesc Psychiatry* 2009; **48**: 155–65.

28 Sallee, FR, Lyne, A, Wigal, T et al.: Long-term safety and efficacy of guanfacine extended release in children and adolescents with attention-deficit/hyperactivity disorder. *J Child Adolesc Psychopharm* 2009; **19**: 215.

29 Spencer TJ. Greenbaum M. Ginsberg LD et al.: Safety and effectiveness of coadministration of guanfacine extended release and psychostimulants in children and adolescents with attention-deficit/hyperactivity disorder. *J Child Adolesc Psychopharm* 2009; **19**: 501–10.

30 Cummings DD, Singer HS, Krieger M et al.: Neuropsychiatric effects of guanfacine in children with mild Tourette syndrome: a pilot study. *Clin Neuropharmacol* 2002; **25**: 325–32.

31 Scahill L, Aman MG, McDougle CJ et al.: A prospective open trial of guanfacine in children with pervasive developmental disorders. *J Child Adolesc Psychopharmacol* 2006; **16**: 589–98.

32 Handen BL, Sahl R, Hardan AY: Guanfacine in children with autism and/or intellectual disabilities. *J Dev Behav Pediatr* 2008; **29**: 303–8.

33 Horrigan JP, Barnhill LJ: Guanfacine and secondary mania in children. *J Affect Disord* 1999; **54**: 309–14.

34 Leckman JF, Ort S, Cohen DJ et al.: Rebound phenomena in Tourette's syndrome after abrupt withdrawal of clonidine: behavioral, cardiovascular and neurochemical effect. *Arch Gen Psychiatry* 1986; **43**: 1168–76.

35 Wilson MF, Haring O, Lewin A et al.: Comparison of guanfacine versus clonidine for efficacy, safety and occurrence of withdrawal syndrome in step-2 treatment of mild to moderate essential hypertension. *Am J Cardiol* 1986; **57**: 43E–49E.

36 Blier P: Pharmacology of rapid-onset antidepressant treatment strategies. *J Clin Psychiatry* 2001; **62**: 12–17.

37 Yudofsky S, Williams D, and Gorman J: Propranolol in the treatment of rage and violent behavior in patients with chronic brain syndromes. *Am J Psychiatry* 1981; **138**: 218–20.

38 Greendyke RM, Schuster DB, and Wooton JA: Propranolol in the treatment of assaultive patients with organic brain disease. *J Clin Psychopharmacol* 1984; **4**: 282–5.

39 Ratey JJ, Morrill R, & Oxenkrug G: Use of propranolol for provoked and unprovoked episodes of rage. *Am J Psychiatry* 1983; **140**: 1356–7.

40 Kuperman S, Stewart MA: Use of propranolol to decrease aggressive outbursts in younger patients. Open study reveals potentially favorable outcome. *Psychosomatics* 1987; **28**: 315–19.

41 Grizenko N, Vida S: Propranolol treatment of episodic dyscontrol and aggressive behavior in children. *Can J Psychiatry* 1988; **33**: 776–8.

42 Williams DT, Mehl R, Yudofsky S et al.: The effect of propranolol on uncontrolled rage outbursts in children and adolescents with organic brain dysfunction. *J Am Acad Child Psychiatry* 1982; **21**: 129–35.

43 Levy M, Berson A, Cook T et al.: Treatment of agitation following traumatic brain injury: a review of the literature. *NeuroRehabilitation* 2005; **20**: 279 –306.

44 Famularo R, Kinscherff R, Fenton T: Propranolol treatment for childhood posttraumatic stress disorder, acute type. A pilot study. *Am J Dis Child* 1988; **142**: 1244–7.

45 Nugent NR, Christopher NC, Crow JP et al.: The efficacy of early propranolol administration at reducing PTSD symptoms in pediatric injury patients: a pilot study. *J Traumatic Stress* 2010; **23**: 282–7.

46 Ipser JC, Kariuki CM, Stein DJ: Pharmacotherapy for social anxiety disorder: a systematic review. *Expert Rev Neurotherapeutics* 2008; **8**: 235–57.

47 Kathol RG, Noyes 'R, Slymen DJ et al.: Propranolol in chronic anxiety disorders. A controlled study. *Arch Gen Psychiatry* 1980; **37**: 1361–5.

48 Schatzberg AF, Cole JO, DeBattista C: *Manual of Clinical Psychopharmacology*, 5th edn. Arlington, VA: American Psychiatric Publishing, 2005.

49 Fleminger S, Greenwood RJ, Oliver DL: Pharmacological management for agitation and aggression in people with acquired brain injury. *Cochrane Database Syst Rev* 2003; **1**: CD003299.

50 Lieberman JA, Stroup TS, McEvoy JP et al.: Effectiveness of antipsychotic drugs in patients with chronic schizophrenia. *N Engl J of Med* 2005; **353**: 1209–23.

51 Poyurovsky M: Acute antipsychotic-induced akathisia revisited. *British J Psychiatry* 2010; **196**: 89–91.

52 Alpert M, Allan ER, Citrome L et al.: A double-blind, placebo-controlled study of adjunctive nadolol in the management of violent psychiatric patients. *Psychopharmacol Bull* 1990; **26**: 367–71.

53 Allan ER, Alpert M, Sison CE et al.: Adjunctive nadolol in the treatment of acutely aggressive schizophrenic patients. *J Clin Psychiatry* 1996; **57**: 455–9.

54 Buitelaar JK, van der Gaag RJ, Swaab-Barnueld H et al.: Pindolol and methylphenidate in children with attention-deficit hyperactivity disorder. Clinical efficacy and side-effects. *J Child Psychol Psychiatry* 1996; **37**: 587–95.

55 Ciraulo DA, Shader RI, Greenblat DJ et al.: *Drug Interactions in Psychiatry*. 3rd edn. Philadelphia, PA: Lippincott Williams & Wilkins, 2006.

CHAPTER 15

Atypical Psychopharmacologic Strategies

Jess Shatkin & Aron Janssen
New York University School of Medicine, New York, USA

Nonstandard psychoactive drugs, such as vitamins, opiate antagonists, exogenous hormones and herbal medications, are gaining increasing attention in adult and childhood psychiatric disorders. Patients and practitioners have become more familiar with data supporting or refuting the use of these agents in children. It is beyond the scope of this chapter to cover the entire range of atypical psychopharmacological agents, as nontraditional medications constitute today a unique and complex segment of clinical pharmacology. Only treatments that have received some degree of experimental scrutiny will be covered in this chapter, including opiate antagonists, memantine, riluzole, secretin, and topiramate. Given the great increase in the use of herbal medications and dietary supplements since the early 1990s, these products will be covered in the second half of this chapter.

Opiate antagonists

The study of opiate antagonists began with the use of nalorphine as an antidote to intoxication with opium derivatives [1]. Later, naloxone was marketed for human use to treat opiate toxicity. However, several behavioral effects suggested other uses for the drug. Animal studies showed that opiate antagonists reverse the hyperphagia and obesity associated with elevations in endogenous opiate levels [2], decrease social aggression and attenuate drug- or stress-induced stereotypy [3, 4]. These observations led to studies of opiate antagonists for the treatment of obesity, eating disorders, autistic disorder, and self-injurious behavior.

Pharmacotherapy of Child and Adolescent Psychiatric Disorders, Third Edition.
Edited by David R. Rosenberg and Samuel Gershon.
© 2012 John Wiley & Sons, Ltd. Published 2012 by John Wiley & Sons, Ltd.

Mechanism of action

Opiate antagonists block the effects of exogenous opiate derivatives [5]. Morphine-like substances (endorphins and enkephalins) are present naturally in the brain and are released during times of physical pain or stress, accounting for the phenomena of post-traumatic analgesia and euphoria following intense exercise. Opiate antagonists block these effects, and it is through this blockade that their psychiatric effects are derived.

Clinical studies and potential indications

Autism spectrum disorders

The presence of social withdrawal, self-injurious behavior, stereotypies, and sensory hyper- or hypo-sensitivity in opiate intoxication led to the hypothesis that endogenous opioids could play an etiologic role in autism [6]. The first systematic study of naltrexone in autistic children [7] indicated improvements in some autistic (withdrawal, unproductive speech and stereotype) and nonautistic (restlessness and tantrums) symptoms. This group expanded their study in 18 autistic children (aged three to eight years) under double-blind conditions. The treatment group improved significantly on a global assessment scale but not on the specific symptom scales previously employed. Social withdrawal and communicative speech were the areas that showed the most consistent improvements [8]. Reviews of subsequent studies [1, 9] showed that, in children with autism, naltrexone may decrease both self-injurious behavior and stereotyped behaviors while increasing pro-social behaviors. However, because of the heterogeneity of the available clinical trials and the low number of patients, there is not yet sufficient evidence to support the use of naltrexone in the treatment of autism [1].

Self-injurious behavior

Self-injurious behavior (SIB) is a symptom that cuts across several psychiatric disorders [10]. The underlying biological mechanism of SIB has been indirectly related to dopaminergic pathways. Several placebo-controlled studies have reported reduction of SIB with naloxone or naltrexone treatment, but these studies have been conducted on small samples and have been of short duration [11]. Controlled [12, 13] and uncontrolled [14] reports ranging from one [15] to six [13] subjects demonstrated equivocal results. The majority of these studies [14] reported a therapeutic effect for the treatment of SIB with opiate antagonists. However, methodological differences and deficiencies prevail, and some reports [16, 17] failed to demonstrate any effect on SIB. In summary, there is equivocal evidence in support of the treatment of SIB in youngsters with opiate antagonists. Demonstration of long-term clinical benefit is essential because

SIB typically persists for years and the possibility of tolerance to opiate antagonism is uncertain.

Alcohol dependence

The use of naltrexone for alcohol dependence is well established among adult patients [18]. Among adolescents, the research into naltrexone as a treatment for alcohol dependence is limited to case reports and open trials. However, these reports [19,20] show encouraging and positive results and appear to support its efficacy among adolescents.

Eating disorders

Opiate antagonists inhibit hyperphagia in some strains of genetically obese rodents and rodents with high endogenous opioid levels. This effect was initially noted in patients with Prader–Willi syndrome [21] and patients with obesity [22] and bulimia [23], but later studies did not support these findings [24, 25]. Several authors have suggested that a subset of bulimics with abnormal endorphin levels may respond to opiate antagonists [26–28], but current data do not support the clinical use of naltrexone to treat these disorders in humans. In addition, recent animal studies involving melanocortin peptide analogues suggest that these peptides may have an anorectic effect [29], justifying further studies to clarify the links between the endogenous opioid system and feeding behavior [30].

Dosage and administration

Two forms of opiate antagonist are used in psychiatry: parenteral naloxone and oral naltrexone. The onset of action from either route is within minutes. Oral naltrexone is variably absorbed and reaches peak concentrations in one hour, with >90% of the drug being converted to active (6-beta-naltrexol) and inactive metabolites. The approximate mean elimination half-lives for naloxone and naltrexone in adults are one and four hours, respectively. Six-beta-naltrexol has a half-life of 12.9 hours in adults; the half-life of naloxone in children has not been well studied. For autism and autism-related self-injurious behavior, naltrexone has been studied in children in a dosage range from 0.5 to 2.0 mg/kg/day. For alcohol dependence in adolescents, the studies recommend a daily dose of 50 mg.

Side effects and contraindications

In the studies cited above, mild sedation was the only adverse effect in children [8, 31] The manufacturer of naltrexone and naloxone (DuPont^{tm}) also reports mild hepatic toxicity at high doses but not at doses which effectively block opioid receptors. As such, liver function tests may be ordered before initiation of treatment and periodically during chronic treatment to monitor for this rare effect. Insomnia, anxiety, and gastrointestinal upset are listed as infrequent side effects but have not been reported in clinical studies. Abuse and dependence to these agents are not described. There are no reported cases of overdose.

Memantine

Memantine works within the glutamatergic system, is FDA approved for the treatment of moderate to severe Alzheimer's disease, and has been investigated for the treatment of a myriad of psychiatric disorders. Among children, its use has been studied for those with autism spectrum disorders.

Mechanism of action

Memantine is an NMDA receptor antagonist that acts as a noncompetitive open-channel blocker, binding at the site for magnesium. Memantine preferentially enters the receptor channel when the channel is excessively open. As such, memantine is theorized to protect against glutamatergic excitotoxicity.

Clinical studies and potential indications

Obsessive compulsive disorder

Several case reports and open-label trials indicated the potential benefit of memantine for use in adults with OCD [32, 33]. A subsequent single-blind case-control study in an intensive residential treatment program demonstrated the efficacy of memantine augmentation for treatment of OCD symptoms. In the study, patients receiving memantine augmentation had a 27% improvement on the Y-BOCS, and matched, non-augmented controls on treatment as usual had a 16.5% improvement [34].

Depression

One randomized controlled trial, an open-label study, and several case reports have been published on the use of memantine for the treatment of depression [32]. Results were equivocal, but the authors noted that discrepancies related to subject characteristics and exclusion criteria may have influenced the results [35].

Bipolar disorder

Data is limited on the efficacy of memantine in the treatment of bipolar disorder, but two cases demonstrated improvement in the depressive and cognitive symptoms of the illness when given memantine [32].

Autism spectrum disorders

Glutamatergic dysfunction has been implicated in autism spectrum disorders, and several open-label studies and a retrospective analysis have been published on the use of memantine. With most using the Children's Global Impressions Scale (CGI) as a primary outcome measure, the studies demonstrated symptomatic improvement (primarily among behavioral symptoms rather than core autistic features) in those taking memantine [32, 36].

Dosage and administration

Memantine is provided in tablets and solution to be administered orally. It is typically administered twice a day. It is well absorbed independent of proximity to meals. In psychiatric studies the dose ranged from 10–40 mg per day. It is partially metabolized by the liver and partially cleared by the kidneys and has a terminal half-life of 60–80 hours. Dosage should be adjusted for those with severe renal impairment.

Side effects and contraindications

Generally, memantine is a well tolerated medication with few patients discontinuing the drug because of side effects. The most common side effects include pain, hypertension, dizziness, and gastrointestinal distress. One study found approximately 10% of patients administered memantine had a fall during the study [36]. There are no absolute contraindications for memantine, but care should be taken for patients with severe hepatic or renal impairment. More studies are needed investigating its safety in children.

Riluzole

Glutamate is the major excitatory neurotransmitter in the CNS. Its extracellular concentrations are tightly regulated, and high glutamatergic states such as those found with trauma and ischemia are associated with neurotoxicity [37]. The role of glutamate in mood and anxiety disorders has been investigated in multiple studies using peripheral or postmortem measures as well as magnetic resonance spectroscopy. Results of these studies [38] implicate the role of the glutamatergic system in the etiology and treatment of mood and anxiety disorders. Riluzole, a glutamate-modulating agent, is used primarily for the treatment of amyotrophic lateral sclerosis and has been investigated for use in many psychiatric illnesses.

Mechanism of action

Riluzole inhibits glutamatergic neurotransmission in the CNS acting as a neuroprotective agent. In addition to inhibition of glutamine release, it inhibits voltage-dependent sodium channels and blocks postsynaptic NMDA- and kainite-type glutamate receptors [39]. *In vivo* it has neuroprotective, sedative and anticonvulsant properties.

Clinical studies and potential indications

Mood disorders

Initial case reports were promising for riluzole's potential benefit for use in treatment-resistant mood disorders. An open-label trial of riluzole for use in treatment-resistant depression followed, showing significant improvement in the Montgomery–Asberg Depression Rating Scale (MADRS) after six weeks of treatment [40]. Additionally, an eight-week open-label trial for riluzole (in combination with lithium) in the treatment of bipolar depression showed significant improvement in the MADRS [41]. No double-blind placebo-controlled trials have been reported in the literature for children, though studies are underway.

Obsessive-compulsive disorder

As with mood disorders, glutamatergic excess has been postulated as a potential etiology of OCD. Evidence of this claim includes elevated levels of glutamate measured in the CSF of medication-naïve OCD subjects. A small open-label trial of riluzole in children with OCD showed promising results with a mean improvement of 19.7% on the CY-BOCS (Children's Yale-Brown Obsessive-Compulsive Scale) after the 12-week study [42].

Generalized anxiety disorder

In an eight-week trial, 18 adults with generalized anxiety disorder (GAD) were enrolled for open-label riluzole monotherapy. In this study, 80% of completers responded to treatment as measured on the Hamilton Anxiety Rating Scale (HAM-A), and 53% had remitted by the end of the trial [43].

Dosage and administration

Riluloze is provided in a tablet to be administered orally. It is typically given twice a day and should be taken either an hour before or two hours after a meal to avoid a food-related decrease in bioavailability. The typical dose for ALS is 50 mg twice a day, and in psychiatric studies the dose has ranged typically from 100–200 mg per day. In the Grant et al. OCD study [42], patients were given a 10 mg capsule up to 120 mg per day maximum. (The 10 mg capsules were formulated by the NIH Clinical Center Pharmacy specifically for this study). The smallest commercially available dose is 50 mg. Riluzole is metabolized in the liver (CYP1A2) and has a half-life of 12–14 h.

Side-effects and contraindications

The most commonly reported side effects include nausea, weakness and elevated liver enzymes. Less common side-effects include diarrhea, dizziness and anorexia. In rare cases, riluzole has been associated with life-threatening hypersensitivity reactions, including reports of hypersensitivity pneumonitis, elevated transaminases and pancreatitis [43].

Secretin

Secretin is a gastrointestinal hormone produced in the intestine, where its role is well described. Secretin receptors have also been found in the brains of rats and pigs, though its role in the central nervous system in not well understood. Anecdotal reports exist about secretin's potential benefit for autism spectrum disorders, but this claim is not supported by current evidence.

Mechanism of action

The role of secretin in gastrointestinal function is well described. It stimulates the secretion of bile from the liver and plays a role in water homeostasis. Additionally, secretin receptors have been identified in the brains of rats and pigs [44]. Secretin infusion was observed to have decreased the activity of rats [45], but its role in the human brain remains unclear.

Clinical studies and potential indications

Secretin has been studied for the treatment of autism spectrum disorders. Initially, anecdotal reports of improvement of the behavioral symptoms of autism when given secretin led to more formal scientific inquiry. Reports in small-scale studies [46] were encouraging and led to larger studies [47] with more equivocal results. A Cochrane Review carried out in 2005 [48] reviewed all the randomized placebo-controlled trials of secretin in the treatment of autism spectrum disorders. The authors concluded that there is inadequate evidence that secretin is effective in the treatment of autism spectrum disorders.

Dosage and administration

Secretin is administered intravenously and has been used at various doses in published studies. The dosage range in the published studies was between 2 CU/kg and 4 CU/kg, given as either a single dose or administered four to six weeks apart.

Side-effects and contraindication

Secretin had a wide variety of side-effects reported in the various studies. These included worsening of aggressive and hyperactivity symptoms, elevated liver function tests, gastrointestinal distress, rash, fever, tachycardia and photosensitivity.

Topiramate

Topiramate is approved for partial onset and generalized tonic-clonic seizures in children and adults. It has been studied for the treatment of various psychiatric disorders in adults, including OCD, bipolar disorder, schizophrenia, PTSD, and alcohol abuse. In children, data is limited primarily to case reports and open label trials for bipolar disorder.

Mechanism of action

The full mechanism of action of topiramate is not well understood at this time. It is hypothesized that topiramate enhances GABAergic transmission, and it may also inhibit glutamate release by inhibition of the AMPA kainite type glutamate receptor. It is also an inhibitor of several specific isozymes of carbonic anhydrase.

Clinical studies and potential indications

Obsessive compulsive disorder

Several case reports and open-label trials [49] and one double-blind placebo controlled trial [50] support the potential benefit of adjunctive topiramate for OCD in adults. Published studies demonstrate an improvement in CGI when maximum dose tolerable of an SSRI was augmented with topiramate, and the double-blind placebo controlled trial demonstrated a significant improvement in the Y-BOCS compulsions scale but not the Y-BOCS obsessions scale.

Bipolar disorder

Many case reports in the adult literature support the use of topiramate as an adjunctive agent in treatment refractory bipolar disorder, but there is some inconsistency [50]. In addition, no clear evidence supports its use in acute mania. Furthermore, a pilot study of topiramate in acute mania in children [51] was terminated early without conclusive results because of adult data demonstrating no efficacy.

Schizophrenia

There is inconclusive evidence to support the use of topiramate in the treatment of schizophrenia, despite some open-label trials showing a decrease in negative symptoms using the PANSS [52]. There is no evidence to support its use in childhood schizophrenia.

Post-traumatic stress disorder

A retrospective review showed significant improvement in nightmares and flashbacks over the study period [53], but more studies are needed to support its use. There are no studies of topiramate for use in childhood PTSD at this time.

Alcohol abuse

A double-blind placebo controlled trial of topiramate for alcohol abuse has shown promising results [54]. Those taking topiramate had fewer drinks per day and fewer days of drinking as compared to placebo-controlled participants. No studies have been performed in adolescents.

Dosage and administration

Topiramate is administered orally with a peak plasma concentration occurring two hours after ingestion. It is metabolized by hydroxylation, hydrolysis and glucuronidation. About 70% of an administered dose is eliminated as unchanged drug in the urine. The half-life is approximately 21 hours. Topiramate is dosed for adults initially at 12.5 mg to 25 mg daily and titrated in 25 mg increments to an effective and tolerated dose. For psychiatric disorders, this generally ranges between 200 mg and 500 mg per day.

Side effects and contraindications

Topiramate is generally well tolerated by patients. Predominant side effects include but are not limited to paresthesias, gastrointestinal distress, dizziness, memory problems, and somnolence. Cases of metabolic acidosis and acute glaucoma have been reported in both children and adults. Topiramate should be used with extreme caution for those with renal and hepatic disease, given post-marketing reports of death from hepatic failure. Because of its inhibitory effect on carbonic anhydrase, topiramate should be used cautiously in patients with nephrolithiasis and should not be combined with any other drugs that inhibit carbonic anhydrase.

Herbal medications and dietary supplements

The use of complementary and alternative medicine (CAM), such as acupuncture, herbal medications and dietary supplements, massage therapy, and macrobiotic diets, has greatly increased in recent years. It is currently estimated that 38% of adults and 12% of children in the United

States use some form of CAM [55] with total expenditures by Americans totaling $34 billion dollars per year or 11% of total out-of-pocket medical expenses [56].

Herbal medications have grown in popularity consonant with their increase in availability. The Dietary Supplement Health and Education Act of 1994 (DSHEA) renamed "food additives" (such as vitamins and minerals, amino acids, tissue extracts, and botanical products) as "dietary supplements," thereby lessening their regulation by the Food and Drug Administration (FDA [57, 58]. Along with this change in nomenclature, the burden of proof was shifted from the manufacturer of the product to demonstrate safety and efficacy (as is required for drugs) to the FDA to demonstrate that the product presents a health risk [59]. To consumers, this means that herbal medications can be produced and distributed without any proof that they are safe and effective, while allowing manufacturers to make unproven claims about how their products affect the human body.

Numerous epidemiological studies have shown that unconventional therapies, including herbal medications, tend to be used disproportionately by those suffering from anxiety, depression, and chronic pain [60–63]. One study found that 20% of children had taken an herbal therapy for ADHD, often concurrent with their prescription medication. Of great concern is the fact that 70% of these children's psychiatrists, 56% of their pediatricians, and 74% of their pharmacists were unaware of their use of herbal treatments [61–64]. Other studies have shown that up to 60% of families with a child with ADHD have tried dietary treatments [65] and that 30% of children diagnosed with autism spectrum disorder have received CAM treatments [66]. Despite the frequent use of CAM in the treatment of psychiatric disorders, there is little objective data available to demonstrate the efficacy of almost all unconventional treatments for adults and less still for children and adolescents [67, 68]. In addition, there remain no national standards for measuring competence among providers of complementary and alternative medicine [69]. Herbal medications and supplements are not strictly regulated by the FDA, so there is little consistency among different manufacturers of these products, particularly regarding quality, dosage, and potency, which only further complicates their use. There are no assurances that a given product actually contains the active ingredients it purports to contain or that it is free from impurities [70]. Finally, the products themselves are most often not benign, and many concerns about their interactions with other drugs, supplements, and herbal medications have been raised.

There are literally hundreds, if not thousands, of herbal medications currently being marketed in the United States, and their presence is ubiquitous at every consumer level, from herbalist boutiques to grocery stores.

Only those treatments that are typically employed for psychiatric purposes and have received some degree of experimental scrutiny will be covered in this chapter. We focus on the more commonly available treatments in the text below and have placed some of the less frequently utilized treatments in Table 15.1.

Ginkgo (*Ginkgo biloba*)

Ginkgo, the maidenhair tree, is one of the oldest species of trees alive today, dating back 200 million years. The leaves of the tree have been valued in China for their medicinal properties for over 4000 years and have been used for a variety of indications, including asthma, vertigo, and tinnitus. More recently, ginkgo has been studied for use in dementia, intermittent claudication, and mountain sickness [2]. Since 1994, when the German government approved a standardized form of leaf extract (EGb 761) for the treatment of dementia, the use of Ginkgo has greatly increased both in Europe and the United States [71].

Mechanism of action

Ginkgo extracts, particularly the flavonoids, terpenoids, and organic acids, are believed to act synergistically as free radical scavengers and antagonists of platelet activating factor. The result of this activity is improved vascular perfusion due to dilatation of arteries and capillaries, a reduction in thrombosis, and a decrease in the release of inflammatory mediators [72].

Clinical studies and potential indications

A Cochrane review [72] of 36 randomized double-blind trials concluded that, due to numerous small studies and study variability, the data supporting gingko for the treatment of dementia is inconsistent and unreliable. In addition, randomized, double-blind placebo-controlled trials have found minimal benefit from standardized dosages of gingko for the treatment of cognitive performance in patients with multiple sclerosis [73], and small improvements in long-term memory and associational learning tasks among healthy older adults with no effects on young adults [74].

However, more recent randomized, double-blind, placebo-controlled studies in patients with Alzheimer's or multi-infarct dementia receiving 120–240 mg of EGb 761 daily have reported significant improvements in cognitive function [75, 76]. Ginkgo may also have a role in the treatment of other psychiatric illnesses, as Kleijnen and Knipschild noted, in a meta-analysis of 40 studies [77], clinically significant improvement in adults treated with ginkgo for symptoms of anxiety, fatigue, and

Table 15.1 Less commonly employed alternative treatments

Product	Mechanism of action	Clinical studies and indications	Dosage and administration	Side-effects and contraindications
D-cycloserine (DCS)	DCS is an antibiotic that has been used for many years for the treatment of *Mycobacterium tuberculosis*. DCS functions as a partial NMDA agonist, and as such may be important in the neural activity underlying learned associations and extinction of fear	Numerous small randomized double-blind placebo controlled studies have suggested at least short-term benefit from the use of DCS taken before exposure therapy in adults with social phobia [139, 140], acrophobia [135], panic disorder [136], and OCD [137, 138]. One randomized double-blind placebo controlled study of children and adolescents, ages eight—17 years, with a diagnosis of OCD compared 30 youth who received either CBT plus DCS or CBT plus placebo [133]. Though not statistically different, those taking DCS experienced moderate improvements compared to placebo on all scales (CYBOCS 72% average reduction vs. 58% with placebo, CGI-S 57% reduction vs. 41% with placebo, and ADIS-CSR 71% reduction vs. 53% with placebo)	For the treatment of tuberculosis, 500–1000 mg of DCS is generally prescribed, divided twice daily. Dosages in the adult anxiety studies have generally ranged from 50–500 mg taken 1 to 4 h before exposure therapy treatment. In the one study of children and adolescents, weight adjusted dosages of 25–50 mg, 1 h before sessions was employed	Few side effects have been reported in the aforementioned studies but are known to include headache, irritability, depression, psychosis, and convulsions

Table 15.1 (*Continued*)

Product	Mechanism of action	Clinical studies and indications	Dosage and administration	Side-effects and contraindications
ginseng (*Panax* family)	Twenty-five ginsenosides, believed to be the active ingredients, have been identified to date [81]. Ginseng inhibits the uptake of numerous neurotransmitters, including norepinephrine, serotonin, dopamine, glutamate, and GABA in rat brain tissue [71]	Randomized double-blind placebo controlled studies of adults have been mixed—improvements in abstract thinking and a tendency toward faster simple reaction times with no differences in concentration, memory, or subjective experience were found in one study [81], while another found no differences in cognitive function [71]. Positive effects were noted in one randomized study on quality of life ratings among menopausal women [134], but, a second randomized trial of ginseng combined with gingko found no effects on menopausal symptoms, mood, anxiety, sleep or cognition [141]. One trial of ginseng in 36 children and adolescents in an open label fashion who were treated with a proprietary blend of ginseng and gingko for the treatment of ADHD found that 53% reported improvement on the Connor's Parent Rating Scale for inattention, 74% reported improvement for hyperactivity/impulsivity, and 62% reported improvement in oppositional measures [142]	Capsules, tablets, and liquid are all available for oral ingestion; 400 mg daily of oral standardized ginseng was useful in improving cognitive function in the aforementioned study of adults [81]	General side-effects are limited to insomnia, headache, epistaxis, anxiety, and vomiting. Ginseng inhibits platelet aggregation and should therefore be used with caution in individuals taking antiplatelet agents or NSAIDS. Ginseng may act as a mild stimulant, possibly capable of potentiating the effects of MAO inhibitors, stimulants (including caffeine), and haloperidol, and should, therefore, probably be avoided in individuals using prescribed stimulants [143]

(continued)

Table 15.1 (*Continued*)

Product	Mechanism of action	Clinical studies and indications	Dosage and administration	Side-effects and contraindications
inositol (vitamin B8)	Inositol is involved in the transportation and metabolism of fatty acids and cholesterol and is an important precursor in the phosphatidyl-inositol second-messenger system, which is used by numerous noradrenergic, serotonergic, and cholinergic receptors [145]. Patients suffering clinical depression have lowered levels of inositol in the CSF [142], a finding which suggested its utility in the treatment of depression	Pharmacologic doses of inositol have been shown to be effective in one double-blind, placebo controlled study of 28 patients with major depression [146]. These results have yet to be replicated, and two double-blind placebo controlled trials (n = 27, n = 42) found no effect when augmenting SSRIs with inositol [147, 150]. In addition, the STAR-D depression study which employed inositol as an augmenting medication found no benefit [151]. Three small double-blind, placebo controlled studies have suggested efficacy for inositol in the treatment of adults with obsessive compulsive disorder, panic disorder and bulimia nervosa [144, 147, 149]. Inositol treatment showed no benefit in a study of nine autistic children, nor in a study of 11 children with ADHD [148, 152]	A therapeutic dosage has not been established for inositol. In the aforementioned studies, oral dosage has ranged from six to 18 g of inositol daily	No consistent side-effects nor contraindications have been reported to date

Table 15.1 (*Continued*)

Product	Mechanism of action	Clinical studies and indications	Dosage and administration	Side-effects and contraindications
kava kava (*Piper methysticum*)	Kavapyrones act as central skeletal muscle relaxants and anticonvulsants; inhibit sodium and calcium channels; and are believed to increase $GABA_A$ receptor density and cause reversible inhibition of MAOB	Six studies, five randomized double-blind (four of which involved use of a placebo comparison group and one of which used two active comparison medications but at typically subtherapeutic dosages) and one observational, support the use of kava; while three randomized double-blind studies (all of which used a placebo comparison group and one of which combined kava with St. John's Wort) found no effect on anxiety [153]. There are no published data describing the use of kava in children and adolescents	Clinical trials have ranged from 100–400 mg of kavalactones per day. Typical recommendations for store bought preparations would be 100 mg of an extract of 70% kavalactones two to three times daily	GI distress, pupil dilation, blurred vision, and somnolence are most common [81]. Rare cases of hepatitis, hematuria, macrocytic anemia, ataxia, and severe eczema have been reported [71, 154]. The FDA has released a consumer advisory warning regarding the risk of severe liver damage from kava [155]
N-acetylcysteine (NAC)	NAC is a metabolite of the amino acid cysteine and best known for its use in treating acetaminophen and paracetamol overdose. Its metabolite, cystine, is known to reduce synaptic release of glutamate and enhance glial clearance of glutamate, protecting against glutamate toxicity and modulating NMDA glutamate receptors in mood and psychotic disorders	Small clinical trials and case reports suggest that NAC may have clinical utility in the treatment of marijuana, nicotine, and cocaine addiction, in addition to pathological gambling [156]. At least one randomized double-blind placebo controlled trial has demonstrated the utility of NAC in reducing negative but not positive symptoms of schizophrenia [157]. Another study by the same group found similar positive results for the treatment of bipolar depression [158]. One randomized double-blind placebo controlled trial of 45 women and five men with trichotillomania assigned 12 weeks of NAC versus placebo, and after 9 weeks of treatment, 54% of those taking NAC demonstrated a reduction in symptoms [159]. There are no published data describing the use of NAC in children and adolescents	Dosages in studies have varied from 600 mg up to 3 g/day	Side-effects of NAC are generally rare but can include nausea, vomiting, diarrhea, and constipation; rarely, rashes, fever, headache, sedation, and hypotension have been reported

(continued)

Table 15.1 (*Continued*)

Product	Mechanism of action	Clinical studies and indications	Dosage and administration	Side-effects and contraindications
SAMe (*s-Adenosyl-methionine*)	SAMe is found in every living cell in the human body and plays a critical role in the metabolic pathways of several systems, including the CNS. It has been hypothesized that SAMe increases the fluidity of cell membranes, thereby facilitating neurotransmission by heightening the density of receptors or by increasing their efficiency [160]. It is also known to be a beta adrenergic and dopamine receptor agonist	Numerous controlled trials have found SAMe to be more effective than placebo and equal in efficacy to tricyclic antidepressants when given parenterally (either intramuscularly or intravenously) for the treatment of major depressive disorder [161]. Fewer trials support its use when given orally, and less evidence still supports its use as an adjunctive medication for those unresponsive to traditional antidepressants [161], although one recent double-blind trial has demonstrated efficacy [162]. Support for the use of SAMe in children and adolescents rests entirely on a very small number of case reports [163]	Standard dosages for SAMe have not been established. In most studies lower doses have been given by parenteral route (200–400 mg/d) and larger doses by oral route (up to 3000 mg/d)	Because SAMe is a naturally occurring substance, relatively few side effects have been reported in studies other than gastrointestinal distress. Of potential concern are reports of SAMe-induced mania in one patient with no history of mania, arguing against the use of SAMe for individuals with a history of bipolar disorder [165]

ADHD = Attention-Deficit/Hyperactivity Disorder; ADIS-CSR = anxiety disorders interview schedule–clinician severity rating; CBT = cognitive behavioral therapy; CYBOCS = children's yale brown obsessive compulsive scale; CGI-S = childrens global impression – severity scale; CSF = cerebrospinal fluid; CNS = central nervous system; FDA = food and drug administration; GABA = gamma-aminobutyric acid; MAOB = Monoamine oxidase B; MAOI = monoamine oxidase inhibitor; NSAIDS = non-steroidal anti-inflammatory agents; NMDA = N-Methyl-D-aspartic acid; OCD = obsessive compulsive disorder; STAR-D = Sequenced Treatment Alternatives to Relieve Depression.

depressed mood. The generalizability of this data, however, is limited as most of the studies suffered from small sample sizes, poorly defined patient populations, and nonstandardized outcome measures. One recent randomized, double-blind placebo controlled study did find statistical benefit for adults treated with gingko for generalized anxiety and adjustment disorders [78].

Studies of children and adolescents have investigated the utility of gingko for the treatment of ADHD and dyslexia. In the former case, one double-blind controlled trial found that gingko was not as effective as methylphenidate for the treatment of ADHD [79]. In contrast, however, one small study of 15 five- to 13-year-old children with dyslexia found that 80 mg/day given over an average of 34 days led to improvements in reading accuracy, although reading speed was unchanged [80].

Dosage and administration
Ginkgo is available in the United States in liquid or solid form for oral ingestion. Typical dosage regimens are 40 mg three times daily or 80 mg twice daily. Preparations should be standardized to contain 24% flavone and 6% terpene lactones, equivalent to the EGb 761 extract [81].

Side-effects and contraindications
Side-effects of ginkgo are generally mild and include gastrointestinal upset and nausea, headache, diarrhea, anxiety, and insomnia. Though admittedly quite rare, subarachnoid hemorrhage, subdural hematomas, and intracerebral hemorrhage have all been reported in individuals receiving concurrent treatment with anticoagulant medications, likely secondary to ginkgo's effect on reducing platelet aggregation [71]. Simultaneous treatment with anticoagulants should probably be avoided, as should treatment in individuals with impairment in blood clotting.

Melatonin

The precise role of melatonin is uncertain. Its synthesis and secretion from the pineal gland are controlled by the suprachiasmatic nucleus of the hypothalamus and synchronized by ambient light. That is, production of melatonin occurs during darkness and is inhibited during daylight. It is known to be an effective free radical scavenger, to reduce oxidative stress in newborns with sepsis, and to have analgesic properties perhaps related to the release of beta-endorphin [82]. Additionally, norepinephrine stimulation is known to regulate the synthesis of melatonin from its precursor, serotonin.

Mechanism of action

While the mechanism of action has yet to be clearly elucidated, this potent hormone is believed to regulate both circadian and reproductive rhythms. Similarly, melatonin itself is synthesized rhythmically, controlled primarily by the light-dark cycle. Other factors, such as genetic regulation, age, diet, and season of the year, however, have also been demonstrated to affect serum melatonin levels in humans [82].

Clinical studies and potential indications

In recent years melatonin secretion has been found to be altered in numerous disorders, including migraine headaches, epilepsy, Alzheimer's disease, jet lag and other sleep disturbances, and a variety of psychiatric disorders [76, 82]. Extensive clinical trials have not been performed, but much observational and anecdotal evidence has been gathered suggesting an important, but probably not causal, role for melatonin. Pineal gland dysfunction, for example, has been hypothesized to induce the photosensitivity observed in seasonal affective disorder [82] as evidenced by the fact that melatonin administration induces a worsening of depressive symptoms and that light therapy is the treatment of choice. Supersensitivity to light has also been suggested as a trait marker for bipolar affective disorder [84]. Significant alterations in melatonin secretion in depression have been suggested to belie the neuroendocrine axis dysfunction observed, and plasma melatonin levels have been found to inversely correlate with violent suicides. In addition, elevated levels of melatonin have been found in anorexia nervosa and in bulimics during active phases of their illness [85]. Phase shifting and higher nocturnal levels of melatonin have been found in individuals suffering from panic disorder, and melatonin secretion has been noted to be blunted in both schizophrenia and obsessive-compulsive disorder [82].

A meta-analysis of 17 randomized double-blind placebo controlled trials involving 284 adult subjects found that melatonin significantly reduced sleep-onset latency and increased sleep efficiency and total sleep duration, although the effects were extremely modest [87]. Another meta-analysis found no convincing evidence suggesting melatonin is effective for treating insomnia in adults [88]. Children with developmental disabilities, such as blindness, deafness, intellectual disability, autism and CNS disorders, are predisposed to disturbances in their sleep-wake cycle because they often misperceive cues necessary for synchronizing their sleep with the environment [89]. Numerous studies have demonstrated the beneficial effects of melatonin in promoting sleep among the vast majority of such children who are treated [89–95]. In addition, a number of studies have found melatonin effective for the treatment of insomnia associated with autism spectrum disorders and ADHD [96–99].

Dosage and administration

In the studies mentioned above, oral dosages of melatonin have varied from 1–15 mg, far in excess of the amount typically found within the human body at any given time (300 mcg). Dosages available for purchase in the U.S. generally range from 300 mcg to 5 mg and are available in immediate release ($t_{1/2}$ of approximately 40 minutes) and extended release. Two types of preparations are available for purchase—natural or animal-grade preparations (including bovine pineal gland extracts) and synthetic or pharmacy-grade melatonin.

Side-effects and contraindications

Melatonin generally appears to be safe, and tolerance has not been observed [89]. The most commonly reported side-effects include nightmares, headaches, morning grogginess, mild depression, and decreased libido. Based upon the fact that high levels of endogenous melatonin have been found in males with hypogonadotropic hypogonadism and delayed puberty, a theoretical suppression of the hypothalamic-gonadal axis has been proposed. In addition, some studies have found a reduced seizure threshold among children with neurologic impairment. Finally, given that melatonin can cause inflammation, children with asthma and those taking corticosteroids should proceed with caution [100].

Though no contraindications to the use of melatonin are found in the literature, use with sedative/hypnotics or alcohol should be discouraged given the potentially synergistic effects. Additionally, recent concerns both in the United States and abroad regarding mad-cow disease and its human variant, Creutzfield–Jakob, would suggest that consumption of bovine products of CNS origin may be unwise.

Omega-3 fatty acids

Omega-3 fatty acids are long-chain, polyunsaturated fatty acids from plant and marine sources. The two most commonly noted are eicosapentaenoic acid (EPA) and docosahexaenoic acid (DHA). Preliminary studies have identified a possible role for omega-3 fatty acids in the treatment of hypertension, asthma, rheumatoid arthritis, and Crohn's disease [101]. They may also decrease risk of cardiac arrest and coronary artery disease and decrease serum triglycerides.

Mechanism of action

Omega-3 fatty acids are thought to inhibit second-messenger systems, as high-dose therapy has been shown to suppress phosphatidylinositol-associated second-messenger activity. Omega-3 fatty acids also have demonstrated anti-inflammatory and immunosuppressive features [101], which may be useful in the treatment of a variety of psychiatric and nonpsychiatric illnesses.

Clinical studies and potential indications

Randomized double-blind placebo controlled trials of omega-3 fatty acids have generally demonstrated positive results for the treatment of depression and bipolar disorder when used as an augmenting medication. Meta-analyses show benefits, although studies have been heterogeneous and have varied in dosage and levels of the various omega-3 products, EPA or DHA, they have used. Two small double-blind placebo controlled trials of omega-3 monotherapy were not positive, although one of the studies trended toward significance. A third study comparing 20 mg of fluoxetine to omega-3 found similar response rates to both treatments but an even more favorable response when the treatments were combined. Small studies of pregnant and postpartum women have revealed mixed results for the treatment of perinatal depression [102]. Finally, one small randomized double-blind placebo controlled pilot study of omega-3 fatty acids for depression in children ages 6–12 years found significant benefit from omega-3 in comparison to placebo with a greater than 50% reduction in the Children's Depression Rating Scale [103].

Dosage and administration

Effective standardized dosages have yet to be determined but have generally ranged between 1 and 9 g/day. In the aforementioned study of children [103], 1 g/day was given in a 2:1 ratio of EPA to DHA, typical of most over-the-counter products.

Side effects and contraindications

Mild gastrointestinal complaints, such as loose stools, comprise the most common side effects. Omega-3 fatty acids may also prolong bleeding time and should be used with caution in patients taking anticoagulants.

St. John's wort (*Hypericum perforatum*)

St. John's wort is the name of a plant (wort in Old English) that produces bright yellow flowers on or about summer solstice, June 24, John the Baptist's birthday. Extracts of the plant have been used for centuries for a wide range of indications, including anxiety, depression, skin inflammation, asthma, wounds and burns [81]. Over the past 20 years, numerous studies have assessed the efficacy of St. John's wort in treating a variety of psychiatric illnesses. Few of these studies, however, have met the gold standard for clinical medication trials (randomized, double-blind, placebo controlled), and even fewer have compared St. John's wort to a control group using a standard antidepressant. In addition, little work to date has focused on children and adolescents.

Mechanism of action

There has been much confusion about the precise active ingredient(s) responsible for the action of St. John's wort. Hypericin is now generally believed to be responsible for the clinical effects of the herb by inhibiting the reuptake of serotonin and other neurotransmitters. Hypericin extracts generally have a half-life of 24 hours and have been found to show affinity for a wide variety of neurotransmitter receptors, including adenosine, $GABA_A$, $GABA_B$, 5-HT, NMDA, and inositol triphosphate. Though initially believed to have a weak MAO-inhibitor effect, recent literature suggests that hypericin is devoid of such activity.

Clinical studies and potential indications

Linde et al.'s 1996 meta-analysis of 23 randomized trials consisting of 1757 outpatients with mild to moderately severe depression determined that St. John's wort was superior to placebo and as effective as standard antidepressants [104]. The studies compared in this analysis were quite heterogeneous, as were the diagnostic criteria, compliance control, duration of treatment, and dosage regimen of St. John's wort and standard antidepressants, thereby limiting the utility of this data. Two additional reports in the *British Medical Journal* found the efficacy of St. John's wort equal to that of imipramine in adults [105,106] but, once again, limitations have made the data somewhat difficult to interpret. Likewise, comparisons of fluoxetine and sertraline with St. John's wort, although limited in scope, have suggested that St. John's wort is effective in the treatment of mild to moderate depression. Given the limitations of prior work, the National Institutes of Health funded a multisite study comparing St. John's wort with sertraline and placebo in an eight-week trial for adults with moderately severe major depressive disorder, which found that St. John's wort did not separate from placebo [110], nor, however, did sertraline separate from placebo on the primary measure (HAM-D rating scale), although sertraline did separate from placebo on the CGI with a modest effect size (0.41). In contrast, one recent randomized double-blind trial found St. John's wort as effective as paroxetine for treatment of moderate to severe depression and in preventing relapse over 16 weeks of treatment [111]. Finally, Linde et al.'s more recent Cochrane review of 37 randomized double-blind trials found that St. John's wort appears to have utility in the treatment of mild to moderate symptoms of depression but is minimally effective in severe depression [112].

One open-label study has suggested that St. John's wort may have utility in the treatment of obsessive compulsive disorder [113], but a double-blind placebo controlled trial of St. John's wort for OCD was negative [114]. Open label studies have also suggested efficacy for St. John's wort in the treatment of premenstrual syndrome [115], but double-blind placebo controlled studies have been mixed; one study found that St. John's wort was statistically superior to placebo for physical and behavioral symptoms but not for mood and pain-related premenstrual symptoms, [116] while an earlier double-blind placebo controlled trial found that St. John's wort trended toward significance but did not statistically separate from placebo [117].

There are no published randomized controlled trials of St. John's wort for the treatment of depression in children and adolescents. However, two open-label trials have reported positive results. In 2003, Findling et al.: [118] treated 33 children and adolescents, aged 6–16 years, with up to 900 mg/day of St. John's wort and found that 25 of the 30 participants completing the study met criteria for response by week eight (83% response rate); and Simeon et al.: [119] treated 26 patients, 12–17 years, with the same dosage and found that of the 11 patients who completed the study, nine (82%) met criteria for response. Finally, one randomized, double-blind placebo controlled trial has found that St. John's wort is as ineffective as placebo on attention-deficit/hyperactivity disorder [120].

Dosage and administration

The dosing of St. John's wort is difficult to determine and has generally varied in clinical trials. Given that there is little uniformity among the different brand-name preparations available, and that the amount of active product (hypericin) may vary greatly, reliable dosage strategies have yet to be devised. In general, a range of 200 to 1000 micrograms/day of hypericin is recommended for the treatment of depression [81]. In the United States this typically translates into 300 mg three times a day of an extract standardized to 0.3% hypericin. If there is no improvement in symptoms after 4–6 weeks, alternative treatment is advised.

Side-effects and contraindications

Most studies have documented fewer side effects with time-limited treatment of St. John's wort than with traditional antidepressants. Still, St. John's wort falls prey to side effects typically associated with serotonin-specific antidepressants, though generally to a lesser extent. Fatigue, restlessness, and headache are perhaps the most common side-effects noted, at 5, 6, and 7%, respectively, in two studies [121, 122]. Gastrointestinal side-effects, such as anorexia, diarrhea, nausea, and dyspepsia, have generally been reported at a lower frequency, although one study reported their occurrence at 5% [121]. Dermatologic effects have also been reported, and direct sunlight exposure has been noted on occasion to produce blisters, rash, and pruritis [123]. Although side-effects have generally been described as minimal, concerns about the potential for St. John's wort to interact with other medications and herbs has received increasing attention.

St. John's wort is known to reduce the efficacy of digoxin via induction of intestinal P-glycoprotein, thereby resulting in dramatic decreases in serum digoxin levels [124]. Concentrations of indinavir, cyclosporin, and combined oral contraceptives are also known to be decreased by concomitant administration of St. John's wort, resulting in drug resistance in HIV-positive patients, transplant rejection, and breakthrough bleeding (with possible contraceptive failure), respectively [125]. St. John's wort has also been suggested as the cause of mania induction in five published cases [59,126] and a possible cause of cardiovascular collapse during anesthesia [127]. Furthermore, St. John's wort may interact with MAO inhibitors [127] and beta-sympathomimetic amines (such as ma huang or pseudoephedrine [128]) leading to a hypertensive crisis, or serotonin-specific reuptake inhibitors (such as fluoxetine), leading to a serotonin syndrome [116].

Valerian (*Valeriana officinalis*)

Valerian is a pink-flowered perennial, whose malodorous root has been used for centuries as a treatment for nervous conditions, insomnia, headache, stress, epilepsy, colic, and a variety of other disparate conditions [81]. Its use has been approved in Germany for nervousness and insomnia, and it is for these indications that it is most commonly used in the United States.

Mechanism of action

Although numerous constituents have been identified, there is as yet no consensus as to the effective ingredient(s) in valerian. $GABA_A$ and $5\text{-}HT_A$ receptor agonism, along with reuptake inhibition and decreased degradation of GABA itself, have been suggested by animal studies as possible mechanisms of action.

Clinical studies and potential indications

A recent meta-analysis of 18 randomized controlled trials of valerian for the treatment of insomnia found that subjects generally reported an improved sleep quality but that there was insufficient objective evidence from these studies to suggest that sleep had actually improved or been lengthened by treatment [129]. Two small studies, one randomized controlled trial comparing valerian to diazepam and placebo in GAD and another open trial combining St. John's wort with valerian for the treatment of anxiety and depression, are also not adequately convincing of valerian's efficacy [130]. One open label study of over 900 children under 12 years of age taking a proprietary blend of valerian and lemon balm for the treatment of dysomnia and restlessness found significant improvements in sleep for the majority of those treated [131], and one randomized double-blind placebo-controlled trial of five children with intellectual disability found that valerian led to significant reduction in sleep latency and increases in total sleep time and sleep quality with greater benefit among those with comorbid hyperactivity [132].

Dosage and administration
Historically, valerian has been made into a tea by steeping 3 to 5 g of dried root in hot water. Valerian is currently available in capsule, tablet, liquid, and tea form. Dosages may vary, but typically 2–3 g of dried root equivalent given three times daily or at bedtime is recommended.

Side-effects and contraindications
Side-effects are typically rare but may include gastrointestinal disturbance, headache, poor sleep quality, contact allergies, and mydriasis [71]. The use of other CNS depressants along with valerian may potentiate its effect.

Conclusion

Countless medications, herbal treatments, and dietary supplements are currently available in the United States for a variety of unproven psychiatric indications. While evidence of the efficacy for some of these medications is established, the few randomized double-blind placebo controlled studies that have been performed have often contained flaws or small sample sizes, which limit the utility of their findings. In addition, the vast majority of studies have included only adult subjects, providing little data on the effects of these treatments in children and adolescents. Herbal medications and dietary supplements, in particular, are often impure, inconsistent in their potency, expensive, and rarely covered by health insurance. Making matters worse, their use is contraindicated with numerous prescribed medications.

Regardless of the fact that there is little scientific data to support the use of these products, consumers are using herbal medications and dietary supplements in ever increasing numbers. Although it is certainly understandable that our patients would prefer a "natural" herb or supplement to a pharmaceutically manufactured medication, it is important to remind our patients that "natural" does not necessarily mean "safe." Our experience in the United States little more than two decades ago with the amino acid, l-tryptophan, which resulted in the deaths of 36 Americans and over 1500 with serious illness due to the eosinophilia-myalgia syndrome, should serve as a warning to those who would blithely recommend or prescribe such treatments.

References

1 Thompson T, Schuster CR: *Behavioral Pharmacology*. Englewood Cliffs, NJ: Prentice-Hall, 1968.

2 O'Brien CP, Stunkard AJ, Ternes JW: Absence of naloxone sensitivity in obese humans. *Psychosomatic Med* 1982; **44**(2): 215–23.

3 Cronin GM, Wiepkema PR, van Ree JM: Endogenous opioids are involved in abnormal stereotyped behaviors of tethered sows. *Neuropeptides* 1985; **6**(6): 527–30.

4 Skorupska M, Langwinski R: Some central effects of opioid antagonists, Part I. *Pol J Pharmacol Pharmacy* 1989; **41**(5): 401–11.

5 Chabane N, Leboyer M, Mouren-Simeoni MC: Opiate antagonists in children and adolescents. *Eur Child Adolesc Psychiatry* 2000; **9**: 144–50.

6 Deutsch SI: Rationale for the administration of opiate antagonists in treating infantile autism. *Am J Mental Deficiency* 1986; **90**(6): 631–5.

7 Campbell M, Adams P, Small AM et al.: Naltrexone in infantile autism. *Psychopharmacol Bull* 1988; **24**: 135–9.

8 Campbell M, Anderson LT, Small AM et al.: Naltrexone in autistic children: a double-blind and placebo-controlled study. *Psychopharmacol Bull* 1990; **26**(1): 130–5.

9 Symons FJ, Thompson A, Rodriguez MC: Self-injurious behavior and the efficacy of naltrexone treatment: a quantitative synthesis. *Ment Retard Dev Disabil Res Rev* 2004; **10**(3): 193–200.

10 Schroeder SR, Oster-Granite ML, Berkson G et al.: Self-injurious behavior: Gene-brain-behavior relationships. *Ment Retard Dev Disabil Res Rev* 2001; **7**(1): 3–12.

11 Szymanski L, Kedesdy J, Sulkes S et al.: Naltrexone in treatment of self injurious behavior: a clinical study. *Res Developmental Disabilities* 1987; **8**(2): 179–90.

12 Barrett RP, Feinstein C, Hole WT: Effects of naloxone and naltrexone on self-injury: a double-blind, placebo-controlled analysis. *Am J Mental Retardation* 1987; **93**(6): 644–51.

13 Kars H, Broekema W, Glaudemans-van Gelderen I et al.: Naltrexone attenuates self-injurious behavior in mentally retarded subjects. *Biol Psychiatry* 1990; **27**(7): 741–6.

14 Herman BH, Hammock MK, Arthur-Smith A et al.: Naltrexone decreases self-injurious behavior. *Annals of Neurology* 1987; **22**(4): 550–2.

15 Beckwith BE, Couk DI, Schumacher K: Failure of naloxone to reduce self-injurious behavior in two developmentally disabled females. *Appl Res Mental Retardation* 1986; **7**(2): 183–8.

16 Walters AS, Barrett RP, Feinstein C et al.: A case report of naltrexone treatment of self-injury and social withdrawal in autism. *J Autism Dev Disord* 1990; **20**: 169–76.

17 Davidson PW, Kleene BM, Carroll M et al.: Effects of naloxone on self-injurious behavior: a case study. *Appl Res Mental Retardation* 1983; **4**(1): 1–4.

18 Garbutt JC, West S, Carey TS et al.: Pharmacological treatment of alcohol dependence, a review of evidence. *JAMA* 1999; **14**: 1318–25.

19 Wold M, Kaminer Y: Naltrexone for alcohol abuse. *J Am Acad Child and Adolesc Psychiatry* 1997; **36**: 6–7.

20 Volpicelli JR, Alterman AI, Hayashida M et al.: Naltrexone in the treatment of alcohol dependence. *Arch General Psychiatry* 1992; **49**: 881–7.

21 Kyriakides M, Silverstone T, Jeffcoate W et al.: Effect of naloxone on hyperphagia in Prader-Willi syndrome. *Lancet* 1980; **1**(8173): 876–7.

22 Atkinson RL, Berke LK, Drake CR et al.: Effects of long-term therapy with naltrexone on body weight in obesity. *Clin Pharmacol Therapeutics* 1984; **38**(4): 419–22.

23 Sternbach HA, Annitto W, Pottash AL et al.: Anorexic effects of naltrexone in man. *Lancet* 1982; **1**(8268): 388–9.

24 Zipf WB, Berntson GG: Characteristics of abnormal food-intake patterns in children with Prader-Willi syndrome and study of effects of naloxone. *Am J Clin Nutrition* 1987; **46**(2): 277–81.

25 Mitchell JE, Christenson G, Jennings J et al.: A placebo-controlled, double-blind crossover study of naltrexone hydrochloride in outpatients with normal weight bulimia. *J Clin Psychopharmacol* 1989; **9**(2): 94–7.

26 Alger SA, Schwalberg MD, Bigaouette JM et al.: Effect of a tricyclic antidepressant and opiate antagonist on binge-eating behavior in normoweight bulimic and obese, binge-eating subjects. *Am J Clin Nutrition* 1991; **53**(4): 865–71.

27 Jonas JM, Gold MS: Treatment of antidepressant-resistant bulimia with naltrexone. *Int J Psychiatry Med* 1986–7; **16**(4): 305–9.

28 Jonas JM, Gold MS: Naltrexone treatment of bulimia: clinical and theoretical findings linking eating disorders and substance abuse. *Advances Alcohol Substance Abuse* 1987; **7**(1): 29–37.

29 Vergoni AV, Bertolini A: Role of melanocortins in the central control of feeding. *Eur J Pharmacol* 2000; **405**: 25–32.

30 Johnson RD: Opioid involvement in feeding behaviour and the pathogenesis of certain eating disorders. *Med Hypotheses* 1995; **45**: 491–7.

31 Campbell M, Overall JE, Small AM et al.: Naltrexone in autistic children: an acute open dose range tolerance trial. *J Am Acad Child and Adolesc Psychiatry* 1989; **28**(2): 200–6.

32 Zdanys K, Tampi R: A systematic review of off-label uses of memantine for psychiatric disorders. *Progress Neuro-Psychopharmacol Bioll Psychiatry* 2008; **32**(6): 1362–74.

33 Aboujaoude E, Barry JJ, Gamel N: Memantine augmentation in treatment-resistant obsessive-compulsive disorder: an open-label trial. *J Clin Psychopharmacol* 2009; **29**(1): 51–5.

34 Stewart SE, Jenike EA, Hezel DM et al.: A single-blinded case-control study of memantine in severe obsessive-compulsive disorder. *J Clin Psychopharmacol* 2010; (1): 34–9.

35 Ferguson JM, Shingleton RN: An open-label, flexible-dose study of memantine in major depressive disorder. *Clin Neuropharmacol* 2007; **30**(3): 136–44.

36 Erickson CA, Posey DJ, Stigler KA et al.: A retrospective study of memantine in children and adolescents with pervasive developmental disorders. *Psychopharmacology (Berl)* 2007; **191**(1): 141–7.

37 Zarate CA, Manji HK: Riluzole in psychiatry: a systematic review of the literature. *Expert Opin Drug Metab Toxicol* 2008; **4**(9): 1223–34.

38 Kugaya A, Sanacora G: Beyond monoamines: glutamatergic function in mood disorders. *CNS Spectr.* 2005; **10**: 808–19.

39 Doble A: The pharmacology and mechanism of action of riluzole. *Neurology* 1996; **47**(6 Suppl 4): 233–41.

40 Zarate CA Jr, Payne JL, Quiroz J et al.: An open-label trial of riluzole in patients with treatment-resistant major depression. *Am J Psychiatry* 2004; **161**(1): 171–4.

41 Zarate CA Jr, Quiroz JA, Singh JB et al.: An open-label trial of the glutamate-modulating agent riluzole in combination with lithium for the treatment of bipolar depression. *Biol Psychiatry* 2005; **57**(4): 430–2.

42 Grant P, Lougee L, Hirschtritt M et al.: An open-label trial of Riluzole, a glutamate antagonist, in children with treatment-resistant obsessive-compulsive disorder. *J Child Adolesc Psychopharmacol* 2007; **17**(6): 761–7.

43 Grant P, Song J, Swedo S: Review of the use of glutamate antagonist Riluzole in psychiatric disorders and a description of recent use in childhood obsessive-compulsive disorder. *J Child Adolesc Psychopharmacol* 2010; **20**(4): 309–15.

44 Charlton CG, O'Donohue TL, Miller RI et al.: Secretin immunoreactivity in rat and pig brain. *Peptides* 1981; **2**(1): 45–49.

45 Charlton CG, Miller RI, Crawley JN et al.: Secretin modulation of behavioural and physiological functions in the rat. *Peptides* 1983; **4**: 739–42.

46 Horvath K, Stefanatos G, Sokolski KN et al.: Improved social and language skills after secretin administration in patients with autistic spectrum disorders. *J Assoc Acad Minor Phys* 1998; **9**: 9–15.

47 Owley T, McMahon W, Cook E et al.: Multisite, double-blind, placebo-controlled trial of porcine secretin in autism. *Journal of the American Academy of Child & Adolescent Psychiatry* 2001; **40**(11): 1293–9.

48 Williams KW, Wray JJ, Wheeler DM: Intravenous secretin for autism spectrum disorder. *Cochrane Database Syst Rev.* 2005; **20**(3): Article No. CD003495.

49 Van Ameringen M, Mancini C, Patterson B et al.: Topiramate augmentation in treatment-resistant obsessive-compulsive disorder: a retrospective, open-label case series. *Depress Anxiety* 2006; **23**(1): 1–5.

50 Berlin HA, Koran LM, Jenike MA et al.: Double-blind, placebo-controlled trial of topiramate augmentation in treatment-resistant obsessive-compulsive disorder. *J Clin Psychiatry* 2011; **72**(5): 716–21.

51 Delbello M, Findling R, Kushner S et al.: A pilot controlled trial of topiramate for mania in children and adolescents with bipolar disorder. *J. Child Adolesc Psychiatry* 2005; **44**(6): 539–47.

52 Drapalski AL, Rosse RB, Peebles RR et al.: Topiramate improves deficit symptoms in a patient with schizophrenia when added to a stable regimen of antipsychotic medication. *Clin Neuropharmacol* 2001; **24**(5): 290–4.

53 Berlant JL, Van Kammen DP: Open label topiramate as primary or adjunctive therapy in chronic civilian posttraumatic stress disorder: a preliminary report. *J Clin Psychiatry* 2002; **63**(1): 15–20.

54 Johnson BA, Ait-Daoud, Bowden CL et al.: Oral Topiramate in the treatment of alcohol dependence: a randomised controlled trial. *Lancet* 2003; **361**: 1677–85.

55 Barnes PM, Bloom B, Nahin R: Complementary and alternative medicine use among adults and children: United States, 2007. *CDC National Health Statistics Report #12*, 2008.

56 Richard L, Nahin P, Barnes M et al.: Costs of complementary and alternative medicine (CAM) and frequency of visits to CAM practitioners: United States. *Natl Health Stat Report* 2007; **18**: 1–14.

57 O'Reilly PO: Nicotinic acid therapy and the chronic schizophrenic. *Dis Nerv Sys* 1955; **16**: 67–72.

58 Slifman NR, Obermeyer WR, Aloi BK: Contamination of botanical dietary supplements by Digitalis Lanata. *New England Journal of Medicine* 1998; **339**: 806–11.

59 Murri NA (ed.): Focus on natural products. *Drug Therapy Topics* 1996; **25**(9).

60 Astin JA: Why patients use alternative medicine: Results of a national study. *JAMA* 1998; **279**: 1548–53.

61 Furnham A, Bhagrath R: A comparison of health beliefs and behaviors of clients of orthodox and complementary medicine. *Br J Clin Psychol* 1993; **32**: 237–46.

62 Davidson, K: Diagnosis of depression in alcohol dependence: changes in prevalence with drinking status. *British Journal of Psychiatry* 1993; **166**: 199–204.

63 Furnham A, Smith C: Choosing alternative medicine: a comparison of the beliefs of patients visiting a general practitioner and a homeopath. *Science Medicine* 1988; **26**(7): 685–9.

64 Cala S, Crismon ML, Baumgartner J: A survey of herbal use in children with attention-deficit-hyperactivity disorder or depression. *Pharmacotherapy* 2003; **23**: 222–30.

65 Stubberfield T, Parry T: Utilization of alternative therapies in attention-deficit hyperactivity disorder. *J Paediatr Child Health* 1999; **35**(5): 450-3.

66 Levy SE, Mandell DS, Merhar S et al.: Use of complementary and alternative medicine among children recently diagnosed with autistic spectrum disorder. *J Dev Behav Pediatr* 2003; **24**(6): 418–23.

67 Ernst E: Harmless herbs? *Am J Med* 1990; **104**: 170–8.

68 Eskinaz D, Hoffman FA: Progress in complementary and alternative medicine: contribution of the national institutes of health and the food and drug administration. *J Altern Complement Med* 1998; **4**: 459–67.

69 Ernst E: Competence in complementary medicine. *Comp Ther Med* 1995; **3**: 6–8.

70 Martineau J, Barthelemy C, Garreau B, Lelord G: Vitamin B6, magnesium, and combined B6-Mg: Therapeutic effects in childhood autism. *Biol Psychiatry* 1985; **20**: 467–78.

71 Fugh-Berman A, Cott JM: Dietary supplements and natural products as psychotherapeutic agents. *Psychosomatic Medicine* 1999; **61**: 712–28

72 Birks J, Grimley Evans J: Ginkgo biloba for cognitive impairment and dementia. *Cochrane Database Syst Rev* 2009; **21**(1): CD003120.

73 Lovera J, Bagert B, Smoot K et al.: Ginkgo biloba for the improvement of cognitive performance in multiple sclerosis: a randomized, placebo-controlled trial. *Mult Scler* 2007; **13**(3): 376–85.

74 Burns NR, Bryan J, Nettelbeck T: Ginkgo biloba: no robust effect on cognitive abilities or mood in healthy young or older adults. *Hum Psychopharmacol.* 2006; **21**(1): 27–37.

75 Napryeyenko O, Sonnik G, Tartakovsky I: Efficacy and tolerability of Ginkgo biloba extract EGb 761 by type of dementia: analyses of a randomised controlled trial. *J Neurol Sci.* 2009; **283**(1–2): 224–9.

76 Yancheva S, Ihl R, Nikolova G et al.: Ginkgo biloba extract EGb 761(R), donepezil or both combined in the treatment of Alzheimer's disease with neuropsychiatric features: a randomised, double-blind, exploratory trial. *Aging Ment Health* 2009; **13**(2): 183–90.

77 Kleijnen J, Knipschild P: Ginkgo biloba. *Lancet* 1992; **340**: 1136–9.

78 Woelk H, Arnoldt KH, Kieser M et al.: Ginkgo biloba special extract EGb 761 in generalized anxiety disorder and adjustment disorder with anxious mood: a

randomized, double-blind, placebo-controlled trial. *J Psychiatr Res.* 2007; **41**(6): 472–80.

79 Salehi B, Imani R, Mohammadi MR et al.: Ginkgo biloba for attention-deficit/hyperactivity disorder in children and adolescents: a double blind, randomized controlled trial. *Prog Neuropsychopharmacol Biol Psychiatry* 2010; **34**(1): 76–80.

80 Donfrancesco R, Ferrante L: Ginkgo biloba in dyslexia: a pilot study. *Phytomedicine* 2007; **14**(6): 367–70.

81 Greenwald J: Herbal healing. Time Magazine. November 1995; **23**: 58–69.

82 Gitto E, Aversa S, Reiter RJ et al.: Update on the use of melatonin in pediatrics. *J Pineal Res* 2011; **50**(1): 21–8.

83 Pies R: Adverse neuropsychiatric reactions to herbal and over-the-counter "antidepressants." *J Clin Psychiatry* 2000; **61**(11): 815–20.

84 Nierenberg AA, Burt T, Matthews J et al.: Mania associated with St. John's wort. *Biol Psychiatry* 1999; **46**(12): 1707–8.

85 Kennedy SH, Garfinkel PE, Parienti V et al.: Changes in melatonin levels but not cortisol levels are associated with depression in patients with eating disorders. *Arch Gen Psychiatry* 1989; **46**(1): 73–8.

86 Tomoda A, Miike T, Uezono K et al.: A school refusal case with biological rhythm disturbance and melatonin therapy. *Brain Dev* 1994; **16**(1): 71–6.

87 Brzezinski A, Vangel MG, Wurtman RJ et al.: Effects of exogenous melatonin on sleep: a meta-analysis. *Sleep Med Rev* 2005; **9**: 41–50.

88 Buscemi N, Vandermeer B, Hooton N et al.: Efficacy and safety of exogenous melatonin for secondary sleep disorders and sleep disorders accompanying sleep restriction: meta-analysis. *BMJ* 2006; **18;332**(7538): 385–93.

89 Jan JE, O'Donnell ME: Use of melatonin in the treatment of pediatric sleep disorders. *J Pineal Res.* 1996; **21**(4): 193–9.

90 Jan JE, Espezel H, Appleton RE: The treatment of sleep disorders with melatonin. *Dev Med Child Neurol* 1994; **36**(2): 97–107.

91 Pillar G, Etzioni A, Shahar E et al.: Melatonin treatment in an institutionalized child with psychomotor retardation and an irregular sleep-wake pattern. *Arch Dis Child* 1998; **79**(1): 63–4.

92 Wasdell MB, Jan JE, Bomben MM et al.: A randomized, placebo-controlled trial of controlled release melatonin treatment of delayed sleep phase syndrome and impaired sleep maintenance in children with neurodevelopmental disabilities. *J Pineal Res* 2008; **44**: 57–64.

93 Ishizaki A, Sugama M, Takeuchi N: Usefulness of melatonin for developmental sleep and emotional/behavior disorders studies of melatonin trial on 50 patients with developmental disorders. *No To Hattatsu* 1999; **31**(5): 428–37.

94 Jan JE, Freeman RD: Melatonin therapy for circadian rhythm sleep disorders in children with multiple disabilities: what have we learned in the last decade? *Dev Med Child Neurol.* 2004; **46**: 776–82.

95 Dodge NN, Wilson GA: Melatonin for treatment of sleep disorders in children with developmental disabilities. *J Child Neurol* 2001; **16980**: 581–4.

96 Weiss MD, Wasdell MB, Bomben MM et al.: Sleep hygiene and melatonin treatment for children and adolescents with ADHD and initial insomnia. *J Am Acad Child Adolesc Psychiatry* 2006; **45**(5): 512–19.

97 Giannotti F, Cortesi F, Cerquiglini A et al.: An open-label study of controlled-release melatonin in treatment of sleep disorders in children with autism. *J Autism Dev Disord.* 2006; **36**(6): 741–52.

98 Andersen IM, Kaczmarska J, McGrew SG et al.: Melatonin for insomnia in children with autism spectrum disorders. *J Child Neurol.* 2008; **23**(5): 482–5.

99 Paavonen EJ, Nieminen-von Wendt T, Vanhala R et al.: Effectiveness of melatonin in the treatment of sleep disturbances in children with Asperger disorder. *J Child Adolesc Psychopharmacol* 2003; **13**(1): 83–95.

100 Owens JA, Moturi S: Pharmacologic treatment of pediatric insomnia. *Child Adolesc Psychiatric Clin N Am* 2009; **18**(4): 1001–16.

101 Freeman MP: Omega-3 fatty acids in psychiatry: a review. *Annals Clin Psychiatry* 2000; **12**(3): 159–65.

102 Freeman MP, Fava M, Lake J et al.: Complementary and alternative medicine in major depressive disorder: the American Psychiatric Association Task Force report. *J Clin Psychiatry* 2010; **71**(6): 669–81.

103 Nemets H, Nemets B, Apter A et al.: Omega-3 treatment of childhood depression: a controlled, double-blind pilot study. *Am J Psychiatry* 2006; **163**(6): 1098–100.

104 Linde K, Ramirez G, Mulrow CD, et al.: St John's wort for depression – an overview and meta-analysis of randomised clinical trials. *BMJ* 1996; **313**: 253.

105 Pfeiffer SI, Norton J, Nelson L et al.: Efficacy of vitamin B6 and magnesium in the treatment of autism: a methodology review and summary of outcomes. *J Autism Dev Disord* 1995; **25**: 481–93.

106 Willemsen-Swinkels SH, Buitelaar JK, Nijhof GJ et al.: Failure of naltrexone hydrochloride to reduce self-injurious and autistic behavior in mentally retarded adults. Double-blind placebo- controlled studies. *Arch Gen Psychiatry* 1995; **52**(9): 766–73.

107 Woelk H: Comparison of St. John's Wort and imipramine for treating depression: randomized controlled trial. *BMJ* 2000; **321**: 536–9.

108 Brenner R, Azbel V, Madhusoodanan S et al.: Comparison of an extract of hypericum (LI 160) and sertraline in the treatment of depression: a double-blind, randomized pilot study. *Clin Ther* 2000; **22**(4): 411–19.

109 Laakmann G, Schule C, Baghai T et al.: St. John's wort in mild to moderate depression: the relevance of hyperforin for the clinical efficacy. *Pharmacopsychiatry,* 1998; **31**(Suppl 1): 54–9.

110 Hypericum Depression Trial Study Group: Effect of *Hypericum perforatum* (St. John's wort) in major depressive disorder: a randomized controlled trial. *JAMA* 2002; **287**: 1807–14.

111 Anghelescu IG, Kohnen R, Szegedi A et al.: Comparison of Hypericum extract WS 5570 and paroxetine in ongoing treatment after recovery from an episode of moderate to severe depression: results from a randomized multicenter study. *Pharmacopsychiatry* 2006; **39**: 213–19.

112 Linde K, Mulrow CD, Berner M et al.: St. John's wort for depression. *Cochrane Database Syst Rev* 2005; (2): CD000448.

113 Taylor LH, Kobak KA: An open-label trial of St. John's Wort (Hypericum perforatum) in obsessive-compulsive disorder. *J Clin Psychiatry* 2000; **61**(8): 575–8.

114 Kobak KA, Taylor LVH, Bystritsky A: St. John's wort versus placebo in obsessive–compulsive disorder: results from a double-blind study. *Int Clin Psychopharmacol* 2005; **20**: 299–304.

115 Stevinson C, Ernst E: A pilot study of Hypericum perforatum for the treatment of premenstrual syndrome. *BJOG* 2000; **107**(7): 870–6.

116 Canning S, Waterman M, Orsi N et al.: The efficacy of *Hypericum perforatum* (St. John's wort) for the treatment of premenstrual syndrome: a randomized, double-blind, placebo-controlled trial. *CNS Drugs* 2010; **24**(3): 207–25.

117 Hicks SM, Walker AF, Gallgaher J et al.: The significance of "nonsignificance" in randomized controlled studies: a discussion inspired by a double-blinded study on St. John's wort (Hypericum perforatum L.) for premenstrual symptoms. *J Altern Complementary Med* 2004; **10**(6): 925–32.

118 Findling RL, McNamara NK, O'Riordan MA: An open-label pilot study of St. John's Wort in juvenile depression. *J Am. Acad. Child Adolesc. Psychiatry* 2003; **42**(8): 908–14.

119 Simeon J, Nixon MK, Milin R: Open-label pilot study of St. John's Wort in adolescent depression. *J Child Adolesc Psychopharmacol* 2005; **15**(2): 293–301.

120 Weber W, Stoep AV, McCarty RL: Hypericum performatum (St. John's wort) for attention-deficit/hyperactivity disorder in children and adolescents. *JAMA* 2008; **299**(22): 2633–41.

121 Vorbach EU, Arnold KH, Hubner WD: Efficacy and tolerability of St. John's Wort extract Hypericum extract LI 160 in patients with severe depressive incidents according to ICD-10. *Pharmacopsychiatry* 1997; **30**(suppl 1): S81–S85.

122 Wheatley D: Hypericum extract. Potential in the treatment of depression. *CNS Drugs* 1998; **9**: 431–40.

123 Lantz MS, Buchalter E, Giambanco V: St. John's wort and antidepressant drug interactions in the elderly. *J Geriatr Psychiatry Neurol* 1999; **12**: 7–10.

124 Cheng TO: St. John's wort interaction with digoxin (let), *Arch Intern Med* 2000; **160**(16): 2548.

125 Bon D, Hartmann K, Kuhn M: Sanz-Strietflicht Nr. 40: Johanniskraut: an enzyme inductor? *Pharmacist Ztg.* 1999; **137**, 535–6.

126 Monmaney T, Roan S: Alternative medicine, the $18 billion experiment. *Los Angeles Times*, 1998; A1.

127 Irefin S, Sprung J: A possible cuase of cardiovascular collapse during anesthesia: use of St. John's Wort. *J Clin Anesth* 2000; **12**(6): 498–9.

128 Menolascino FJ, Donaldson JY, Gallagher TF: Orthomolecular therapy: its history and applicability to psychiatric disorders. *Child Psychiatry Hum Dev* 1988; **18**(3): 133–50.

129 Fernández-San-Martín MI, Masa-Font R, Palacios-Soler L et al.: Effectiveness of Valerian on insomnia: a meta-analysis of randomized placebo-controlled trials. *Sleep Med* 2010; **11**(6): 505–11.

130 Saeed SA, Bloch RM, Antonacci DJ: Herbal and dietary supplements for treatment of anxiety disorders. *Am Fam Physician* 2007; **76**(4): 549–56.

131 Müller SF, Klement S: A combination of valerian and lemon balm is effective in the treatment of restlessness and dyssomnia in children. *Phytomedicine* 2006; **13**(6): 383–7.

132 Francis AJ, Dempster RJ: Effect of valerian, Valeriana edulis, on sleep difficulties in children with intellectual deficits: randomised trial. *Phytomedicine* 2002; **9**(4): 273–9.

133 Guastella AJ, Richardson R, Lovibond PF: A randomized controlled trial of D-cycloserine enhancement of exposure therapy for social anxiety disorder. *Biol Psychiatry* 2008; **63**(6): 544–9.

134 Hofmann SG, Meuret AE, Smits JA: Augmentation of exposure therapy with D-cycloserine for social anxiety disorder. *Arch Gen Psychiatry* 2006; **63**(3): 298–304.

135 Ressler KJ, Rothbaum BO, Tannenbaum L: Cognitive enhancers as adjuncts to psychotherapy: use of D-cycloserine in phobic individuals to facilitate extinction of fear. *Arch Gen Psychiatry* 2004; **61**(11): 1136–44.

136 Otto MW, Tolin DF, Simon NM et al.: Efficacy of d-cycloserine for enhancing response to cognitive-behavior therapy for panic disorder. *Biol Psychiatry* 2010; **67**(4): 365–70.

137 Wilhelm S, Buhlmann U, Tolin DF: Augmentation of behavior therapy with D-cycloserine for obsessive-compulsive disorder. *Am J Psychiatry* 2008; **165**(3): 335–41.

138 Kushner MG, Kim SW, Donahue C: D-cycloserine augmented exposure therapy for obsessive-compulsive disorder. *Biol Psychiatry* 2007; **62**(8): 835–8.

139 Storch EA, Murphy TK, Goodman WK: A preliminary study of D-cycloserine augmentation of cognitive-behavioral therapy in pediatric obsessive-compulsive disorder. *Biol Psychiatry* 2010; **68**(11): 1073–6.

140 Wiklund IK, Mattsson LA, Lindgren R: Effects of a standardized ginseng extract on quality of life and physiological parameters in symptomatic postmenopausal women: a double-blind, placebo-controlled trial. *Int J Clin Pharmacol Res* **19**(3): 89–99.

141 Hartley DE, Elsabagh S, File SE: Gincosan (a combination of Ginkgo biloba and Panax ginseng): the effects on mood and cognition of 6 and 12 weeks' treatment in post-menopausal women. *Nutr Neurosci* 2004; **7**(5–6): 325–33.

142 Lyon MR, Cline JC, Totosy de Zepetnek J et al.: Effect of the herbal extract combination Panax quinquefolium and Ginkgo biloba on attention-deficit hyperactivity disorder: a pilot study. *J Psychiatry Neurosci* 2001; **26**(3): 221–8.

143 Devlin TM (ed.): *Textbook of Biochemistry with Clinical Correlations*, 3rd Edition. New York, NY: Wiley-Liss, 1992.

144 Benjamin J, Agam G, Levine J et al.: Inositol treatment in psychiatry. *Psychopharmacol Bull* 1995; **31**: 167–75.

145 Barkai A, Dunner DL, Gross HA et al.: Reduced myo-inositol levels in cerebrospinal fluid from patients with affective disorder. *Biol Psychiatry* 1978; **13**: 65–72.

146 Levine J: Controlled trials of inositol in psychiatry. *Eur Neuropsychopharmacol* 1997; **7**(2): 147–55.

147 Nemets B, Mishory A, Levine J et al.: Inositol addition does not improve depression in SSRI treatment failures. *J Neural Transm* 1999; **106**: 795–8.

148 Levine J, Mishori A, Susnosky S: Combination of inositol and serotonin reuptake inhibitors in the treatment of depression. *Biological Psychiatry* 1999; **45**: 270–3.

149 Warden D, Rush AJ, Trivedi MH: The STAR*D Project results: A comprehensive review of findings. *Curr Psychiatry Rep.* 2007; **9**: 449–59.

150 Fux M, Levine J, Aviv A et al.: Inositol treatment of obsessive-compulsive disorder. *Am J Psychiatry* 1999; **153**(9): 1219–21.

151 Gelber D, Levine J, Belmaker RH: Effect of inositol on bulimia nervosa and binge eating. *Int J Eat Disord* 2001; **29**(3): 345–8.

152 Levine J, Aviram A, Holan A: Inositol treatment of autism. *J Neural Transm* 1997; **104**(2–3): 307–10.

153 Lakhan SE, Vieira KF: Nutritional and herbal supplements for anxiety and anxiety-related disorders: systematic review. *Nutrition Journal* 2010; **9**: 42.

154 Escher M, Desmeules J, Giostra E et al.: Hepatitis associated with Kava, a herbal remedy for anxiety. *BMJ* 2001; **322**: 139.

155 Consumer Advisory: Kava-Containing Dietary Supplements May be associated with Severe Liver Injury. http://www.fda.gov/Food/ResourcesForYou/Consumers/ucm085482.htm.

156 Dean O, Giorlando F, Berk M: N-acetylcysteine in psychiatry: current therapeutic evidence and potential mechanisms of action. *J Psychiatry Neurosci* 2010; **35**(6): 78–86.

157 Berk M, Copolov D, Dean O et al.: N-acetyl cysteine as a glutathione precursor for schizophrenia—a double-blind, randomized, placebo-controlled trial. *Biol Psychiatry* 2008; **64**(5): 361–8.

158 Berk M(a), Copolov D, Dean O: N-Acetyl Cysteine for Depressive Symptoms in Bipolar Disorder—A Double-Blind Randomized Placebo-Controlled Trial. *Biol Psychiatry* 2008; **64**(6): 468–7.

159 Grant JE, Odlaug BL, Kim SW: N-acetylcysteine, a glutamate modulator, in the treatment of trichotillomania: a double-blind, placebo-controlled study. *Arch Gen Psychiatry* 2009; **66**(7): 756–63.

160 Bressa GM: S-adenosyl-l-methionine (SAMe) as antidepressant: meta-analysis of clinical studies *Acta Neurol Scand* 1994; (154): 7–14.

161 Papakostas GI: Evidence for S-adenosyl-L-methionine (SAM-e) for the treatment of major depressive disorder. *J Clin Psychiatry* 2009; **70**(Suppl 5): 18–22.

162 Papakostas GI, Mischoulon D, Shyu I et al.: S-adenosyl methionine (SAMe) augmentation of serotonin reuptake inhibitors for antidepressant nonresponders with major depressive disorder: a double-blind, randomized clinical trial. *Am J Psychiatry* 2010; **167**(8): 942–8.

163 Schaller J, John T, Bazzan AJ: SAMe use in children and adolescents. *Eur Child Adolesc Psychiatry* 2004; **13**: 332–4.

164 Kagan BL, Sultzer DL, Rosenlicht N: Oral S-adenosylmethionine in depression: a randomized, double-blind, placebo-controlled trial. *Am J Psychiatry* 1990; **147**(5): 591–5.

165 Carney MW, Chary TK, Bottiglieri T: The switch mechanism and the bipolar/unipolar dichotomy. *Br J Psychiatry* 1989; **154**: 48–51.

CHAPTER 16

Psychopharmacology in Preschool Children*

Mini Tandon & Joan Luby
Washington University School of Medicine, St. Louis, USA

Introduction

The preschool period, characterized by a very steep developmental curve, gives rise to unique mental-health assessment and treatment challenges. Rapid progression of expressive language and socio-emotional skills characterize this age period (for review, see [1]). More specifically, preschoolers are developing an awareness of self-concept and their own emotional states, and are also starting to perceive and understand the mental and emotional states of others. The young child's emotional style, capacities, and competencies are rapidly shaped through experiences such as play exploration, peer interactions, and the relationship with a primary caregiver. This developing comprehension of self and others helps guide social and emotional competence. Conversely, delays or impairments in this domain have been associated with psychopathology [2, 3].

In the context of these developmental issues, the use of psychotropic medication must be preceded by a thorough and comprehensive assessment by a clinician skilled in the mental health assessment of this age group. Once the assessment has been completed, and if psychotropic medications are considered, a frank discussion with caregivers should include review of the principle that pharmacology is not used in the preschool period in most cases unless psychotherapy has been attempted, and all other feasible psychosocial interventions have failed or proven insufficient [4]. The reasons for this position include the unclear effects of psychotropic medications on the rapidly developing brain, the under-studied general

*Preparation of this manuscript is supported by K12 DA 000357 to Dr. Tandon and R01MH 64769-01 to Dr. Luby. The authors have no conflicts of interest or other disclosures to report.

Pharmacotherapy of Child and Adolescent Psychiatric Disorders, Third Edition.
Edited by David R. Rosenberg and Samuel Gershon.

medical safety and efficacy of these medications in children younger than age six, and some evidence that preschoolers may have greater sensitivity to the side-effects of some psychotropics [4–6]. The following chapter aims to review the specific considerations for use of pharmacologic agents during this early and rapid period of development, along with empirically-based psychotherapeutic interventions to be tried prior to or in conjunction with pharmacologic treatments.

Developmental considerations

The necessity of age-appropriate assessment

To capture adequately the complexities of this early developmental period, a comprehensive assessment conducted over several sessions is recommended [7]. Several variations on this approach may be feasible and useful, but a four-part assessment over four consecutive weeks, involving observation of the child with more than one caregiver, has been described and has numerous advantages. It may also be useful to send information packets prior to the assessment for caregivers to complete, including basic symptom checklists such as the 0–5 version of the Child Behavior Checklist (CBCL), any Teacher Report Forms (TRF), the Health and Behavior Questionnaire (HBQ), or other measures of symptoms, behavioral style, and various developmental parameters. Any surveys or questionnaires are scored prior to the first session, so that clues about pertinent symptom domains can be gleaned prior to obtaining the history from caregivers. In the first session, it is useful to take a detailed history from caregivers without the preschooler present to facilitate full disclosure and efficient history-taking. A complete ascertainment of perinatal and developmental history, family history, social history, current symptoms, and chief complaint should be obtained. Although there is often pressure from families for immediate changes in treatment, such changes are not made until the assessment is complete, including any medication changes, if the child comes to the evaluation already on medication. Exceptions to this might be if a child is clearly taking inappropriate medication for which the clinician cannot find justification. Given the central role of the relationship between child and primary caregiver at this stage of development, even when medication is the main consideration, no assessment is considered complete or appropriate without inclusion of the caregiver and observation of dyadic play to ascertain an accurate mental status exam.

During the second session, observation of child and caregiver in unstructured free play is recommended. The secondary caregiver is invited to engage in free play with the preschooler in a play room with age-appropriate toys while clinicians observe in the room and/or behind a two-way mirror. The aim is to note, by gross clinical observation, the quality and tone of the relationship between child and caregiver, the child's play skill and themes of interest, mental status, and overall development. In the third session, a semi-structured assessment is done with the child and primary caregiver. In this session, which has mild stressors similar to those experienced in daily life, the dyad is asked to have a snack, complete a set of block design patterns together, then engage in free play as they would at home. A separation and reunion is also observed. A clinician observes the interpersonal and play dynamics from behind a two-way mirror. Again, a mental status exam is gleaned from this observation of dyadic play. When possible, a team of clinicians discusses the cases weekly during the evaluation process as part of a case conference. Observation of the child with two different caregivers is important to determine if there is relationship specificity to the child's symptoms (a phenomenon well known in some forms of early childhood psychopathology).

The fourth and final session involves the caregivers and clinician meeting again without the child. In this session, the psychodynamic formulation and differential diagnosis is discussed in detail. A comprehensive treatment plan is recommended, including specialty referrals for developmental services if needed.

The benefit of this four-part evaluation is the longitudinal view and the opportunity for a comprehensive assessment that allows observation of the preschooler and their caregiver(s) over time and in different contexts. This allows for a more accurate view of stable underlying features of the child's mental state, and minimizes the risk of pathologizing transient and normative extremes of mood and behavior characteristic of this developmental period. While this format is less convenient for families and more time and cost intensive, it is important for obtaining a more accurate clinical impression. This assessment process is emphasized, because it is necessary prior to prescription of medication in a preschool child. The absence of such an assessment is likely a major reason why medications are inappropriately prescribed, as family and contextual issues may be more salient and should be addressed first and/or in concert with medications.

Factors unique to preschoolers

Empirical investigations of the clinical characteristics of mental disorders during the preschool period continue to emerge. However, the literature in this area still lags significantly behind that of older children and adolescents. The Diagnostic and Statistical Manual IV (DSM-IV-TR) [8] was not specifically developed to apply to this early childhood stage. The increasing availability of age-appropriate instruments such as the

Preschool Age Psychiatric Assessment (PAPA) [9] has contributed to valid and reliable mental health assessments of preschoolers in research settings [10].

In addition to unique dyadic, relational, and contextual issues, the preschool child presents multiple clinical challenges. The rapid neurodevelopment characteristic of this period is pertinent when considering any psychopharmacologic use. Brain development during the preschool period is not as well understood as later developmental periods, such as adolescence. The complex and rapid emergence of language, motor, social, and emotional development give rise to multiple unique considerations for the use of psychopharmacology. More specifically, pruning and synaptogenesis occur rapidly during this period [11]. Early exposure to psychopharmacologic agents can change neurotransmitter systems into adulthood as shown in animal models that used selective serotonin reuptake inhibitors (SSRIs) during the neonatal period in rats [12]. Any decision to use psychotropics at this stage would need careful consideration, given the overall dearth of knowledge on their impact on human brain development [13, 14].

In contrast to concerns about neurotoxicity, the important question about whether exposure to psychopharmacologic agents in the preschool period can be neuroprotective when warranted has been largely under-investigated. Psychosocial and psychotherapeutic data emerging in older children show positive effects on cognitive development but this is an area in which more investigation of psychopharmacologic effects is needed [15]. The prospect of neuroprotection raises very exciting possibilities about the potential protective role of psychopharmacolgic agents in the developmental psychopathology of specific mental disorders. This is an area in which future investigation is necessary.

Rise in psychopharmacology use

This dearth of available trained providers who administer empirically proven therapies may be one possible factor in the rise of psychotropic use in preschoolers [16, 17]. Psychotropic use in preschoolers has continued to rise in the Medicaid population [5, 18, 19], as well as in privately insured preschool populations [20]. Most concerning is the rise in psychotropic use despite the lack of developmentally informed mental health services available to this age group. One startling statistic is that fewer than 50% of privately insured preschoolers who were treated with antipsychotics in 2007 had a mental health assessment [21]. This represents a very serious and highly correctable public health problem.

Psychotherapy before psychopharmacology

Given the dearth of available FDA-approved psychopharmacologic agents, need for off-label use, and as the increased risks outlined above, age-appropriate, empirically informed psychotherapy and psychosocial interventions should precede any plans for psychopharmacologic intervention in most circumstances. Exceptions to this include persistent patterns of aggression or self-harm that endanger the child or others. Because inpatient hospitalization is rarely appropriate or available for a child of this age, the risks and benefits of medication for these intense levels of aggression require careful consideration [22].

Empirically supported psychotherapies continue to emerge for preschoolers. Perhaps one of the most frequently used and widely validated dyadic psychotherapies is Parent Child Interaction Therapy (PCIT) [23]. This empirically supported therapy aims to diminish disruptive behavior by enhancing the quality of the parent–child relationship and the parent's ability to set firm and nurturing limits. The goals of competency in child directed interaction and parent directed interaction are achieved after a series of weekly one-hour therapy sessions. These dyadic sessions involve *in vivo* learning from a trained clinician-therapist communicating unobtrusively with the primary caregiver from behind a two-way mirror via a "bug" in the caregiver's ear. This therapy has been validated in preschoolers with disruptive disorders and has also been adapted for other disorders in early childhood [24]. Examples include adaptations for Separation Anxiety Disorder [25], depression [26], and attention-deficit/hyperactivity disorder (ADHD) [27]. Adaptations for children with prenatal exposure to nicotine and caregivers that smoke are also in progress [28].

In addition to PCIT and its many adaptations, other therapies and psychosocial interventions that have been well validated for other disorders in older children have been systematically investigated for use in early childhood including Cognitive Behavioral Therapy for Post Traumatic Stress Disorder [29] and Child Parent Psychotherapy for Trauma [30]. In the case of autism spectrum disorders, interventions such as applied behavioral analysis (ABA) [31] have been used for decades, along with newer interventions such as the Early Start Denver Model [32]. As noted, while much progress has been made for nonpsychopharmacologic options in the treatment of early childhood mental disorders, many additional options are in progress, and more are still needed. Despite the current limitations of nonpsychopharmacologic interventions and available clinical providers with expertise in early childhood, the choice of psychotherapy and psychosocial interventions is still warranted prior to, or in addition to, psychopharmacology [4, 17].

When psychopharmacology may be considered as a first line: pragmatic considerations

Psychotherapies designed for this age group continue to emerge and are described below but they are still not widely available in many communities. Mental health professionals who specialize in this age group and can provide empirically evidenced therapies are still lacking in the majority of settings, including urban settings with relatively good mental health services in general. This lack of providers for therapy makes the implementation of therapy as first line less feasible in many communities. In such circumstances, prescribing psychotropics should be based on those with the most evidence and efficacy for use. For example, methylphenidate has been well investigated for preschoolers with ADHD as described below and effect sizes of 0.4–0.8 have been found [33]. Risperidone has been FDA-approved for the treatment of irritability and aggression in Autism and is well-investigated compared to other medications in this very young age [4]. Of course, the need for careful consideration and monitoring overall, and especially in preschool children, cannot be overemphasized and is detailed below [5, 17].

Psychopharmacology in preschool disorders: administration and monitoring

Extrapolation of findings on the efficacy of medications as used in older children or adults should not be generalized to younger children, given the developmental specificity and sensitivities described. One classic example of the need for separate investigation of psychotropic efficacy in childhood was provided by Geller et al. [34] forewarning of the safety of tricyclics, and Hazell et al. [35] showing no efficacy for tricyclic antidepressants over placebo for the treatment of depression in children, unlike in adults.

Also of unique importance is the need for frequent monitoring of young children on psychotropic medication, given concerns for appropriate dosing, greater sensitivity to side-effects or paradoxical effects, metabolic side-effects, and growth [36]. Monitoring at frequent intervals, as detailed below, is essential for any preschooler on a psychotropic. This may be one important area in need of change in practice, especially when psychotropics are given in primary care settings. Consideration should be given to the severity of the illness in determining frequency of visits, since no pre-established parameters exist [4]. Given the need to start low and go slow, preschoolers will need frequent visits until stabilized. Visits every two weeks, or more frequently if feasible, are often indicated during the initial titration. Once the preschooler is stabilized on a medication regimen, the need for frequent followup continues in an attempt to achieve the lowest possible dosage or attempt a med-free trial. Gleason et al. [4] suggest the clinician develop a method for systematically tracking symptoms and functional impairment to guide treatment. Of course, any use of psychotherapy in child and caregiver should be ongoing or re-implemented as soon as it is feasible [4, 5, 17].

While not specific to preschool children, weight gain and lipid monitoring are key considerations when using atypical antipsychotics. Martin et al. [37] found a mean weight gain of 7 kg after six months of exposure to risperidone in a sample of n = 37 children and adolescent inpatients compared to those not taking atypical antipsychotics. Monitoring guidelines for children on antipsychotics, but not specific to preschoolers, include baseline fasting blood glucose, lipids, vital signs, BMI percentile, and detailed personal and family medical histories, along with three- and six-month follow-up lab work. A prolactin level is recommended if symptoms such as lactation are evident. Any attempt at reducing dosage and weight neutral psychotropics (an area of current debate) should be carefully considered while weighing the risks and benefits and determining the necessity of its use [38, 39].

While weight *gain* is more of a consideration in use of atypical antipsychotics, weight *loss* is a well-known concern with the use of stimulants. If a child is a good responder but weight loss is a concern, high calorie diets may be considered as dietary supplements. Vital signs and growth-curve charts, maintained on each visit, should help guide treatment decisions. Working in conjunction with primary care providers offers optimal benefit for monitoring and is strongly recommended [17]. In addition to weight concerns, a thorough cardiac history should be obtained prior to initiating a stimulant. An EKG is not required for all patients, but any cardiac disease history or concerns that arise after treatment is implemented should prompt input from a pediatric cardiologist [40] (see Figure 16.1).

Also of key importance in the consideration of psychopharmacology in preschoolers is the feasibility of the actual administration of the psychotropic, when medications are prescribed. Some preschoolers are challenged by swallowing pills. One alternative is to use liquid forms. A few agents come in liquid formulations (methylphenidate and fluoxetine), sprinkles (methylphenidate and mixed amphetamine salt brands), or patches (clonidine) for ease of dosing in very young children [5]. In addition to nonpill formulations, pill-swallowing educational techniques, including age-appropriate explanations for children, have been published and may be useful [41, 42]. Another method that has been used successfully is crushing of tablets when appropriate (not long-acting formulations) for administration with soft food (such as applesauce or pudding).

ADHD

Trial parent management training x 2mnths or PCIT

Methylphenidate trial ⟹fails ⟹d-amphetamine/mixed amphetaminee ⟹ fails

Works

atomoxetine or

alpha agonist

works

Medication free trial at 6mnths

Re-assess diagnosis

ODD/CD/DISRUPTIVE NOS

Trial parent child interaction therapy and parent management

Continued impairment: add risperidone trial with lab monitoring[1]

Med-free trial at 6 mnths, reassess diagnosis

AUTISM/PERVASIVE DEVELOPMENTAL DISORDER

Behavioral therapy (e.g. Applied Behavioral Analysis or Early Start Denver Model),
parent psychoeducation, speech and language skills, social skills

Persistent and severe aggression?

Add risperidone trial x 6 months as tolerated with lab monitoring[1]
and med-free trial

MDD/DEPRESSION NOS/DYSTHYMIA

Trial dyadic psychotherapy with focus on emotion regulation skills x 3-6 months

Persistent, severe and debilitating depression?

Add trial fluoxetine x 6 months as tolerated

Med free trial and reassess diagnosis

BIPOLAR DISORDER

Trial dyadic psychotherapy with focus on emotion regulation skills x 3-6 months

Persistent, severe and debilitating symptoms with aggression?

Add risperidone trial x 6 months with lab monitoring[1] then medication free trial, reassess diagnosis

Trial risperidone fails

Consult sub-specialist , who may consider another atypical antipsychotic or
Augmentation with mood stabilizer (eg lithium or valproate);

Med free trial and reassess diagnosis

[1] labs include fasting blood glucose, lipid profiles, body mass index, vital signs, monitor for EPS

Figure 16.1 Preschoolers and psychopharmacology: a clinically guided algorithm.
(Reprinted with permission from Psychopharmacology in Pre-schoolers: a Brief Guide
to Clinicians, Tandon, M. and Luby, J. in Child and Adolescent Psychopharmacology
News, Findling R, (ed), Copyright © 2009, Guilford Press.)

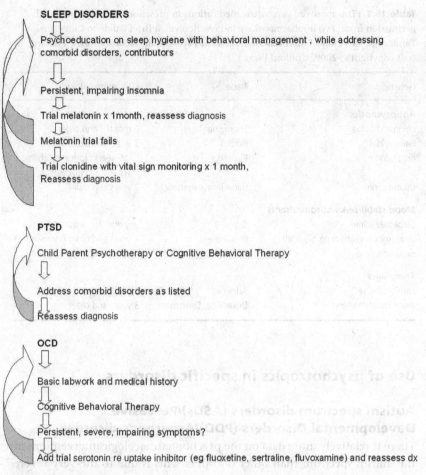

SLEEP DISORDERS

Psychoeducation on sleep hygiene with behavioral management , while addressing comorbid disorders, contributors

Persistent, impairing insomnia

Trial melatonin x 1month, reassess diagnosis

Melatonin trial fails

Trial clonidine with vital sign monitoring x 1 month, Reassess diagnosis

PTSD

Child Parent Psychotherapy or Cognitive Behavioral Therapy

Address comorbid disorders as listed

Reassess diagnosis

OCD

Basic labwork and medical history

Cognitive Behavioral Therapy

Persistent, severe, impairing symptoms?

Add trial serotonin re uptake inhibitor (eg fluoxetine, sertraline, fluvoxamine) and reassess dx

Figure 16.1 (*Continued*)

Off-label prescribing: special considerations

The few psychotropic medications that are FDA approved for use in preschool aged children, but not for use in mental disorders specifically, include those that have been investigated for use in young children with seizure disorders (for example, carbamazepine, valproic acid). Therefore, most prescribing of psychiatric medications in young children must be done off label. The reason for this is likely due in part to the pharmaceutical industry's lack of interest in testing the safety and efficacy of agents for this age group, given their small part of the market as well as their higher risk. Implications of this are that a very thorough informed consent should be done for families of preschool children that includes explicit discussion of lack of FDA approval, as well as the appropriate need for trials of psychotherapy (see Table 16.1).

Table 16.1 FDA-approved psychiatric medications in preschoolers. (Reprinted with permission from: Psychopharmacology in Preschoolers: a Brief Guide to Clinicians. Tandon, M and Luby, J. in: Child & Adolescent Psychopharmacology News, Findling, R. (ed) copyright © 2009, Guilford Press.)

Generic	Trade	FDA-approved age
Antipsychotics		
chlorpromazine	Thorazine	6 months and older
haloperidol	Haldol	3 years and older
risperidone	Risperdal	5–16 years old for irritability associated with autism
thioridazine	thioridazine (generic)	2 years and older
Mood stabilizers/anticonvulsants		
carbamezapine	Tegretol	any age (for seizures)
divalproex sodium (valproic acid)	Depakote	2 years and older (for seizures)
oxcarbazepine	Trileptal	4 years and older
Stimulants		
amphetamine	Adderall	3 years and older
dextroamphetamine	Dexedrine, Dextrostat	3 years and older

Use of psychotropics in specific disorders

Autism spectrum disorders (ASDs)/Pervasive Developmental Disorders (PDD)/Asperger's disorder

There is relatively more data on the psychopharmacologic interventions in the autism spectrum than other disorders. This is due to the very severe and impairing nature of these disorders and the potential for aggression and self-harming behaviors. It is important to ensure that psychosocial interventions, including parent education and ABA, are in place along with special education services emphasizing language, communication, and social skills [31,43]. Psychotropics should only be initiated in addition to the ongoing listed psychosocial interventions when severe aggression or irritability causes impairment or a threat to safety [4]. Children with autism may be more sensitive to the side-effects of some medications. In general, children are more susceptible than adults to sedation, weight gain and extrapyramidal symptoms but less susceptible than adults to those adverse effects that are associated with longer term use and greater dosages, such as tardive dyskinesia [38]; while investigations were not specific to preschoolers, the incidence of tardive dyskinesia occurred 0.4% annually in a meta-analyses of children ages 4–18 on antipychotics, which is about half the rate found in adults [44]. Nonetheless, all younger children should be monitored routinely for adverse events as described previously, and parents should be educated about early signs of these adverse effects [4, 45].

Risperidone has been shown to reduce aggression and irritability associated with autism in children as young as age 5 (see Table 16.1). Luby [46] demonstrated tolerability of low-dose risperidone (0.5–1.5 mg total daily) in a placebo-controlled investigation of n = 24 preschoolers with ASDs. A baseline to six-month autism severity change of 8% was found in the risperidone group versus placebo (3%). Weight gain, sedation, hypersalivation, and elevated prolactin levels were the most commonly reported side-effects [46]. Similar findings were replicated in a larger (n = 40) and older (2–9 year old) sample by Nagaraj et al. [47]. Other double-blind, placebo-controlled studies of risperidone have included children as young as 5 years in adolescent samples, and found improvements in irritability, stereotypies and even hyperactivity in doses ranging from 0.5 to 2 mg per day [48]. Cardiac effects, namely increased QT interval, found with antipsychotic use in older children, were not found to be associated with antipsychotic use in a naturalistic study of n = 12 preschoolers [49].

Co-morbid symptoms, such as those of ADHD, remain challenging to treat in autism spectrum disorders [50]. In a double-blind, placebo-controlled study of methylphenidate (mean dosage 5–20 mg/day) in n = 12 preschoolers with pervasive developmental disorder, Ghuman et al. [51] found improved parent-rated ADHD symptoms; however, it is notable that 50% of the preschoolers reported side-effects, including but not limited to stomach upset, increased stereotypies, and sleeping problems, which require slower titrations and lower dosages given increased sensitivities.

Selective serotonin reuptake inhibitors have shown some effectiveness in reducing repetitive behaviors or irritability associated with the autism spectrum [48]. Fluoxetine, but not escitalopram or citalopram, has shown some reduction in repetitive behaviors in studies which have included few children as young as age 5 years [52, 53]; however, monitoring of activation and agitation associated with SSRIs is critical [54].

Attention-deficit hyperactivity disorder

Attention-deficit hyperactivity disorder is one diagnostic domain in which there is relatively more empirical data to inform the use of psychotropic treatments for preschool children. Increased sensitivities to the side-effects of some psychotropics with known efficacy and widely used in older children, including stimulants for ADHD, have been described in preschoolers [6]. The strongest evidence for treatment of ADHD for older children remains the stimulant class of medications, and, in this domain, preschoolers have also been shown to respond. However, one clinical consideration is that younger children appear to be more sensitive to side-effects as elucidated by findings from the Preschool ADHD Treatment Study (PATS) [6, 55]. The PATS was a multisite study that has provided the largest available database to inform the efficacy of methylphenidate for the treatment of preschool ADHD. The PATS study enrolled n = 303 young children ages 3 to 5.5 who met criteria for DSM-IV ADHD to investigate five-week and 40-week efficacy of methylphenidate. This study had multiple phases, including, but not limited to, parent training, double-blind crossover titration, efficacy and discontinuation. Due to concerns about investigating a pharmacologic agent in very young children, multiple layers of protection including multiple raters, informants, clinicians, and impairment scales were added to ensure that only those children who were reliably diagnosed with DSM-IV ADHD, and who failed parent management, were exposed to stimulant medication. Consequently, only the more severe cases were included in this study. Children with other serious Axis I disorders were also excluded. Therefore, the study population represented preschoolers with severe and noncomorbid ADHD—not the most common manifestation of the disorder seen in the general population as ADHD is often comorbid with other psychiatric disorders [56]. Other methodological limitations included not maximizing dosages, and use of only the short-acting product. To summarize, despite these limitations, the PATS filled an important research gap in stimulant treatment among preschoolers. However, the multiple ethical concerns that guided the study made study findings more challenging to interpret and generalize. The PATS safety data show that, overall, 30% of subjects reported moderate to severe adverse events to methylphenidate including loss of appetite, irritability, initial insomnia, emotional outbursts, and perseveration of thoughts or behaviors, and 11% discontinued the study related to adverse events [33, 57].

The treatment of first choice in preschoolers with mild to moderate ADHD is parent management training and/or PCIT, described previously. However, in circumstances where parenting appears appropriate and the ADHD diagnosis is clear, and PCIT is not available, a stimulant can be cautiously tried. Ironically, although methylphenidate is not FDA-approved for this age range, it has been the subject of more empirical investigations as in PATS than dextro-amphetamine, which has been FDA-approved in preschoolers. Regardless of the discrepancies in FDA-approval, parent management training, careful monitoring and frequent re-assessment is a necessary part of the comprehensive treatment plan. A mean daily dosage of 14 mg of methylphenidate was found to be optimal in PATS, after sensitivities and side-effects were considered in preschoolers. Kratochvil et al. [58] recommend that objective measures, such as Conners forms validated in children as young as age 3 years, be completed by both teachers and parents frequently in this very young population to monitor treatment response. Very severe, treatment refractory cases, which do not respond to psychotherapy or stimulants, can be cautiously tried on alpha agonists or atomoxetine, both of which have clinical efficacy in older children, but limited safety data in preschoolers [4,5,17]. More recently, Kratochvil [59] et al. reported that atomoxetine (at a mean final dose of 1.25 mg/kg/day) successfully reduced ADHD symptoms in an open-label study of n = 22 children ages 5 and 6. Of note, mood lability was the most commonly reported side-effect in 54.5% of the sample [59].

Disruptive behavior disorders (DBD)

The disorders of oppositional defiant disorder (ODD) and conduct disorder (CD) are included in this category. In this case, the first-line treatment is parent management training and PCIT, as it directly addresses the underlying phenomenology [5,60]. Serious attempts at implementation of such treatments should be made for preschoolers in this diagnostic category, as they are known to have enduring efficacy [61,62]. Frequent reassessment for comorbid conditions, such as ADHD, is also critical and should be addressed. Given the larger body of evidence available for the treatment of ADHD and its high comorbidity with ODD, the comorbidity should first be targeted with a stimulant [5,63]. A trial of guanfacine or clonidine may be used to target comorbid ADHD symptoms if stimulants fail, though clonidine has FDA approval only in children aged 12 and older [45,64,65]. Although there is less data to support the specific treatment of ODD and CD with guanfacine or clonidine, it is common clinical practice to attempt a trial of guanfacine as a first line of treatment for disruptive disorders given its favorable safety profile [66,67]. The advantage is the relative safety of such medications, although caution should be used in children with a history of cardiac problems. A trial of risperidone may be justified under circumstances in which the child is so aggressive or defiant that they endanger themselves or others, and in which the other, lower risk pharmacological interventions previously mentioned have failed [4,68]. Risperidone has been relatively well studied in children as young as age 5 years for treatments of aggression and irritability associated with autism [69]; bipolar disorder [70], and aggression in young children [71]. Frequent monitoring of side-effects, bloodwork, including fasting lipid profile, and vital signs should help guide treatment to prevent metabolic side-effects. Any preschooler on psychotropics should be both frequently assessed and provided with a med-free trial at feasible intervals to make sure the medication is still needed. The lowest effective dosage should always be attempted. Diagnostic re-evaluation, which is of key consideration to any child, is critically important in preschoolers, given rapid changes in development and co-morbid conditions [17].

Major depressive disorder (MDD)

Depression has been shown to arise as early as 3 years of age and can be detected clinically using age appropriate interview techniques [46, 72, 73]. The first line of treatment is dyadic therapy focusing on relational issues and emotion development. A novel form of dyadic psychotherapy that is an adaptation of PCIT has been developed and is currently undergoing testing, with promising findings emerging from an open trial [26]. In cases in which psychosocial interventions have been tried and proven ineffective or insufficient, and depression remains severe and impairing, a very cautious trial of medication may be considered although safety and efficacy remain unclear. Fluoxetine, a SSRI, has been used in preschoolers given the extrapolation of its efficacy in older children and adolescents, although caution is advised given the greater propensity toward activating side-effects [74]. High rates of adverse effects, including activation, were noted in a retrospective chart review of 39 children under age 7 years [74]. Activation is speculated to be more common in preschoolers than in older children in general, and this is a key consideration in the use of SSRIs [75]. Regardless of frequency or prevalence of adverse effects, in preschoolers, periodic trials of dose reduction or medication-free trials are warranted. Further, in most cases, developmentally appropriate ongoing psychotherapy should be implemented. As in any disorder, psychiatric and psychotherapeutic treatment of caregivers is also a key component of a comprehensive treatment plan when applicable.

Bipolar disorder

The diagnosis of this disorder remains highly controversial and clinically ambiguous in preschoolers despite some suggestive empirical data and case reports [76–79]. Despite these diagnostic ambiguities, and the question of whether true bipolar disorder can arise this early in childhood, severe and impairing mood instability is common in young children presenting to mental health settings. Preschoolers referred for intense mood lability, often associated with irritability and periods of elevated mood, are often severely impaired and may be in need of more rapid and intense symptom amelioration in conjunction with psychotherapies. When dyadic treatment that is focused on emotion regulation fails or proves insufficient, use of agents such as risperidone may be cautiously tried at low doses and with slow titration [4, 5, 80]. There are several additional atypical antipsychotic medications that may be used; however, risperidone has the advantage of being FDA approved for younger children with autism spectrum disorders. Of key importance are significant concerns about weight gain and metabolic risks of risperidone [81]. Aripiprazole is another atypical agent for pediatric bipolar disorder, but it has only been approved in children as young as age 10 years [82]. When atypicals are used, it is recommended that they should start at low doses with slow upward titrations in an attempt to achieve symptom amelioration at the lowest possible dose. Close monitoring is also critical as outlined below. A clinical consultation with a specialist in early childhood disorders is warranted prior to additional psychopharmacology implementation with mood stabilizing agents. For example, lithium has approval for use in pediatric bipolar disorder for children age 12 years and older, but interference with potty training and frequent bloodwork make its use in preschoolers not recommended as a first or second line of treatment [83,84]. Frequent monitoring (to include weight and height) and bloodwork described previously, along with a med-free trial, should be part of any treatment plan, along with re-assessment for comorbid conditions such as ADHD [4,45].

Anxiety disorders

Obsessive compulsive disorder (OCD)

Multiple studies exist for the treatment of OCD in older children and adults, and have included both cognitive behavioral therapy (CBT) along with selective serotonin reuptake inhibitors (SSRI), but there has been little investigation of the nosology or treatment of the disorder in preschoolers. Based on this, and the availability of empirically proven psychotherapies for other preschool anxiety disorders, therapy alone remains the first choice in preschoolers [85]. In severely refractory cases, and after failure to improve with CBT, an SSRI may be considered. It is advisable to review with a clinician who specializes in early childhood disorders, if possible. Data are limited to a case study, which showed resolution of OCD symptoms in n = 3 preschoolers with 25 mg of sertraline daily, though activation occurred and was treated with additional risperidone [86]. If indicated, lowest dosages of SSRIs, including fluoxetine 2.5 mg or sertraline 5 mg daily, have been suggested [5]. Treatment of comorbid disorders and a complete medical workup may be particularly important with OCD given organic etiologies of these symptoms. Though the evidence remains somewhat controversial, concerns for Pediatric Autoimmune Neuropsychiatric Disorders Associated with Streptococcus (PANDAS) would warrant that any recent strep infection be fully treated and lab work for strep titers be examined, especially in new and relatively sudden onset cases of OCD. However, the association between streptoccal infection and OCD remains controversial with some failure to replicate the data [87–89]. Activation and side-effects must be carefully monitored, and as always, a med-free trial must occur with ongoing efforts at CBT. Cognitive behavioral therapy has been successfully implemented in preschoolers with other conditions described below.

Post-traumatic stress disorder (PTSD)

Current recommendations do not support psychopharmacologic interventions for PTSD in preschoolers. Cognitive behavioral therapy has been implemented effectively for use in preschoolers [29]. Age-appropriate techniques have been applied to modify CBT used in adults for this young population [85, 90]. Furthermore, child parent psychotherapy (CPP), as previously referenced, has been utilized in other manifestations of trauma, such as exposure to domestic and marital violence [30]. Clonidine has been shown to reduce hyperarousal, sleep, and anxiety in an open trial of n = 7 preschoolers with PTSD and aggression, but the small sample size and nonspecificity of treatment did not provide direct support for use in this young age group [91].

Generalized anxiety disorder (GAD)/separation anxiety disorder (SAD)/anxiety NOS

Currently medications are not recommended as a first line of treatment for anxiety in preschoolers. Preschoolers may respond to dyadic play therapy by conquering their fears in play (for review see Tandon et al. 2009) [92]. More recently, Pincus et al. investigated an adaptation of PCIT for separation anxiety [25]. In severely refractory cases, clinical consultation with a specialist in early childhood disorders is recommended, if feasible, prior to initiating any psychopharmacologic trials such as fluoxetine as in depression. Again, given limited investigation of use of psychotropics in preschoolers as a whole, and more specifically, for anxiety, a med-free trial is the focus if initiated, in combination with ongoing dyadic psychotherapy [4]. A few case reports have shown improvements in anxiety symptoms in severe instances of impairing specific phobia and panic attacks using fluoxetine at 5 mg daily in a 2.5-year-old child [93]. Another case study of a 4.1-year-old child treated with fluoxetine at 4–8 mg daily showed improvement of selective mutism in combination with psychotherapy [94]. Nevertheless, psychotherapy remains the treatment of choice in preschoolers [4, 5].

Sleep disorders

Regulation of sleep is a critical developmental issue in the preschool period. In general, pharmacologic agents should not be used for sleep in young children. Psychoeducation and sleep hygiene techniques should be completely exhausted prior to any consideration of a psychopharmacologic intervention. In very refractory cases, a two-week trial of melatonin could be recommended along with ongoing psychoeducation. Limited data are available in the form of case studies extrapolated from older children [95]. In more severe cases, clonidine may be helpful on a short-term basis but safety issues and hypotension must be monitored. In conjunction with a primary care physician, routine physical exam and labwork is appropriate to rule out other anatomical or physiological contributions to poor sleep [5].

Summary

The use of psychotropic medication in preschool children must be preceded by a comprehensive assessment by a clinician skilled in the mental health assessment of this age group. Pharmacology is not typically used in the preschool period unless psychotherapy has been attempted and failed or proven insufficient. In some circumstances, severity of illness and risk of safety prompt cautious psychotropic trials with frequent monitoring and the lowest effective dosages. Psychostimulants have demonstrated efficacy in lower doses in severe forms of ADHD in the preschool period. Early attempts at reduction of dosage or med-free trials, while reattempting psychotherapy for the child and caregiver, are warranted. A number of developmental issues should be considered prior to prescribing and should guide careful monitoring. The lack of mental health clinicians available and specializing in early childhood psychotherapies makes psychotherapy less feasible in many communities. Future empirical investigations of the safety and efficacy of psychopharmacology in specific preschool disorders are critically needed.

References

1 Shaffer D: Development of language and communication skillls: language learning during the preschool period. In: Shaffer D (ed.) *Developmental Psychology*. Pacific Grove, CA: Wadsworth/Thompson Learning, Inc., 2002, pp. 362–7.

2 Denham S: Emotional competence: implications for social functioning. In: Luby J (ed.) *Handbook of Preschool Mental Health*. New York, NY: Guilford Press, 2006, pp. 23–44.

3 Thompson R, Goodvin R, Meyer S: Social development: psychological understanding, self-understanding, and relationships. In Luby J (ed.) *Handbook of Preschool Mental Health*. New York, NY: Guilford Press, 2006.

4 Gleason MM, Egger HL, Emslie GJ et al.: Psychopharmacological treatment for very young children: contexts and guidelines. *J Am Acad Child Adolesc Psychiatry* 2007; **46**: 1532–72.

5 Fanton J, Gleason MM: Psychopharmacology and preschoolers: a critical review of current conditions. *Child Adolesc Psychiatr Clin N Am.* 2009; **18**: 753–71.

6 Greenhill L, Kollins S, Abikoff H et al.: Efficacy and safety of immediate-release methylphenidate treatment for preschoolers with ADHD. *J Am Acad Child Adolesc Psychiatry* 2006; **45**: 1284–93.

7 Luby J, Tandon M: Assessing the preschool-age child. In : Dulcan M (ed.) *Dulcan's Textbook of Child and Adolescent Psychiatry*. Arlington, VA: American Psychiatric Publishing, Inc., 2010.

8 APA: *Diagnostic and Statistical Manual of Mental Disorders, Fourth Edition, Text Revision*. Washington, DC: American Psychiatric Association., 2000

9 Egger H, Ascher B, Angold A: Preschool Age Psychiatric Assessment (PAPA): Version 1.1. Durham, NC: Center for Developmental Epidemiology, Department of Psychiatry and Behavioral Sciences, Duke University Medical Center, 1999.

10 Egger H, Erkanli A, Keeler G et al.: Test-retest reliability of the Preschool Age Psychiatric Assessment (PAPA). *J Am Acad Child Adolesc Psychiatry* 2006; **45**: 538–49.

11 Shonkoff JP, Phillips DA: *From Neurons to Neighborhoods: The Science of Early Childhood Development*. Washington, DC: National Academy Press, 2000.

12 Maciag D, Simpson KL, Coppinger D et al.: Neonatal antidepressant exposure has lasting effects on behavior and serotonin circuitry. *Neuropsychopharmacology* 2006; **31**: 47–57.

13 Vitiello B: Pediatric psychopharmacology and the interatction between drugs and the developing brain. *Canadian Journal of Psychiatry* 1998; **43**: 582–4.

14 Vitiello B: Psychopharmacology for young children: Clinical needs and research opportunities. *Pediatrics*. 2001; **104**: 983–9.

15 Nelson CA, Zeanah CH, Fox NA et al.: Cognitive recovery in socially deprived young children: the Bucharest Early Intervention Project. *Science*. 2007; **318**: 1937–40.

16 Gleason M, Froehlich W: Preschoolers and psychopharmacological interventions. *Child Adolesc Psychopharmacol News* 2008; **13**(2): 1–5.

17 Tandon M, Luby J: Psychopharmacology in preschoolers: a brief guide to clinicians. *Child Adolesc Psychopharmacol News* 2009; **14**(4): 5–7.

18 Cooper WO, Hickson GB, Fuchs C et al.: New users of antipsychotic medications among children enrolled in TennCare. *Arch Pediatr Adolesc Med*. 2004; **158**: 753–9.

19 Zito JM, Safer DJ, Valluri S et al.: Psychotherapeutic medication prevalence in Medicaid-insured preschoolers. *J Child Adolesc Psychopharmacol* 2007; **17**: 195–203.

20 Olfson M, Crystal S, Huang C et al.: Trends in antipsychotic drug use by very young, privately insured children. *J Am Acad Child Adolesc Psychiatry* 2010; **49**: 13–23.

21 Egger H: A perilous disconnect: antipsychotic drug use in very young children. *J Am Acad Child Adolesc Psychiatry* 2010; **49**: 3–6.

22 Staller JA: Psychopharmacologic treatment of aggressive preschoolers: a chart review. *Prog Neuropsychopharmacol Biol Psychiatry* 2007; **31**: 131–5.

23 Eyberg S: Parent-child interaction therapy: integration of traditional and behavioral concerns. *Child Behav Therapy* 1988; **10**: 33–46.

24 Eyberg S: Tailoring and adapting the parent-child interaction therapy to new populations. *Education and Treatment of Children*. 2005; **28**: 197–201.

25 Pincus D, Santucci L, Ehrenreich J et al.: The implementation of modified parent-child interaction therapy for youth with separation anxiety disorder. *Cognitive Behav Practice* 2008; **15**: 118–25.

26 Lenze SN, Pautsch J, Luby J: Parent-child interaction therapy emotion development: a novel treatment for depression in preschool children. *Depress Anxiety* 2010; **28**: 153–9.

27 Wagner SM, McNeil CB: Parent-child interaction therapy for ADHD: a conceptual overview and critical literature review. *Child Fam Behav Ther* 2008; **30**: 231–56.

28 Tandon M: Prenatal Cigarette Exposure and Course of Childhood ADHD. American Academy of Child and Adolecent Psychiatry and National Institute on Drug Abuse; 2010–2014. Funded grant.

29 Scheeringa MS, Salloum A, Arnberger RA et al.: Feasibility and effectiveness of cognitive-behavioral therapy for posttraumatic stress disorder in preschool children: two case reports. *J Trauma Stress* 2007; **20**: 631–6.

30 Lieberman AF, Van Horn P, Ippen CG: Toward evidence-based treatment: child-parent psychotherapy with preschoolers exposed to marital violence. *J Am Acad Child Adolesc Psychiatry* 2005; **44**: 1241–8.

31 Ferster CB, Demyer MK: The development of performances in autistic children in an automatically controlled environment. *J Chronic Dis* 1961; **13**: 312–45.

32 Smith C, Rogers S, Dawson G: The Early Start Denver Model: a comprehensive early intervention approach for toddlers with autism. In: Handleman JS, Harris S (eds) *Preschool Education Programs for Children with Autism.* Austin, TX: Pro-ed, 2007.

33 Wigal T, Greenhill L, Chuang S et al.: Safety and tolerability of methylphenidate in preschool children with ADHD. *J Am Acad Child Adolesc Psychiatry* 2006; **45**: 1294–303.

34 Geller B, Reising D, Leonard HL et al.: Critical review of tricyclic antidepressant use in children and adolescents. *J Am Acad Child Adolesc Psychiatry* 1999; **38**: 513–16.

35 Hazell P, O'Connell D, Heathcote D et al.: Efficacy of tricyclic drugs in treating child and adolescent depression: a meta-analysis. *BMJ.* 1995; **310**: 897–901.

36 Vitiello B: Research in child and adolescent psychopharmacology: recent accomplishments and new challenges. *Psychopharmacology (Berl).* 2007; **191**: 5–13.

37 Martin A, Landau J, Leebens P et al.: Risperidone-associated weight gain in children and adolescents: a retrospective chart review. *J Child Adolesc Psychopharmacol* 2000; **10**: 259–68.

38 Correll CU: Monitoring and management of antipsychotic-related metabolic and endocrine adverse events in pediatric patients. *Int Rev Psychiatry.* 2008; **20**: 195–201.

39 Correll CU, Carlson HE: Endocrine and metabolic adverse effects of psychotropic medications in children and adolescents. *J Am Acad Child Adolesc Psychiatry* 2006; **45**: 771–91.

40 Perrin JM, Friedman RA, Knilans TK: Cardiovascular monitoring and stimulant drugs for attention-deficit/hyperactivity disorder. *Pediatrics* 2008; **122**: 451–3.

41 Beck MH, Cataldo M, Slifer KJ et al.: Teaching children with attention deficit hyperactivity disorder (ADHD) and autistic disorder (AD) how to swallow pills. *Clin Pediatr (Phila).* 2005; **44**: 515–26.

42 Ghuman JK, Cataldo MD, Beck MH et al.: Behavioral training for pill-swallowing difficulties in young children with autistic disorder. *J Child Adolesc Psychopharmacol.* 2004; **14**: 601–11.

43 Aman MG: Treatment planning for patients with autism spectrum disorders. *J Clin Psychiatry* 2005; **66**(Suppl 10): 38–45.

44 Correll CU, Kane JM: One-year incidence rates of tardive dyskinesia in children and adolescents treated with second-generation antipsychotics: a systematic review. *J Child Adolesc Psychopharmacol.* 2007; **17**: 647–56.

45 Rappley MD: Actual psychotropic medication use in preschool children. *Infants and Young Children* 2006; **19**: 154–63.

46 Luby J: Early childhood depression. *Am J Psychiatry* 2009; **166**: 974–9.

47 Nagaraj R, Singhi P, Malhi P: Risperidone in children with autism: randomized, placebo-controlled, double-blind study. *J Child Neurol.* 2006; **21**: 450–5.

48 Canitano R, Scandurra V: Psychopharmacology in autism: an update. *Prog Neuropsychopharmacol Biol Psychiatry* 2011; **35**: 18–28.

49 Nahshoni E, Spitzer S, Berant M et al.: *QT Interval and Dispersion in Very Young Children Treated with Antipsychotic Drugs: A Retrospective Chart Review.* New York, NY: Mary Ann Liebert, Inc, 2009.

50 Lecavalier L: Behavioral and emotional problems in young people with pervasive developmental disorders: relative prevalence, effects of subject characteristics, and empirical classification. *J Autism Dev Disord* 2006; **36**: 1101–14.

51 Ghuman JK, Aman MG, Lecavalier L et al.: Randomized, placebo-controlled, crossover study of methylphenidate for attention-deficit/hyperactivity disorder symptoms in preschoolers with developmental disorders. *J Child Adolesc Psychopharmacol* 2009; **19**: 329–39.

52 Hollander E, Phillips A, Chaplin W et al.: A placebo controlled crossover trial of liquid fluoxetine on repetitive behaviors in childhood and adolescent autism. *Neuropsychopharmacology* 2005; **30**: 582–9.

53 King BH, Hollander E, Sikich L et al.: Lack of efficacy of citalopram in children with autism spectrum disorders and high levels of repetitive behavior: Citalopram ineffective in children with autism. *Arch Gen Psychiatry* 2009; **66**: 583–90.

54 Kolevzon A, Mathewson KA, Hollander E: Selective serotonin reuptake inhibitors in autism: a review of efficacy and tolerability. *J Clin Psychiatry.* 2006; **67**: 407–14.

55 Kollins S, Greenhill L, Swanson J et al.: Rationale, design, and methods of the Preschool ADHD Treatment Study (PATS). *J Am Acad Child Adolesc Psychiatry* 2006; **45**: 1275–83.

56 Wilens TE, Biederman J, Brown S et al.: Patterns of psychopathology and dysfunction in clinically referred preschoolers. *J Dev Behav Pediatr* 2002; **23**: S31–6.

57 Riddle M: *New Findings from the Preschoolers with ADHD Treatment Study (PATS)*. New York, NY: Mary Ann Liebert, Inc., New York, 2009.

58 Kratochvil CJ, Egger H, Greenhill LL et al.: Pharmacological management of preschool ADHD. *J Am Acad Child Adolesc Psychiatry* 2006; **45**: 115–18.

59 Kratchivil C, Vaughan B, Mayfield-Jorgensen M et al.: *A Pilot Study of Atomoxetine in Young Children with ADHD*. New York, NY: Mary Ann Liebert, Inc., 2009.

60 Eyberg SM, Nelson MM, Boggs SR: Evidence-based psychosocial treatments for children and adolescents with disruptive behavior. *J Clin Child Adolesc Psychol* 2008; **37**: 215–37.

61 Hood KK, Eyberg SM: Outcomes of parent-child interaction therapy: mothers' reports of maintenance three to six years after treatment. *J Clin Child Adolesc Psychol* 2002; **32**: 419–29.

62 Kaminski JW, Valle LA, Filene JH et al.: A meta-analytic review of components associated with parent training program effectiveness. *J Abnorm Child Psychol* 2008; **36**: 567–89.

63 Spencer TJ, Wilens TE, Biederman J et al.: Efficacy and safety of mixed amphetamine salts extended release (Adderall XR) in the management of attention-deficit/hyperactivity disorder in adolescent patients: a 4-week, randomized, double-blind, placebo-controlled, parallel-group study. *Clin Ther.* 2006; **28**: 266–79.

64 Connor DF, Barkley RA, Davis HT: A pilot study of methylphenidate, clonidine, or the combination in ADHD comorbid with aggressive oppositional defiant or conduct disorder. *Clin Pediatr (Phila).* 2000; **39**: 15–25.

65 Lee B: Clinical experience with guanfacine in 2-and 3-year-old children with attention deficit hyperactivity disorder. *Infant Mental Health Journal.* 1997; **18**: 300–5.

66 Ipser J, Stein DJ: Systematic review of pharmacotherapy of disruptive behavior disorders in children and adolescents. *Psychopharmacology (Berl)* 2007; **191**: 127–40.

67 Hazell PL, Stuart JE: A randomized controlled trial of clonidine added to psychostimulant medication for hyperactive and aggressive children. *J Am Acad Child Adolesc Psychiatry* 2003; **42**: 886–94.

68 Reyes M, Buitelaar J, Toren P et al.: A randomized, double-blind, placebo-controlled study of risperidone maintenance treatment in children and adolescents with disruptive behavior disorders. *Am J Psychiatry* 2006; **163**: 402–10.

69 Luby J, Mrakotsky, C., Stalets et al.: Risperidone in preschool children with autistic spectrum disorders: an investigation of safety and efficancy. *J Child Adolesc Psychopharmacol* 2006; **16**: 1–13.

70 Biederman J, Mick E, Hammerness P et al.: Open-label, 8-week trial of olanzapine and risperidone for the treatment of bipolar disorder in preschool-age children. *Biol Psychiatry* 2005; **58**: 589–94.

71 Cesena M, Gonzalez-Heydrich J, Szigethy E et al.: A case series of eight aggressive young children treated with risperidone. *J Child Adolesc Psychopharmacol* 2002; **12**: 337–45.

72 Egger HL, Angold A: Common emotional and behavioral disorders in preschool children: presentation, nosology, and epidemiology. *J Child Psychol Psychiatry.* 2006; **47**: 313–37.

73 Klein DN, Dougherty LR, Olino TM: Toward guidelines for evidence-based assessment of depression in children and adolescents. *J Clin Child Adolesc Psychol* 2005; **34**: 412–32.

74 Zuckerman ML, Vaughan BL, Whitney J et al. (eds): Tolerability of selective serotonin reuptake inhibitors in 39 children under age 7: a retrospective chart review. *J Child Adolesc Psychopharmacol* 2009; **17**: 165–74.

75 Safer DJ, Zito JM: Treatment-emergent adverse events from selective serotonin reuptake inhibitors by age group: children versus adolescents. *J Child Adolesc Psychopharmacol.* 2006; **16**: 159–69.

76 Luby J, Tandon M, Nicol G: Three clinical cases of DSM-IV mania symptoms in preschoolers. *J Child Adolesc Psychopharmacol* 2007; **17**: 237–43.

77 Danielyan A, Pathak S, Kowatch RA et al.: Clinical characteristics of bipolar disorder in very young children. *J Affect Disord* 2007; **97**: 51–9.

78 Luby J, Belden A: Defining and validating bipolar disorder in the preschool period. *Developmental Psychopathology* 2006; **18**: 971–88.

79 Luby J, Belden A, Tandon M (eds) *Bipolar Disorder in the Preschool Period: Development and Differential Diagnosis.* New York: Guilford Press, 2010.

80 Luby J, Tandon M, Belden A: Preschool bipolar disorder. *Child Adolesc Psychiatr Clin N Am.* 2009; **18**: 391–403.

81 Morrato EH, Nicol GE, Maahs D et al.: Metabolic screening in children receiving antipsychotic drug treatment. *Arch Pediatr Adolesc Med.* 2010; **164**: 344–51.

82 Birmaher B, Brent D, Bernet W et al.: Practice parameter for the assessment and treatment of children and adolescents with depressive disorders. *J Am Acad Child Adolesc Psychiatry.* 2007; **46**: 1503–26.

83 Nandagopal JJ, DelBello MP, Kowatch R: Pharmacologic treatment of pediatric bipolar disorder. *Child Adolesc Psychiatr Clin N Am.* 2009; **18**: 455–69.

84 Hagino OR, Weller EB, Weller RA et al.: Untoward effects of lithium treatment in children aged four through six years. *J Am Acad Child Adolesc Psychiatry* 1995; **34**: 1584–90.

85 Scheeringa M WC, Cohen JA, Amaya-Jackson L, Guthrie D: Trauma-focused cognitive-behavioral therapy for posttraumatic stress disorder in three through six year-old children: a randomized clinical trial. *J Child Psychol Psychiatry* 2010; **52**: 853–60.

86 Oner O, Oner P: Psychopharmacology of pediatric obsessive-compulsive disorder: three case reports. *J Psychopharmacol* 2008; **22**: 809–11.

87 Kurlan R, Johnson D, Kaplan EL: Streptococcal infection and exacerbations of child-hood tics and obsessive-compulsive symptoms: a prospective blinded cohort study. *Pediatrics* 2008; **121**: 1188–97.

88 Schrag A, Gilbert R, Giovannoni G et al.: Streptococcal infection, Tourette syndrome, and OCD: is there a connection? *Neurology* 2009; **73**: 1256–63.

89 Gilbert DL, Kurlan R: PANDAS: horse or zebra? *Neurology* 2009; **73**, 1252–3.

90 Scheeringa MS, Zeanah CH, Cohen JA: PTSD in children and adolescents: toward an empirically based algorithm. *Depress Anxiety* 2010; **0**: 1–13.

91 Harmon RJ, Riggs PD: Clonidine for posttraumatic stress disorder in preschool chil-dren. *J Am Acad Child Adolesc Psychiatry* 1996; **35**: 1247–9.

92 Tandon M, Cardeli E, Luby J: Internalizing disorders in early childhood: a review of depressive and anxiety disorders. *Child Adolesc Psychiatr Clin N Am.* 2009; **18**: 593–610.

93 Avci A, Diler RS, Tamam L: Fluoxetine treatment in a 2.5-year-old girl. *J Am Acad Child Adolesc Psychiatry* 1998; **37**: 901–2.

94 Wright HH, Cuccaro ML, Leonhardt TV et al.: Case study: fluoxetine in the multi-modal treatment of a preschool child with selective mutism. *J Am Acad Child Adolesc Psychiatry* 1995; **34**: 857–62.

95 Weiss MD, Wasdell MB, Bomben MM et al.: Sleep hygiene and melatonin treatment for children and adolescents with ADHD and initial insomnia. *J Am Acad Child Adolesc Psychiatry* 2006; **45**: 512–19.

CHAPTER 17

Combination Pharmacotherapy for Psychiatric Disorders in Children and Adolescents

Gagan Joshi & Anna M. Georgiopoulos
Harvard Medical School and Massachusetts General Hospital, Boston, USA

Like the use of combination or adjunctive pharmacotherapy in the treatment of congestive heart failure and epilepsy [1], medication combinations are being increasingly used for the treatment of child psychiatric disorders [2–4]. In one population of older adolescents leaving foster care, 10% were prescribed three or more simultaneous psychotropic medicines—most frequently an antidepressant, antipsychotic, and a mood stabilizer [5]. An analysis of over 27 000 medical office visits documented an increase over time in the use of more than one psychotropic medication in children from 22.2% (in 1996–9) to 32.2% (in 2004–7) of visits in which a mental disorder was diagnosed. Specifically, co-administration of antidepressants and antipsychotics or attention-deficit hyperactivity disorder (ADHD) medications and antipsychotics increased during the study period [4].

There are multiple reasons that clinicians may opt for combination pharmacotherapy. When one medication is partially effective but not tolerated in higher doses, augmentation with a second agent may be tried. For example, buprorion might be added to a selective serotonin reuptake inhibitor (SSRI) to achieve full remission of depression. A medication may be added to indirectly raise the levels or boost the effect of an existing medication, as in the case of using relatively lower doses of clomipramine plus an SSRI in the treatment of OCD. Sometimes, medication may be added to offset an adverse effect, as with the addition of cyproheptadine to stimulate appetite in children treated with stimulants for ADHD who are losing weight [6]. Occasionally when children have comorbid conditions, a single agent may be used to treat both, as in the case of desipramine for children with ADHD and depression [7]. Often, however, more than one class of medication is required to address multiple psychiatric

Pharmacotherapy of Child and Adolescent Psychiatric Disorders, Third Edition.
Edited by David R. Rosenberg and Samuel Gershon.
© 2012 John Wiley & Sons, Ltd. Published 2012 by John Wiley & Sons, Ltd.

disorders, as in children with the triad of tic disorders, ADHD and OCD. Sometimes, combination pharmacology is required in children with psychiatric and medical comorbidities, with the differential tolerability to psychotropic agents that may occur in these complex children. For example, in one case series, the best achieved treatment regimen for some children with cystic fibrosis and comorbid ADHD—in order to achieve benefit for ADHD without exacerbating weight loss or other problems caused by their cystic fibrosis—involved the concurrent use of a stimulant and a nonstimulant or two nonstimulant medications [8].

However, there are also scenarios in which the rationale for combination pharmacotherapy may be less clear. This may occur in cases of diagnostic uncertainty or an evolving diagnostic picture. For example, in a case of rapidly worsening anxiety and functional impairment in which prodromal psychosis is suspected, the clinician may consider the risks and benefits of adding an atypical antipsychotic to the patient's anti-anxiety agent in an attempt to prevent further clinical deterioration, versus waiting for more definitive psychotic symptoms to occur first. In other cases, the prescribing clinician or treatment setting has changed, and pertinent treatment history, including presenting symptoms and other factors influencing previous medication initiation decisions, have not been communicated in sufficient detail. In this context, it can be uncertain whether continued combination pharmacotherapy is warranted, and a medication originally intended for short-term use or for symptoms that are no longer of clinical concern is at risk of being unnecessarily continued. In this chapter we review the child psychiatric disorders that may require combinations of pharmacotherapeutic agents and the evidence available to guide our use of combination pharmacotherapy.

Bipolar disorder

Combination pharmacotherapy has increasingly been used to manage pediatric onset bipolar disorder (BPD) in clinical practice. In a recent retrospective chart review, more than three-fourths (77%) of young people diagnosed with bipolar spectrum disorder (n = 53) were receiving active combination psychopharmacological treatment under the care of child psychiatrists practicing in a pediatric psychopharmacology specialty clinic [9].

Controlled studies [10] have shown that a combination of mood stabilizers may be more efficacious than monotherapy for the acute [1] and maintenance [11] treatment of adult patients with bipolar disorder (BPD). This trend is reflected in a reported increase in the average number of medications prescribed for a large sample of adult patients with BPD discharged from the Clinical Center Research Unit of the Biological Psychiatry Branch of the National Institute of Mental Health (NIMH) between 1974 and 1995 [1]. Children with BPD may also be only partially responsive to lithium monotherapy [12], warranting initiation of a so-far small number of pediatric combination pharmacotherapy studies [13].

In adults, the BALANCE [14] study showed that combination therapy with lithium plus valproate prevented relapse better than valproate monotherapy. However, it was unclear whether this combination therapy was superior to lithium monotherapy [14], and it was possible to conclude that the addition of valproate to lithium monotherapy may be of minimal benefit [15]. Findling et al. [16, 17] conducted a series of trials examining the acute and maintenance efficacy and safety of combination therapy with lithium and divalproex sodium in young people with BPD. Young people (n = 90; 5–17 years old) who met the diagnostic criteria for BPD type I or II and had experienced a manic or hypomanic episode within the three months prior to baseline were treated with both lithium and divalproex for a mean duration of 11 weeks in an open fashion [16]. Target doses of 20 mg/kg/day of divalproex and 30 mg/kg/day of lithium were achieved by the end of 2 weeks—unless drug-related adverse effects precluded further dose increase—with doses adjusted to achieve serum divalproex levels between 50 and 100 µg/mL and serum lithium levels between 0.6 and 1.2 mmol/L. At the end of the trial, participants received a divalproex mean dose of 863 (±398) mg/day with a mean serum level of 79.8 (±25.9) µg/mL and a lithium mean dose of 923 (±380) mg/day with a mean serum level of 0.9 (±0.3) mmol/L. Significant response for mania and depression was observed by eight weeks of this combination treatment and nearly half of the participants (47%) achieved biphasic sustained remission (mood stabilization for four consecutive weeks). A history of psychosis was more common in the nonremitters. Combination therapy was well tolerated. Gastrointestinal disturbance, enuresis, tremors, headache, and increased thirst were the most common adverse effects experienced by more than a third of the participants. Adverse effects were generally of mild severity and transient. Treatment-limiting adverse effects, which were mostly attributable to lithium, were experienced by a substantial minority (17%) of the young people with BPD. The response rate achieved by eight weeks on combined divalproex and lithium therapy in this trial was superior to the response rate observed with short-term (eight-week) monotherapy of divalproex or lithium in young people with BPD [18]. These findings suggest that the use of combination divalproex and lithium may be reasonably well tolerated in young people with BPD. Nearly two-thirds of the young people with BPD (n = 38) who achieved sustained remission (n = 60) on combination therapy experienced relapse in their mood symptoms upon double-blind randomization to treatment with a single mood stabilizer (either lithium or divalproex) [19]. Unlike in the BALANCE study, survival time to relapse did not differ between lithium and divalproex treatment groups in this pediatric population [19]; it is possible that lithium does not carry the same advantage over divalproex in children, or that the Findling study was not powerful enough to detect a relatively small difference. Those who relapsed on a single mood stabilizer were subsequently retreated in an open-label manner for eight weeks with the combination of lithium and divalproex [17]. Ninety percent of the young people with BPD responded to a mean total daily lithium dose of 872 mg (22.2 mg/kg) and divalproex dose of 833 mg (21.0 mg/kg). Overall, re-initiation of combination therapy was well tolerated with no subjects discontinuing due to a medication-related adverse event. It appears that most young people with BPD who stabilize on combination lithium and divalproex therapy and subsequently relapse during monotherapy can safely and effectively be re-stabilized with the re-initiation of lithium and divalproex combination treatment. Notably there were no significant differences in the serum levels of lithium and divalproex prior to re-initiation and upon re-stabilization on combination therapy. This series of studies has the advantage of answering the clinically relevant question of whether pediatric patients prescribed this combination therapy who destabilize following removal of one agent are likely to re-stabilize when it is re-introduced. However, a study directly comparing treatment arms randomized to each monotherapy, combination therapy, and placebo would significantly add to the evidence base regarding lithium and divalproex combination therapy.

In two studies by Kafantaris et al. [20, 21], antipsychotic agents in combination with lithium were found to be therapeutic in adolescents with BPD (either acutely manic or mixed with psychotic features), and early withdrawal resulted in relapse. In the first study [20], young people (n = 5) with BPD experienced resolution of psychotic features on a combination of haloperidol and lithium. These young people experienced a re-emergence of their psychotic symptoms within 1 week after withdrawal of haloperidol. In an extension of this study [21], 64% of the adolescents with BPD (n = 42) responded to a four-week treatment with lithium in combination with an antipsychotic agent. The responders were more likely to be medication naive and to be experiencing their first psychotic episodes. When responders to the combination therapy were subsequently treated with lithium monotherapy, nearly half of the BPD adolescents experienced re-emergence of symptoms. Adolescents who had had a prior psychotic episode could not tolerate discontinuation of their antipsychotic medication. However, the design of these studies did not make it possible to determine whether antipsychotic alone would be as effective as the combination of lithium plus antipsychotic in this population.

In a six-week, controlled trial of divalproex monotherapy compared to divalproex and quetiapine combination therapy in acutely manic, hospitalized adolescents, DelBello et al. [22] found a significantly greater symptom reduction and higher response rates for divalproex and quetiapine (mean dose: 432 mg/day) combination treatment than for divalproex alone (87% versus 53%) at a mean serum divalproex level of 102 mg/dL in the divalproex monotherapy group and 104 mg/dL in the divalproex and quetiapine combination group. Again, while suggestive that antipsychotic augmentation may be useful and tolerable, it cannot be determined from this study whether quetiapine alone would be as effective as the combination of divalproex plus quetiapine. In a six-month, uncontrolled trial of combination treatment with either risperidone and lithium or risperidone and divalproex in 37 acutely manic or mixed young people with BPD, Pavuluri et al. [23] reported similar rates of response (defined as ≥50% decline from baseline on the Young Mania Rating Scale (YMRS)) and remission (defined as ≥50% change from baseline YMRS, Clinical Global Improvement ≤2, and Children's Global Assessment Scale ≥51). For the two groups, they reported 80% response and 60% remission for the combination of risperidone and divalproex, and 82% response and 65% remission for the combination risperidone and lithium, with large effect sizes (2.82 and 4.36, respectively). Mean risperidone doses were 0.75 (±0.75) mg in combination with lithium and 0.70 (±0.67) mg in combination with divalproex. The divalproex sodium mean dose was 925 (±325) mg (serum level: 106 μg/dl) and the lithium carbonate mean dose was 750 (±400) mg (serum level: 0.9 mEq/l). Overall, combination therapy was well tolerated in both groups. The majority of side-effects were mild to moderate. The two subjects who withdrew from the lithium and risperidone group cited enuresis and fatigue as reasons. All subjects gained weight over six months. The mean weight increase for lithium and risperidone was 6 (±3.8) kg and for the combination of divalproex and risperidone, the mean weight increase was 6.8 (±4.2) kg.

Summary of combination therapy with adjunctive mood stabilizers or antipsychotics

These studies, taken together, suggest that combination therapy with adjunctive mood stabilizers or antipsychotic agents with the goal of improving response rates merits further study, particularly in those children with moderate to severe symptomatology for whom the possibility of additional benefit may outweigh the risk of additional side-effects. Further randomized controlled trials with larger sample sizes and direct

comparisons of both monotherapies to each other and to the correspond-
ing combination therapy are needed to conclusively determine that a
combination therapy is more efficacious than monotherapy in pediatric
BPD.

Weight gain associated with atypical antipsychotic medications

As weight gain is associated with the use of atypical antipsychotic
medications, combination therapy with agents that are associated with
weight loss could be beneficial in offsetting weight gain. This notion was
empirically examined by Wozniak et al. [24] in an eight-week uncontrolled trial of olanzapine with and without topiramate for the treatment of
BPD in young people (6–17 years old). Although there was no difference
in tolerability and antimanic response, the weight gain in young people
with BPD who received topiramate (70.5 ±30.5 mg/day) in combination
with olanzapine was significantly lower than with olanzapine treatment
alone (5.3 ± 2.1 kg versus 2.6 ± 3.6 kg). In an attempt to study the
mitigating effect of stimulant medications on the weight gain, metabolic
abnormalities, sleep disturbance, prolactin abnormalities, and therapeutic effects that are associated with atypical antipsychotics, Penzner et al.
[25] examined the hypothesis that stimulants have an opposing dopamine
receptor activity and adverse effects, through a large (n = 153) naturalistic study of young people (4–19 years old) who required treatment with
atypical antipsychotics (risperidone, aripiprazole, quetiapine, olanzapine,
ziprasidone, or clozapine) for clinically significant aggression or oppositionality associated with diverse psychiatric conditions (oppositional
defiant disorder, conduct disorder, disruptive behavior disorder-NOS,
impulse control disorder-NOS, intermittent explosive disorder, Tourette's
disorder, autism spectrum disorders). Contrary to expectation, co-
treatment of atypical antipsychotics with stimulants did not seem to
significantly reduce antipsychotic effects on body composition (body
weight, body mass index, fat mass, and waist circumference), metabolic
parameters (total cholesterol, low-density lipoprotein cholesterol, high-
density lipoprotein-cholesterol, triglycerides, triglycerides/ high-density
lipoprotein ratio, glucose, insulin and homeostasis model assessment of
insulin resistance), prolactin, sedation, or broad efficacy.

Attention-deficit hyperactivity disorder is highly comorbid with juvenile
onset BPD. Systematic studies of pediatric populations with BPD show that
the rates of comorbid ADHD range from 60% to 90% [26–28]. Whereas a
high prevalence of ADHD is reported in young people with BPD, a modest rate (22%) of comorbid BPD is reported in pediatric populations with
ADHD [29]. In young people with BPD and ADHD whose mood is well stabilized, ADHD symptoms often become the second most severe presenting
complaint [30].

In youngsters with BPD, comorbid ADHD could be addressed selectively with the anti-ADHD armamentarium but only after mood stabilization.

ADHD agents in mood-stabilized young people with BPD

The anti-ADHD agents (stimulants and nonstimulants) have been studied in mood-stabilized young people with BPD and most often reported to be efficacious in treating comorbid features of ADHD without precipitating (hypo)-mania. A controlled trial of stimulants as an adjunctive therapy for ADHD in young people with mania stabilized on divalproex found mixed amphetamine salts (AMP) to be safe and efficacious for the treatment of ADHD in the context of BPD [31]. In this two-stage trial, young people with comorbid BPD and ADHD who achieved significant improvement in mania, but no improvement of ADHD symptoms (80%; 32/40) in the first phase of an eight-week open trial of divalproex sodium were treated with AMP at a dose of 5 mg twice daily (n = 30; 8–17 years old) for four weeks in a controlled crossover fashion. Significant improvement in ADHD symptoms was observed with combined AMP and divalproex treatment. AMP was considered safe and effective without promoting destabilization of BPD. The adverse effects were few, transient, and mild to moderate in severity. Young people with BPD and comorbid ADHD continued to benefit from the combined therapy in the follow-up maintenance phase (12-week) although nearly half of them (45%) required an increase in the dose of AMP for sustaining the treatment benefits achieved in the acute phase of the trial, even though the overall doses used to successfully treat concurrent ADHD were less than expected.

The role of methylphenidate (MPH) as an anti-ADHD agent in mood-stabilized young people with BPD has been studied through three placebo-controlled trials in relatively small sample sizes with conflicting results. Two placebo-controlled trials suggest benefit of combining MPH with mood stabilizer(s) in treating ADHD in young people with BPD [32, 33] but one trial concluded otherwise [34]. Carlson et al. [32] conducted a crossover study in psychiatrically hospitalized prepubertal children (n = 7; 6–9 years old) diagnosed with both a mood disorder (BPD or major depressive disorder) and a disruptive behavior disorder who were compared on MPH monotherapy, lithium monotherapy, and the combination treatment of MPH and lithium. Results suggested that the combination therapy with low doses of MPH (5 or 10 mg) and lithium (600–1500 mg/day; serum levels between 0.7 and 1.1 mEq/L) was more effective in ameliorating symptoms of ADHD than the monotherapy with either agent.

Findling et al. [33] conducted a four-week, controlled crossover trial of MPH in a sample of young people with BPD with comorbid ADHD (n = 16; 5–17 years old) who achieved euthymia on a stable dose of at least one mood stabilizer, and reported that concomitant treatment with MPH in a dose dependent manner (5 mg/10 mg/15 mg twice daily) significantly improved symptoms of ADHD without destabilization of mood. The majority (75%) of the participants in this trial were on a combination of divalproex and lithium for mood stabilization. Combination treatment was generally well tolerated and the adverse events were as typically expected and generally did not worsen quantitatively on addition of MPH to the ongoing treatment with mood stabilizer(s).

Zenia et al. [34] examined the effect of MPH adjunctive therapy for the treatment of ADHD in young people with BPD by conducting a four-week controlled crossover trial with MPH in young people (n = 16; 8–17 years old) who had a significant response in manic symptoms with aripiprazole (range: 5 to 20 mg/day; mean: 12.8 ± 6.3 mg/day) but continued to experience clinically significant symptoms of ADHD. MPH adjunctive therapy (0.3 and 0.7 mg/kg/day) was not effective in treating symptoms of ADHD, however was effective in treating features of depression and was well tolerated with the exception of one subject who developed severe mood destabilization on MPH.

Uncontrolled trials of nonstimulant anti-ADHD agents have been conducted in comorbid BPD and ADHD populations. Chang et al. [35] examined the role of atomoxetine as an adjunctive therapy for the treatment of ADHD in a small sample of young people with BPD and comorbid ADHD (n = 12; 6–17 years old) who were euthymic on antimanic agent(s) (lithium, anticonvulsants, and atypical antipsychotics). The acute (eight-week) trial of atomoxetine at a mean dose of 60 mg/day was well tolerated and effective in treating the symptoms of ADHD. More importantly none of the participants experienced a (hypo)-manic switch during the course of the trial.

In practice, treatment for BPD typically takes clinical priority over ADHD treatment. The studies reviewed above provide preliminary evidence that once BPD is well controlled using a mood-stabilizing medication, stimulants or nonstimulants may be introduced cautiously. However, because of the small number of participants represented by the available data, even in the aggregate, additional studies of treatments for ADHD in the setting of BPD are needed to draw conclusions regarding the optimal strategy for this common clinical scenario.

Thyroid augmentation

Despite the documented efficacy of thyroid hormone augmentation of mood stabilizers and antidepressants [36] in adults with affective disorders [37], especially patients with rapid-cycling BPD [36], no controlled studies of this potential treatment have been published in children and adolescents.

One case report has described the potential benefit of combining thyroxine (T4) with valproate [38]. A 13-year-old male adolescent with refractory rapid cycling BPD was stabilized for nine months after levothyroxine (125 μg/day titrated over 10 days) was added to valproate 1000 mg/day. In this case report, the patient's pretreatment (baseline) free T4 level was 1.5 ng/dL, and his thyrotropin (TSH) level was 2.1 mI/mL. After six weeks of thyroid augmentation treatment, his free T4 level was 1.4 ng/dL, and his TSH level was less than 0.1 mI/mL. The potential risks and benefits of thyroid augmentation in bipolar children [38] and adolescents have not been studied. Hospitalized adolescents with comorbid BPD and attention-deficit hyperactivity disorder (ADHD) reportedly have lower mean serum T4 concentration compared with patients with BPD alone [39]. This and other observed differences in basal thyroid hormone levels in depressed and manic adolescents [40] may underlie important implications regarding the potential benefits of thyroid supplementation in adolescents with BPD and comorbid ADHD who do not respond to mood stabilizers alone [39].

Major depressive disorder

There is minimal systematic evidence to date replicating antidepressant augmentation strategies typically used in adults with treatment resistant depression in pediatric populations. However, a variable response augmentation rate of SSRIs with lithium in adults with major depressive disorder (MDD) [41] has been replicated in two pediatric studies of augmentation of antidepressant therapy with lithium [42, 43].

In Ryan et al.'s [42] retrospective chart review of the efficacy of lithium augmentation of tricyclic antidepressants (TCAs) in children, 14 adolescents with nonbipolar depression who did not respond adequately to a trial of TCAs and received subsequent augmentation with lithium were reviewed retrospectively by two research nurses not blind to treatment. The majority of the subjects had received at least six weeks of TCA treatment (and no further clinical improvement after week 8) before the addition of lithium for a period of at least six weeks. The mean age of this sample was 17 years. Five patients (36%) required hospitalization over the course of their illness. Six of 14 (43%) patients were considered responders (defined as patients improved to the point of being no more than mildly symptomatic or better) following the addition of lithium, five of 14 (36%) patients had little or no improvement after the addition of lithium, and three of 14 (21%) patients were considered partial responders (i.e., evidenced "some additional improvement") after lithium augmentation. The severity of illness did not differ between the groups, nor did the mean serum lithium level for the responders, (0.65 mEq/L) compared to the nonresponders (0.64 mEq/L). The groups' mean severity rating at four weeks had improved significantly by six weeks following the addition of lithium. Most responders experienced a gradual improvement in symptoms over the first month of lithium treatment. The most common side-effects for patients on TCAs alone were anticholinergic side-effects (n = 12) and dizziness (n = 10) and for the combination of lithium with TCAs, were hand tremors (n = 5), dizziness (n = 5), nausea (n = 5), and dry mouth (n = 5). The conclusion drawn by the authors of this case report is that certain adolescents, previously unresponsive to TCAs, may respond to augmentation with lithium. The duration of the prior TCA treatment was longer (eight weeks) than the described length of TCA treatment in adults (three weeks), leading the authors to conclude that the therapeutic response was indeed a consequence of lithium augmentation rather than a time effect of the TCA treatment alone. The data do not preclude the possibility that some patients might have improved with the passage of time alone, given the fluctuating course of the illness. This study merits controlled replication, especially considering the high switch rate of children with prepubertal MDD to prepubertal bipolarity [44].

Ryan et al.'s [42] report was followed by an open trial of lithium augmentation in adolescent nonresponders to imipramine published by Strober [43]. In this three-week open trial, 24 adolescents classified as nonresponders (less than 50% reduction on Hamilton Depression (HAM-D) scores and final score >10 after six weeks of treatment with imipramine) were compared with a case-control group of ten adolescent nonresponders to imipramine who continued to receive imipramine monotherapy. Lithium was started at 900 mg in three divided doses and subsequently increased, depending on clinical response, to 0.7–1.2 mEq/L. The absolute magnitude of the HAM-D change within each group was modest (i.e., an average of 14% reduction from baseline), as was the non-significant difference between the two groups in average HAM-D scores at the end of the trial. Nevertheless, the average HAM-D score for patients on lithium augmentation decreased from 18 points at the start of the trial to 13.4 points at the end of week 3, compared to a drop of 18.5 to 15.4 in the imipramine monotherapy group. The differential effect examined by computing the percentage of improvement in depression scores for each patient was significant between groups (the average percentage of improvement of 26% for the lithium group compared to 6% for controls, $p < 0.05$, by r-test). Eight subjects in the treatment group showed partial improvement during the three-week trial, in contrast to only one of the ten controls. Lithium augmentation in this study was associated with few side-effects, mainly polyuria and tremor (n = 7). The final estimates of an 8% rate of clinically significant improvement and 33% rate of partial improvement, a much lower rate compared to adult studies of lithium augmentation (65%) [13], suggests that lithium may have a potential use as an adjunctive strategy in some tricyclic-resistant adolescents with MDD, albeit less efficaciously than in adults with tricyclic-resistant MDD.

In addition, there is some evidence regarding the treatment of depression in children with comorbid ADHD. A small case series found the combination of stimulant added to fluoxetine or sertraline for comorbid MDD and ADHD to be well tolerated in children [45]. As is typical in clinical practice, treatment of MDD was prioritized, with the antidepressant started first, followed by addition of a stimulant for persisting ADHD symptoms. Similarly, an open trial of 32 children treated with fluoxetine augmentation of MPH for comorbid ADHD and depressive disorders showed generally positive treatment responses with good tolerability [46].

Kratochvil et al. [47] investigated whether the presence of ADHD moderated outcomes in the Treatment for Adolescents with Depression Study (TADS), in which adolescents with MDD (n = 439) were randomized to fluoxetine, cognitive- behavioral therapy, a combination of these two treatments, or placebo. Sixty-two (14.1%) subjects had comorbid ADHD, and those on stable doses of stimulant (n = 20) were allowed to continue this concomitant treatment during the trial. The presence of ADHD was found to moderate MDD treatment, with improved response to CBT or fluoxetine monotherapy in this cohort compared to those with MDD but without ADHD.

Another study randomized pediatric subjects (n = 173) with ADHD and comorbid depression/anxiety to double blind fluoxetine or placebo, with open label concomitant atomoxetine treatment for the final five of eight weeks. Tolerability for combined atomoxetine and fluoxetine was good and symptoms of both ADHD and depression improved and tolerability for combined atomoxetine and fluoxetine was generally good. However, in the combined group, greater increases in pulse and blood pressure than subjects receiving monotherapy were noted, and there was a trend toward more frequent complaints of decreased appetite. Of note, atomoxetine is metabolized via the cytochrome P-450 2D6 (CYP2D6) pathway, and the dose of atomoxetine may require downward adjustment when co-administered with SSRI antidepressants that inhibit CYP2D6 such as fluoxetine. In addition, a later double-blind randomized controlled trial did not find benefit for atomoxetine in improving MDD symptoms in children with comorbid ADHD and MDD [48].

Attention-deficit hyperactivity disorder

The use of single agents in the treatment of ADHD may not be effective in 30–40% of children [49]. Although desipramine was often prescribed in the past for children with stimulant-resistant ADHD or in combination pharmacotherapy [50, 51], cases of sudden death associated with desipramine [52] have diminished the enthusiasm for the prescription of desipramine in youngsters with ADHD or MDD.

Nortriptyline has seen a resurgence as a second- (or third)-line agent [53] for the treatment of comorbid or stimulant-refractory ADHD [54]. Its benefit in the treatment of ADHD was retrospectively evaluated by Wilens et al. [55] who noted that 47% of a sample of 37 children and 21 adolescents with treatment-refractory, highly comorbid ADHD were receiving adjunctive medications in addition to nortriptyline. Nortriptyline treatment ranging from 0.4 to 4.5 mg/kg (average 2 mg/kg/daily) may have had an independent effect because no association was found between response and concurrent pharmacotherapy. Mild adverse effects were reported in 20 subjects (34%) [55].

More recently, there has been increasing interest in combination therapy for the management of ADHD symptoms in young people who experience partial response to an anti-ADHD agent. Wilens et al. [56] evaluated the effectiveness of giving OROS methylphenidate (OROS-MPH) to young people who were partial responders to atomoxetine in the treatment of ADHD. Significant improvement in the severity of ADHD features and executive functioning was observed following a three-week addition of up to 54 mg OROS-MPH in young people (n = 50) who experienced partial response to a four-week treatment with atomoxetine therapy. The mean weight-corrected doses of atomoxetine and OROS-MPH in the combination therapy were 1.1 mg/kg/day and 1 mg/kg/day, respectively. Combination therapy was generally well tolerated with insomnia, headache, appetite loss, and irritability the most commonly reported adverse effects.

Two nonstimulant alpha-2 adrenergic receptor agonists—extended release guanfacine and extended release clonidine—now have Food and Drug Administration approval for use either as monotherapy or in combination therapy with a stimulant for the treatment of ADHD in children. Spencer et al. [57] added extended release guanfacine for treating ADHD in young people with partial response to stimulant (MPH or AMP). Significant improvement in ADHD severity (56% decrease in severity) was observed with guanfacine combination therapy in young people (6–17 years; mean age = 11.4 years old) treated with MPH (n = 42) and AMP (n = 33). Guanfacine was titrated up to maximum dose of 4 mg/day (mean dose 3.1 mg/day; 0.07 mg/kg). Combination therapy was well tolerated with fatigue (34.7%), headache (33.3%), upper abdominal pain (32.0%), irritability (32.0%), somnolence (18.7%), and insomnia (16.0%) as the most common adverse effects. In a 16-week controlled trial of clonidine, MPH, and combination therapy with MPH (25.4 ± 18.2 mg/day) and clonidine, (0.23 ± 0.13 mg/day) in young people with ADHD (n = 122;

7–12 years old), the magnitude of improvement in the severity of ADHD was observed to be the largest with combination treatment than with monotherapy with either agent [58]. The most frequent adverse effects included nervousness, somnolence, apathy, depression, dyspepsia, insomnia, fatigue, and headache. The rates of adverse effects experienced in the combination therapy were not different than those noted with either agent alone.

Taken together, these findings suggest that combination therapy with a stimulant plus nonstimulant for ADHD is a promising strategy for treating symptoms of ADHD that are partially responsive to monotherapy.

Obsessive-compulsive disorder

Many children with obsessive compulsive disorder (OCD) are partial responders to SSRIs. In a retrospective chart review of 38 pediatric patients with OCD treated with fluoxetine, Geller and et al. [26] reported that combination pharmacotherapy was required for treatment success in 42% of the sample [26]. A common approach in low treatment-response cases would be the combination of clomipramine with an SSRI, which is more effective than monotherapy with either agent.

In a case series on combination treatment with SSRI and clomipramine for the treatment of OCD in young people (n = 5) and young (n = 2) adults (predominantly males), Figueroa and colleagues [59] reported improvement in OCD with the addition of most often clomipramine (5/7) to partially SSRI (sertraline, fluoxetine, fluvoxamine, paroxetine) treatment responsive OCD symptoms. Treatment effects persisted through 5 to 22 months of follow-up from the onset of combination therapy. Combination therapy was reasonably well tolerated with cardiovascular (tachycardia, QTc prolongation) concerns being the most common adverse effects. In this case series, due to the potential of SSRI and clomipramine to increase the blood levels of both the medications, lower than expected doses of both the medications were tolerated and needed in combination therapy for achieving therapeutic response in individuals with OCD. This case series suggests that clomipramine and SSRI combinations may be more effective for patients who cannot tolerate high doses of either medication or who remain significantly impaired on one drug. In the only other published augmentation strategy in pediatric OCD, Simeon et al. [60] openly treated six adolescent OCD patients who failed to respond to clomipramine at a mean daily dose of 92 mg for three to 32 weeks. Fluoxetine was then added at 20–40 mg, and the clomipramine dosage reduced. This combination resulted in marked clinical global improvement in five patients and moderate improvement in one patient after eight to 24 weeks of combined treatment. Therapeutic effects persisted during follow-up of 8 to 44 weeks. Combination therapy resulted in more effective responses at lower doses of both medications, with fewer overall side-effects. Clonazepam was also shown to be helpful in children [61] with OCD, but sedation, as well as behavioral disinhibition in children in particular, may limit the use of clonazepam and lorazepam, which should be used with caution.

The other most commonly used pharmacotherapeutic combinations for the treatment of juvenile OCD–SSRI plus benzodiazepine, SSRI plus TCA, and SSRI plus mood stabilizers or atypical antipsychotics—have not been systematically evaluated in open or controlled pediatric studies [26].

Tics and Tourette's syndrome

It is well known that stimulants can exacerbate tics [54]. Conversely, it has been estimated that approximately 50% of patients with Tourette's syndrome may also meet the diagnostic criteria for ADHD [54]. Tricyclic antidepressants have been successfully used in children with this comorbidity. There is minimal data on combination therapy in pediatric patients with tic disorders. One small open label trial of haloperidol plus trazodone in patients with tic disorders found good tolerability and response; in this case, augmentation was used in hopes of reducing the required dose of haloperidol [62].

Pervasive developmental disorders

The treatment of pervasive developmental disorder (PDD) requires appropriate behavioral and pharmacological interventions [63]. Combination pharmacotherapy (the simultaneous use of two or more medications) was used in 16% of a sample of 109 children, adolescents, and adults (mean age: 13.9 years) diagnosed with higher functioning PDD [64]. None of these pharmacological combinations has yet been systematically evaluated in open or controlled pediatric studies for the treatment of children and adolescents with PDD.

Conclusion

The treatment of comorbid child psychiatric disorders requires a knowledge of the neurochemical correlates of each disorder and medication under consideration for use. While combination pharmacotherapy is increasingly being used as a strategy to treat children with complex or difficult-to-manage psychiatric illness, caution should be used when combining medications in children. It is important to be aware of possible medication interactions that may warrant dose adjustments (for instance, reduction of atomoxetine dose when used with fluoxetine) or contraindicate certain treatments (the use of a monoamine oxidase inhibitor simultaneously with an SSRI). Adding or adjusting psychopharmaceutic agents one at a time in a systematic fashion whenever clinically feasible will facilitate a clearer assessment of the benefits and adverse effects of each agent, and decrease the likelihood that agents that are minimally effective or poorly tolerated in a given child will be continued longer than necessary. Use of evidence-based psychotherapies to augment the effects of medications, while outside the scope of this chapter, should also be strongly considered in children with complex or treatment resistant psychiatric profiles. Controlled studies assessing the safety and effectiveness of combined pharmacotherapy in child psychiatric disorders are needed to assist in the development of effective treatment strategies and practice guidelines for children and adolescents presenting with psychiatric comorbidity or with severe psychiatric illness resistant to monotherapy treatment approaches.

References

1 Frye MA, Ketter TA, Leverich GS et al.: The increasing use of polypharmacotherapy for refractory mood disorders: 22 years of study. *J Clinical Psychiatry* 2000; **61**: 9–15.

2 Wilens TE, Spencer T, Biederman J et al.: Combined pharmacotherapy: an emerging trend in pediatric psychopharmacology. *J Child Adolesc Psychopharmacol* 1995; **34**: 110–12.

3 Wilens TE: Combined pharmacotherapy in pediatric psychopharmacology: friend or foe? *J Child Adolesc Psychopharmacol* 2009; **19**: 483–4.

4 Comer JS, Olfson M, Mojtabai R: National trends in child and adolescent psychotropic polypharmacy in office-based practice, 1996–2007. *J Child Adolesc Psychopharmacol* 2010; **49**: 1001–10.

5 Raghavan R, McMillen JC: Use of multiple psychotropic medications among adolescents aging out of foster care. *Psychiatr Serv* 2008; **59**: 1052–5.

6 Daviss WB, Scott J: A chart review of cyproheptadine for stimulant-induced weight loss. *J Child Adolesc Psychopharmacol* 2004; **14**: 65–73.

7 Biederman J, Baldessarini RJ, Wright V et al.: A double-blind placebo controlled study of desipramine in the treatment of attention deficit disorder: III. Lack of impact of comorbidity and family history factors on clinical response. *J Child Adolesc Psychopharmacol* 1993; **32**: 199–204.

8 Georgiopoulos A, Hua L: The diagnosis and treatment of attention deficit-hyperactivity disorder in children and adolescents with cystic fibrosis: a retrospective study. *Psychosomatics* 2011; **52**: 160–6.

9 Potter MP, Liu HY, Monuteaux MC et al.: Prescribing patterns for treatment of pediatric bipolar disorder in a specialty clinic. *J Child Adolesc Psychopharmacol* 2009; **19**: 529–538.

10 Small JG, Klapper MH, Marhenke JD et al.: Lithium combined with carbamazepine or haloperidol in the treatment of mania. *Psychopharmacol Bull* 1995; **31**: 265–72.

11 Denicoff KD, Smith-Jackson EE, Disney ER et al.: Comparative prophylactic efficacy of lithium, carbamazepine, and the combination in bipolar disorder. *J Clin Psychiatry* 1997; **58**: 470–8.

12 Alessi N, Naylor M, Ghaziuddin M et al.: Update on lithium carbonate therapy in children and adolescents. *J Child Adolesc Psychopharmacol* 1994; **33**: 291–304.

13 Thase ME, Kupfer DJ, Frank E et al.: Treatment of imipramine-resistant recurrent depression: II. An open clinical trial of lithium augmentation. *J Clin Psychiatry* 1989; **50**: 413–17.

14 The BALANCE Investigators and Collaborators: lithium plus valproate combination therapy versus monotherapy for relapse prevention in bipolar 1 disorder (balance): a randomised open-label trial. *Thelancet.com* 2010; **375**: 385–95.

15 Alda M, O'Donovan C: A much needed BALANCE. *Bipolar Disord* 2010; **12**: 678–80.

16 Findling RL, McNamara NK, Gracious BL et al.: Combination Lithium and Divalproex Sodium in Pediatric Bipolarity. *J Am Acad Child Adolesc Psychiatry* 2003; **42**: 895–901.

17 Findling RL, McNamara NK, Stansbrey R et al.: Combination lithium and divalproex sodium in pediatric bipolar symptom re-stabilization. *J Am Acad Child Adolesc Psychiatry* 2006; **45**: 142–8.

18 Kowatch RA, Suppes T, Carmody TJ et al.: Effect size of lithium, divalproex sodium, and carbamazepine in children and adolescents with bipolar disorder. *J Child Adolesc Psychopharmacol* 2000; **39**: 713–20.

19 Findling RL, McNamara NK, Youngstrom EA et al.: Double-Blind 18-Month Trial of Lithium Versus Divalproex Maintenance Treatment in Pediatric Bipolar Disorder. *J Am Acad Child Adolesc Psychiatry* 2005; **44**: 409–17.

20 Kafantaris V, Dicker R, Coletti DJ et al.: Adjunctive antipsychotic treatment is necessary for adolescents with psychotic mania. *J Child Adolesc Psychopharmacol* 2001; **11**: 409–13.

21 Kafantaris V, Coletti DJ, Dicker R et al.: Adjunctive antipsychotic treatment of adolescents with bipolar psychosis. *J Am Acad Child Adolesc Psychiatry* 2001; **40**: 1448–56.

22 Delbello MP, Schwiers ML, Rosenberg HL et al.: A double-blind, randomized, placebo-controlled study of quetiapine as adjunctive treatment for adolescent mania. *J Am Acad Child Adolesc Psychiatry* 2002; **41**: 1216–23.

23 Pavuluri, MN, Henry DB, Carbray JA et al.: Open label prospective trial of risperidone in combination with lithium or divalproex sodium in pediatric mania. *J Affective Disorders* 2004; **82**: S103–111.

24 Wozniak J, Mick E, Waxmonsky J et al.: Comparison of open-label, 8-week trials of olanzapine monotherapy and topiramate augmentation of olanzapine for the treatment of pediatric bipolar disorder. *J Child Adolesc Psychopharmacol* 2009; **19**: 539–45.

25 Penzner JB, Dudas M, Saito E et al.: Lack of effect of stimulant combination with second-generation antipsychotics on weight gain, metabolic changes, prolactin levels, and sedation in youth with clinically relevant aggression or oppositionality. *J Child Adolesc Psychopharmacol* 2009; **19**: 563–73.

26 Geller DA, Biederman J, Reed ED et al.: Similarities in response to fluoxetine in the treatment of children and adolescents with obsessive-compulsive disorder. *J Child Adolesc Psychopharmacol* 1995; **34**: 36–44.

27 West S, McElroy S, Strakowski S et al.: Attention deficit hyperactivity disorder in adolescent mania. *Am J Psychiat* 1995; **152**: 271–3.

28 Wilens T, Biederman J, Forkner P et al.: Patterns of comorbidity and dysfunction in clinically referred preschoolers with bipolar disorder. *J Child Adolesc Psychopharmacol* 2003; **13**: 495–505.

29 Biederman J, Faraone S, Mick et al.: Attention-deficit hyperactivity disorder and juvenile mania: an overlooked comorbidity? *J Am Acad Child Adolesc Psychiatry* 1996; **35**: 997–1008.

30 Wozniak J, Biederman J: A pharmacological approach to the quagmire of comorbidity in juvenile mania. *J Am Acad Child Adolesc Psychiatry* 1996; **35**: 826–8.

31 Scheffer RE, Kowatch RA, Carmody T et al.: Randomized, placebo-controlled trial of mixed amphetamine salts for symptoms of comorbid ADHD in pediatric bipolar disorder after mood stabilization with divalproex sodium. *Am J Psychiatry* 2005; **162**: 58–64.

32 Carlson G, Rapport M, Kelly K et al.: The effects of methylphenidate and lithium on attention and activity level. *J Am Acad Child Adolesc Psychiatry* 1992; **31**: 262–70.

33 Findling RL, Short EJ, McNamara NK et al.: Methylphenidate in the treatment of children and adolescents with bipolar disorder and attention-deficit/hyperactivity disorder. *J Am Acad Child Adolesc Psychiatry* 2007; **46**: 1445–53.

34 Zenia C, Tramontina S, Ketzer C et al.: Methylphenidate combined with aripiprazole in children and adolescents with bipolar and attention-deficit/hyperactivity disorder: a randomized crossover trial. *J Child Adolesc Psychopharacol* 2009; **19**: 553–61.

35 Chang K, Nayar D, Howe M et al.: Atomoxetine as an adjunct therapy in the treatment of co-morbid attention-deficit/hyperactivity disorder in children and adolescents with bipolar I or II disorder. *J Child Adolesc Psychopharacol* 2009; **19**: 547–51.

36 Bauer MS, McBride L, Chase C et al.: Manual-based group psychotherapy for bipolar disorder: a feasibility study. *J Clin Psychiatry* 1998; **59**: 449–55.

37 Joffe R, Singer W, Levitt A et al.: A placebo-controlled comparison of lithium and triiodothyronine augmentation of tricyclic antidepressants in unipolar refractory depression. *Arch Gen Psychiat* 1993; **50**: 387–94.

38 Weeston TF, Constantino J: High-dose T4 for rapid-cycling bipolar disorder. *J Am Acad Child Adolesc Psychiatry* 1996; **35**: 131–2.

39 West SA, Strakowski SM, Sax KW et al.: Phenomenology and comorbidity of adolescents hospitalized for the treatment of acute mania. *Biol Psychiat* 1996; **39**: 458–60.

40 Sokolov ST, Kutcher SP, Joffe RT: Basal thyroid indices in adolescent depression and bipolar disorder. *J Am Acad Child Adolesc Psychiatry* 1994; **33**: 469–75.

41 Fava G, Grandi S, Zielezny M et al.: Cognitive behavioral treatment of residual symptoms in primary major depressive disorder. *Am J Psychiat* 1994; **151**: 1295–9.

42 Ryan ND, Meyer V, Dachille S: Lithium antidepressant augmentation in TCA-refractory depression in adolescents. *J Child Adolesc Psychopharmacol* 1988; **27**: 371–6.

43 Strober M: Relevance of early age-of-onset in genetic studies of bipolar affective disorder. *J Child Adolesc Psychopharmacol* 1992; **31**: 606–10.

44 Geller B, Fox LW, Fletcher M: Effect of tricyclic antidepressants on switching to mania and on the onset of bipolarity in depressed 6- to 12-year-olds. *J Child Adolesc Psychopharmacol* 1993; **32**: 43–50.

45 Findling R: Open-label treatment of comorbid depression and attentional disorder with co-administration of SRIs and psychostimulants in children, adolescents, and adults: a case series. *J Child Adolesc Psychopharmacol* 1996; **6**: 165–75.

46 Gammon GD, Brown TE: Fluoxetine and methylphenidate in combination for treatment of attention deficit disorder and comorbid depressive disorder. *J Child Adolesc Psychopharmacol* 1993; **3**: 1–10.

47 Kratochvil CJ, Newcorn JH, Arnold LE et al.: Atomoxetine alone or combined with fluoxetine for treating ADHD with comorbid depressive or anxiety symptoms. *J Am Acad Child Adolesc Psychiatry* 2005; **44**: 915–24.

48 Bangs ME, Emslie GJ, Spencer TJ et al.: Efficacy and safety of atomoxetine in adolescents with attention-deficit/hyperactivity disorder and major depression. *J Child Adolesc Psychopharmacol* 2007; **17**: 407–20.

49 Wilens T, Biederman J: The stimulants. In: Schaffer D (ed.), *Psychiatric Clinics of North America*. Philadelphia: W. B. Saunders, 1992, pp. 191–222

50 Pataki C, Carlson G, Kelly K et al.: Side effects of methylphenidate and desipramine alone and in combination in children. *Am J Psychiatry* 1993; **32**: 1065–72.

51 Rapport M, Carlson G, Kelly K et al.: Methylphenidate and desipramine in hospitalized children: I. Separate and combined effects on cognitive function. *J Child Adolesc Psychopharmacol* 1993; **32**: 333–42.

52 Riddle M, Geller B, Ryan N: Case study: another sudden death in a child treated with desipramine. *J Child Adolesc Psychopharmacol* 1993; **32**: 792–7.

53 Prince JB, Wilens TE, Biederman J et al.: A controlled study of nortriptyline in children and adolescents with attention deficit hyperactivity disorder. *J Child Adolesc Psychopharmacol* 2000; **10**: 193–204.

54 Spencer T, Biederman J, Wilens T et al.: Nortriptyline in the treatment of children with attention deficit hyperactivity disorder and tic disorder or Tourette's syndrome. *J Child Adolesc Psychopharmacol* 1993; **32**: 205–10.

55 Wilens TE, Biederman J, Geist DE et al.: Nortriptyline in the treatment of attention deficit hyperactivity disorder: A chart review of 58 cases. *J Child Adolesc Psychopharmacol* 1993; **32**: 343–9.

56 Wilens TE, Hammerness P, Utzinger L et al.: An open study of adjunct OROS-methylphenidate in children and adolescents who are atomoxetine partial responders: I Effectiveness. *J Child Adolesc Psychopharmacol* 2009; **19**: 485–92.

57 Spencer TJ, Greenbaum M, Ginsberg LD et al.: Safety and effectiveness of coadministration of guanfacine extended release and psychostimulants in children and adolescents with attention-deficit/hyperactivity disorder. *J Child Adolesc Psychopharmacol* 2009; **19**: 501–10.

58 Palumbo DR, Sallee FR, Pelham WE et al.: Clonidine for attention-deficit/hyperactivity disorder: I. Efficacy and tolerability outcomes. *J Am Acad Child Adolesc Psychiatry* 2008; **47**: 180–8.

59 Figueroa Y, Rosenberg DR, Birmaher B et al.: Combination treatment with clomipramine and selective serotonin reuptake inhibitors for obsessive-compulsive disorder in children and adolescents. *J Child Adolesc Psychopharmacol* 1998; **8**: 61–7.

60 Simeon JG, Thatte S, Wiggins D: Treatment of adolescent obsessive-compulsive disorder with a clomipramine-fluoxetine combination. *Psychopharmacol Bull* 1990; **26**: 285–90.

61 Leonard HL, Topol D, Bukstein O et al.: Clonazepam as an augmenting agent in the treatment of childhood-onset obsessive-compulsive disorder. *J Am Acad Child Adolesc Psychiatry* 1994; **33**: 792–4.

62 Saccomani L, Rizzo P, Nobili L: Combined treatment with haloperidol and trazodone in patients with tic disorders. *J Child Adolesc Psychopharmacol* 2000; **10**: 307–10.

63 Gilman JT, Tuchman RF: Autism and associated behavioral disorders: pharmacotherapeutic intervention. *Ann Pharmacother* 1995; **29**: 47–56.

64 Martin A, Scahill L, Klin A et al.: Higher-functioning pervasive developmental disorders: rates and patterns of psychotropic drug use. *J Am Acad Child Adolesc Psychiatry* 1999; **38**: 923–31.

Index

Pharmacotherapy of Child and Adolescent Psychiatric Disorders, Third Edition.
Edited by David R. Rosenberg and Samuel Gershon.
© 2012 John Wiley & Sons, Ltd. Published 2012 by John Wiley & Sons, Ltd.